Ravi Kumar Sharma • Amit Kumar
Surinder Singh Rana
Editors

Differential Diagnosis and Management of Pancreatic Cystic Lesions

Springer

Editors
Ravi Kumar Sharma
Department of Biotechnology
Chandigarh University
Mohali, Punjab, India

Amit Kumar
Department of Gastroenterology
Command Hospital (Southern Command)
Pune, Maharashtra, India

Surinder Singh Rana
Department of Gastroenterology
Postgraduate Institute of Medical Education
and Research (PGIMER)
Chandigarh, India

ISBN 978-981-92-0653-7 ISBN 978-981-92-0654-4 (eBook)
https://doi.org/10.1007/978-981-92-0654-4

This Springer imprint is published by the registered company Springer Nature Singapore Pte Ltd.
The registered company address is: 152 Beach Road, #21-01/04 Gateway East, Singapore 189721, Singapore

Preface

The advancement and widespread availability of cross-sectional imaging have led to a significant increase in the detection of pancreatic cystic lesions (PCLs), which are now frequently encountered in clinical practice. What was once considered a rare and incidental finding is now a common diagnostic challenge faced by gastroenterologists, radiologists, surgeons, and pathologists alike. The heterogeneity of these lesions—ranging from benign, indolent cysts to premalignant and overtly malignant neoplasms—demands a nuanced understanding that integrates clinical judgment with evolving scientific evidence.

This textbook, *Pancreatic Cystic Lesions*, was conceived to address the need for clear, practical, and clinically relevant information in this complex area of gastroenterology. While numerous resources exist, there remains a demand for a concise guide that assists clinicians in making informed decisions regarding the management of PCLs. This book aims to present essential knowledge in a structured and accessible format, making it a valuable resource for practicing gastroenterologists, pancreatologists, surgeons, and trainees in the field. The strength of this book lies in the contributions of a distinguished group of leading gastroenterologists and experts in the field from India. Their collective wisdom, drawn from extensive clinical experience and academic excellence, is intricately embedded within each chapter. We sincerely acknowledge and appreciate their dedication and generosity in sharing their expertise, which has shaped this volume into a resource that is both authoritative and accessible.

The decision-making process in management of these cystic lesions is often complex, involving multiple variables such as cyst morphology, size, growth dynamics, patient comorbidities, and the presence of high-risk features. This textbook seeks to bring clarity to this complexity by presenting evidence-based recommendations along with practical tips that can be readily applied in clinical settings. In addition to clinical insights, this book emphasizes the importance of a multidisciplinary approach in managing pancreatic cystic lesions. Collaboration among gastroenterologists, radiologists, and pathologists is essential for optimal patient care. The integration of perspectives from gastroenterology, radiology, pathology, surgery, and oncology reflects the real-world approach necessary for managing these lesions effectively. Special attention has also been given to emerging technologies, including artificial intelligence and advanced endoscopic imaging, which hold promise for further transforming the field.

In conclusion, managing pancreatic cysts is both an art and a science and requires a careful approach that combines scientific evidence with sound clinical judgment. Ultimately, the goal of this book is to enhance patient care by promoting informed, evidence-based, and patient-centered decision-making. As our understanding continues to evolve and technologies advance, the management of these lesions will undoubtedly progress—underscoring the need for a thoughtful and individualized approach, where one strategy does not fit all. It is our hope that this book serves as a reliable guide in your clinical practice, helping you deliver the best possible care to your patients.

Mohali, Punjab, India — Ravi Kumar Sharma
Pune, Maharashtra, India — Amit Kumar
Chandigarh, India — Surinder Singh Rana

Contents

Blood and Cyst Fluid Biomarkers in Pancreatic Cystic Lesions

1

Tiwonge Jason Nyirenda, Rituraj Singh, Hunny Khurana, and Puneet Chhabra

Abstract

Pancreatic cystic lesions (PCLs) present a diagnostic challenge due to their heterogeneous nature and variable malignant potential. Accurate differentiation between benign and malignant cysts is critical for guiding management and preventing overtreatment. This chapter reviews the current landscape of blood and cyst fluid biomarkers for the risk stratification of PCLs. Blood-based markers such as CA 19-9, CEA, circulating cell-free DNA, and microRNAs offer noninvasive diagnostic options, though their clinical utility remains limited by sensitivity and specificity constraints. Cyst fluid analysis, particularly carcinoembryonic antigen (CEA), glucose, and amylase, continues to play a pivotal role in distinguishing mucinous from nonmucinous cysts. Advances in molecular diagnostics, including next-generation sequencing for KRAS and GNAS mutations, and emerging biomarkers such as Das-1 and microRNA panels, promise improved accuracy in identifying high-risk lesions. Despite these developments, no single biomarker reliably predicts malignancy, underscoring the need for integrated approaches combining imaging, cytology, and molecular analysis. Future research should focus on validating novel biomarkers and developing cost-effective algorithms to enhance preoperative risk stratification and optimize patient management.

T. J. Nyirenda
Department of Gastroenterology, Hull Teaching Hospital, Hull, UK

R. Singh
University of Illinois College of Medicine Peoria, Peoria, IL, USA

H. Khurana
Department of Medicine, Calderdale and Huddersfield NHS Trust, Huddersfield, UK

P. Chhabra (✉)
Department of Gastroenterology, Calderdale and Huddersfield NHS Trust, Huddersfield, UK

R. K. Sharma et al. (eds.), *Differential Diagnosis and Management of Pancreatic Cystic Lesions*, https://doi.org/10.1007/978-981-92-0654-4_1

Keywords
Pancreatic cystic lesions · Biomarkers · Cyst fluid analysis · CA 19-9 · Carcinoembryonic antigen · Glucose · Amylase · Next-generation sequencing · KRAS · GNAS · microRNAs · Liquid biopsy · Risk stratification · Intraductal papillary mucinous neoplasm · Mucinous cysts · Pancreatic adenocarcinoma

1.1 Introduction

Since Werner Korte first differentiated pancreatic cysts into true cysts, pseudocysts, and cystic tumors in 1898, distinguishing between benign and malignant pancreatic cystic lesions has remained a challenging and debated topic [1]. Detecting mucinous pancreatic cysts provides an opportunity for early screening of pancreatic adenocarcinoma, potentially allowing for curative surgery. Although most pancreatic cysts have a low risk of malignant transformation, approximately 15% of mucinous cysts progress to pancreatic adenocarcinoma [2].

Currently, there is no cost-effective screening tool for pancreatic adenocarcinoma, whether population-based or targeted. However, incidentally discovered pancreatic cysts can be risk-stratified for their malignant potential. Two critical questions arise upon discovering a pancreatic cyst:

1. Is the cyst mucinous or nonmucinous (e.g., pseudocysts and serous cystadenomas)? Nonmucinous cysts generally have a low risk of malignant transformation and do not require surveillance or treatment unless symptomatic.
2. How can we cost-effectively stratify pancreatic cysts into high and low risk and identify those harboring high-grade dysplasia or pancreatic adenocarcinoma?

Diagnosing a mucinous cyst cannot be confidently achieved based solely on imaging (cross-sectional or endosonographic) findings. Endoscopic ultrasound-guided fine-needle aspiration (EUS-FNA) offers a minimally invasive and safe method to obtain cyst fluid for testing various biomarkers, in addition to cytology. Despite recent advances in novel molecular markers in pancreatic cyst fluid, the diagnosis of mucinous cysts still relies on EUS imaging features, cytology, and biochemical analysis using CEA and amylase.

1.2 Blood-Based Biomarkers

Blood-based biomarkers can offer a noninvasive means of diagnosing high-risk pancreatic cysts [3]. These biomarkers become even more important when obtaining pancreatic cyst fluid is challenging, due to the location of the cyst or due to a lack of available expertise. While none of these biomarkers have been established for use in clinical practice due to poor sensitivity, there are novel molecular markers under investigation that have the potential for future clinical use. Most of these biomarkers share the concepts of cyst fluid analysis, and a combination of markers provides the best sensitivity and accuracy.

1.3 Tumor Markers

CA 19-9 is a glycoprotein associated with cancers of the colon, stomach, and bile ducts. It is the most evaluated tumor marker for pancreatic adenocarcinoma and plays a crucial role in the risk stratification of pancreatic cysts. However, using CA 19-9 as a screening tool has limitations. Approximately 10% of the population has a CA 19-9-associated monoclonal antibody that reacts with sialylated lewis antigen, resulting in undetectable levels of the tumor marker [4].

While serum CA 19-9 is widely used as a prognostic marker for predicting the stage and survival of pancreatic ductal adenocarcinoma (PDAC), it has limited utility in differentiating benign from malignant pancreatic lesions [5]. Studies have shown poor sensitivity of serum CA 19-9 in predicting invasive disease or high-grade dysplasia in pancreatic cysts.

For instance, Fritz et al. reported a sensitivity of 74% and a specificity of 86% in differentiating invasive from benign intraductal papillary mucinous neoplasms (IPMNs) using a cutoff value of 35 U/mL [5]. However, other studies have reported much lower sensitivity for CA 19-9 in identifying invasive pancreatic cysts. A meta-analysis of nine retrospective studies, mostly from Asia, found that a CA 19-9 level above 35 U/mL has a sensitivity of 40–50% and a specificity of 88% in differentiating invasive from benign IPMN [6].

Despite its high specificity, CA 19-9 levels can be influenced by confounding factors such as gallstones, cholestasis, and chronic pancreatitis. A retrospective study demonstrated improved sensitivity of cyst fluid CA 19-9 in combination with CA 125 in predicting the future development of PDAC. However, the utility of combining these serum tumor markers is primarily limited to the prognostication of pancreatic adenocarcinoma.

1.3.1 CEA

Carcinoembryonic antigen (CEA) is a glycoprotein present in healthy individuals at a low level and elevated in various gastrointestinal malignancies. While CEA is one of the most common tumor markers in differentiating mucinous from nonmucinous cysts, it has poor sensitivity, lower than CA 19-9 at risk stratifying pancreatic cystic lesions. At levels above 5 ng/mL, CEA has a high specificity in identifying invasive IPMN; however, the sensitivity is abysmal, with studies reporting sensitivity as low as 20% in detecting invasive disease [6]. A retrospective study found sensitivity and specificity of 80% for the combination of CEA (>5 μg/L) and CA 19-9 (>37 U/mL) at differentiating invasive from benign IPMN [5]. Nonetheless, as a serum biomarker for pancreatic neoplasm, CEA has poor performance in the diagnosis or prognosis of invasive pancreatic neoplasms including PDAC.

1.4 DNA-Based Biomarkers

Invasive tumors release circulating cell-free DNA (cfDNA) into the bloodstream, offering a noninvasive "liquid biopsy" for disease monitoring. cfDNA from blood samples often mirrors the mutations found in the primary tumor [7]. Observational studies have detected circulating pancreatic epithelial cells in patients with pancreatic cystic lesions, even without invasive pancreatic adenocarcinoma [8]. However, the diagnostic utility of liquid biopsy is limited by poor sensitivity due to the extremely low number of cfDNA, with less than one mutant template molecule per milliliter of plasma in early-stage cancer patients [9].

A retrospective study evaluated five different cohorts ranging from healthy adults, patients with serous cystadenoma, IPMN to metastatic pancreatic adenocarcinoma and demonstrated a high diagnostic accuracy at discriminating healthy controls and IPMN, and IPMN and pancreatic adenocarcinoma. Using a cutoff of 0.208 ng/mL, the sensitivity and specificity for discriminating IPMN from healthy controls was 81% and 84%, respectively [10]. Mutations in the GNAS gene can identify high-risk pancreatic cysts. Compared to non-neoplastic pancreatic cystic lesions, GNAS mutations are observed more commonly in cfDNA for IPMN [11]. However, there is a low concordance rate between the resected samples and peripheral blood samples. A high degree of mutational heterogeneity is observed in the GNAS mutations [10]. Pancreatic adenocarcinomas associated with IPMN are more frequently associated with KRAS mutations than GNAS mutations [12].

CancerSEEK is a blood test that combines two components—genetic mutational testing and protein biomarker—to detect early-stage cancers. It can detect eight common cancer types through the assessment of the levels of cell-free DNA and eight circulating proteins. Cohen et al. demonstrated a concordance of 100% between primary tumor and plasma in patients with pancreatic adenocarcinoma [9]. Despite the encouraging results, there are two major limitations to its application in pancreatic cancer screening—CancerSEEK is unable to discriminate tumor types and plays an unknown role in the identification of neoplastic or invasive pancreatic cystic lesion.

1.5 RNA-Based Biomarkers

MicroRNAs (miRNAs) are small, noncoding RNAs, 17 to 25 nucleotides in length, that regulate mRNA expression. Most tumors exhibit downregulation of miRNAs, as shown in expression profiling, suggesting their role in tumorigenesis and cancer progression [13]. Circulating miRNAs have been extensively studied as biomarkers for invasive disease and disease progression in patients with pancreatic adenocarcinoma. Various miRNA panels have been used to identify pancreatic adenocarcinoma, but significant heterogeneity exists among these panels, and they have not been well validated.

Schultz et al. utilized the BIOPAC (biomarkers in patients with pancreatic cancer) study cohort to conduct a case–control study evaluating the expression of 754 miRNAs. The study identified two miRNA panels (comprising four and ten miRNAs) that could distinguish pancreatic adenocarcinoma from healthy controls [14]. The addition of CA 19-9 improves diagnostic accuracy; however, this combination panel has not been validated [15].

While emerging evidence supports the diagnostic role of miRNAs in the early detection of pancreatic adenocarcinoma, further consolidation of this evidence is needed before clinical application. Major limitations include the lack of well-powered prospective studies, heterogeneity in miRNA panels, diagnostic thresholds, and the lack of validation of various miRNA panels. Nonetheless, miRNAs represent a potential noninvasive biomarker, especially when combined with other blood-based markers, for risk stratification of neoplastic pancreatic cysts.

1.6 Proteomics

Amylase has traditionally been used as a marker for diagnosing acute pancreatitis. Its potential as a marker for pancreatic cystic lesions was demonstrated in a cross-sectional study involving 146 patients, where low levels of amylase were associated with a higher risk of invasive intraductal papillary mucinous neoplasm (IPMN) [16].

The advent of tandem mass spectrometry and microarray technologies has paved the way for new diagnostic approaches in the early detection of neoplasms. Numerous proteins have been identified in various cross-sectional studies as potential biomarkers for malignant pancreatic cystic lesions. Among these, two notable biomarkers are TSP-1 and CEMIP. However, neither has proven suitable as an independent predictor of high-risk features in pancreatic cystic lesions [17].

1.7 Neutrophil-to- Lymphocyte Ratio (NLR)

Tumor-associated neutrophils enhance tumor survival by releasing cytokines and chemokines that promote tumorigenesis and hinder antitumor therapies. This results in a systemic shift in the neutrophil-to-lymphocyte ratio (NLR), which has been shown in studies to be an indicator of high-grade dysplasia and invasive disease, particularly in intraductal papillary mucinous neoplasm (IPMN). The NLR decreases after treatment and has been demonstrated to complement other biomarkers due to its moderate sensitivity and specificity [18–21].

1.8 Cyst Fluid Biomarkers

For the past two decades, cyst fluid biomarkers have been pivotal in predicting the risk of malignancy or identifying high-risk features in pancreatic cysts. When imaging results are inconclusive, endoscopic ultrasound-guided fine needle aspiration (EUS-FNA) is the next step to determine if the findings will influence management decisions [22]. At this stage, carcinoembryonic antigen (CEA) is considered the gold standard biomarker for mucinous cysts. However, research into other biomarkers, such as amylase and glucose, has demonstrated comparable sensitivity and specificity in distinguishing different cyst subtypes [23, 24]. The primary goal of cyst fluid molecular evaluation is to identify the cyst type and decide whether resection or surveillance is necessary for ongoing management [25].

1.8.1 Cyst Fluid Carcinoembryonic Antigen (CEA)

Carcinoembryonic antigen (CEA) is the most widely used cyst fluid biomarker. It is a glycoprotein secreted from embryonic endoderm epithelium, part of the columnar epithelial cells lining mucinous cysts. A cyst fluid CEA level of ≥192 ng/mL supports the diagnosis of a mucinous cyst, with a sensitivity of 52–78% and a specificity of 63–91% [23]. Variations in results are attributed to the different assays used to process CEA. Other studies have suggested a cutoff value of 800 ng/mL to be highly specific (98%) for mucinous cysts [26]. The various interpretations of CEA levels create confusion and debate over the best cutoff value. Additionally, CEA assays are validated for serum samples rather than cyst fluid [27].

Brugge et al. found that CEA alone was more accurate than EUS and cytology in diagnosing mucinous cysts [28]. However, CEA is not reliable for identifying cysts with high-grade dysplasia or associated invasive carcinoma, nor for distinguishing benign mucinous cysts when used alone. For analysis, 0.5 to 1 cc of fluid is required, which can limit testing in smaller pancreatic cysts.

Ngamruengphong's meta-analysis of seven studies showed that the sensitivity and specificity of CEA in distinguishing benign from malignant pancreatic cysts were quite poor, with pooled estimates reporting a sensitivity and specificity of 63%. It is important to note that the CEA cutoff levels varied from 109.9 to 6000 ng/mL across studies [29].

Some studies limit the usefulness of cyst CEA levels to predicting mucin production only. A recent updated meta-analysis on the utility of cyst CEA levels in differentiating mucinous from nonmucinous cysts showed that a CEA cutoff value of 192 ng/mL had a pooled specificity of 88.6% and a sensitivity of 60.4% [30].

1.8.2 Cyst Fluid Amylase

Amylase, produced and excreted by the exocrine pancreatic gland, has been used to help identify pseudocysts [31]. It can also indicate a communication with the pancreatic duct system, a feature not present in mucinous cystadenomas. A cutoff level of >479 U/L for amylase has shown a sensitivity of 73% and a specificity of 90% in differentiating pseudocysts from other pancreatic cysts [32]. However, other studies have found that low amylase levels have a very high specificity for excluding pseudocysts, while high levels lack diagnostic usefulness. This is because high amylase levels are also found in benign intraductal papillary mucinous neoplasms (IPMNs) and benign mucinous cysts. One hypothesis suggests this may be due to small connections between an IPMN cyst and the ductal system, or that low amylase levels in malignant mucinous cysts could result from uncontrolled cellular growth leading to the occlusion of microscopic ductal connections. A low amylase level (<250 U/L) combined with a low glucose level can help rule out the diagnosis of pseudocyst [33].

Amylase has largely fallen out of favor for diagnosing pancreatic cystic lesions unless there is a clear history of recent pancreatitis, and pseudocyst remains a differential diagnosis

1.8.3 Cyst Fluid Glucose Levels

The reason for low glucose levels in mucinous cysts is not well understood, but it is thought to be related to an increased cell turnover rate [34]. A study involving 78 patients demonstrated a strong correlation between lab-based and on-site glucometer testing, with on-site measurements generally being higher [34]. This finding can be applied in clinical practice to provide real-time data during procedures. A glucose level of <50 mg/dL has been identified as an optimal cutoff for diagnosing mucinous cysts [34]. Low glucose levels have shown a diagnostic accuracy of 84%, sensitivity of 94%, and specificity of 64% for mucinous cysts, comparable to CEA when using a cutoff of 66 mg/dL [24]. However, pseudocysts can also present with low glucose levels [33].

McCarty et al.'s systematic review and meta-analysis of 609 lesions concluded that low pancreatic cyst fluid glucose significantly improves diagnostic accuracy compared to CEA alone [35]. However, it is not effective in detecting degenerate IPMN with dysplasia or invasive carcinoma. Interestingly, elevated glucose levels have also been shown to identify serous cystadenomas with the same cutoff level, achieving a diagnostic accuracy of 89%, sensitivity of 88%, and specificity of 89% [24]. Although not currently included in published guidelines, this method may prove useful in identifying SCAs that do not require imaging surveillance [24].

A recent meta-analysis compared the utility of intra-cystic glucose levels with CEA levels in differentiating mucinous from nonmucinous cysts. Six studies involving 506 patients showed that glucose had a sensitivity of 91% and specificity of 85% for predicting mucinous PCL, while CEA had a sensitivity and specificity of 61% and 93%, respectively. The authors concluded that cyst fluid glucose levels are an easy and useful tool for predicting mucinous cysts compared to CEA [35].

The advantages of using glucose include the need for only small sample volumes and the availability of processing capabilities in most hospital laboratories [24]. This can even be done bedside with a conventional glucometer. Additionally, the cost of intra-cystic glucose testing is significantly lower, at $1–2, compared to $150 for CEA.

1.9 DNA Analysis

Next-generation sequencing (NGS) has emerged as a promising tool for diagnosing cyst subtypes and assessing the risk of high-grade dysplasia [36]. Cystic fluid, which contains DNA from lysed or exfoliated epithelial cells, can be analyzed for genetic abnormalities [37]. Specifically, KRAS and GNAS mutations exhibit 90% sensitivity and 100% specificity for mucinous cysts [36]. When combined with alterations in TP53, SMAD4, CTNNB1, and the mammalian target of rapamycin (mTOR), these mutations maintain high sensitivity and specificity for diagnosing high-grade dysplastic cysts or early adenocarcinoma [36]. Mucinous cystic neoplasms (MCNs) with both KRAS and TP53 mutations are considered more aggressive, increasing the likelihood of progression to pancreatic ductal adenocarcinoma. KRAS and GNAS mutations are also commonly found in intraductal papillary mucinous neoplasms (IPMNs) [38].

A meta-analysis of six studies reported that the presence of KRAS and GNAS mutations diagnosed mucinous pancreatic cystic lesions (PCLs) with 94% sensitivity and 91% specificity [39]. In a study by Ren et al., the diagnostic accuracy of NGS was compared with cytological and carcinoembryonic antigen (CEA) analysis. Among 31 patients with available surgical pathology, NGS demonstrated 88.5% sensitivity and 100% specificity for diagnosing mucinous cysts, while diagnostic cytology and elevated CEA were observed in 46.8% and 50.9% of cases, respectively. Additionally, uncommon hotspot BRAF mutations were identified in 6 out of 10 patients with negative KRAS mutations [40].

Von Hippel-Lindau (VHL) and MEN1/loss of heterozygosity alterations can diagnose serous cystadenomas with 71% sensitivity and 100% specificity. This test also aids in diagnosing cystic pancreatic neuroendocrine tumors, with 68% sensitivity and 98% specificity [36]. When measured alone, MEN1 alterations have 27% sensitivity and 100% specificity for cystic pancreatic neuroendocrine tumors [41]. VHL alterations, along with mutations in TP53 or the TERT promoter, are frequently seen in serous cystadenomas [41]. CTNNB1 mutations are found in solid papillary neoplasms and interestingly do not co-occur with KRAS, GNAS, VHL, or RNF43 mutations [38].

Further studies are necessary to assess and map the progression of patients with low mean allele frequencies of TP53, SMAD4, and mTOR mutations. Additionally, DNA analysis should focus on identifying low-risk patients who can be discharged from long-term surveillance, thereby contributing to cost savings [42].

The monoclonal antibody Das-1 has shown promise in early studies for detecting high-risk mucinous cysts, with a sensitivity of 88.2% and specificity of 99% [43]. Developed using a colon epithelial protein, Das-1 is strongly expressed during preneoplastic and intestinal phenotypic changes [44]. It is not reactive to normal gastric or duodenal mucosa, reducing the risk of contamination during sampling [43]. Das-1 may also help distinguish high-risk from low-risk IPMNs through a combination of immunohistochemistry, western blot analysis, and ELISA [44]. It can be analyzed in acellular and small-volume samples due to the high amounts of colon epithelial protein, as demonstrated in the study by Das et al. [44].

Given its high diagnostic accuracy, molecular analysis is likely to enhance our ability to diagnose malignant pancreatic cystic lesions. However, its widespread use may be limited by the availability and cost of molecular testing.

1.10 Cytology

The assessment of tumor cells within cytology is crucial for diagnosing pancreatic neoplasms. Accurate diagnosis requires detailed analysis of both tumor cells and background features. A significant limitation of cytology is the insufficient material available for diagnosis. The presence of a mucinous background is a hallmark of mucin-producing neoplasms. High-grade dysplasia and invasive carcinoma often appear similar in cyst fluid aspirates [45].

According to all guidelines, positive cytology indicates the need for surgical resection, with a sensitivity of 64.8% and a high specificity of 90.6% [32]. However, negative results cannot reliably rule out high-risk lesions, possibly due to gastrointestinal tract contamination during sampling [31].

Historically, cytology has struggled to provide a high diagnostic yield due to the challenges of interpreting a low number of useful cells. Recently, especially for IPMNs, cytological diagnosis has improved with the use of five new criteria for high-grade dysplasia in IPMNs: smaller cell size compared to an enterocyte, increased nucleo-cytoplasmic ratio, nuclear membrane irregularities, abnormal chromatin pattern, and background cellular necrosis. A study found that using increased NC ratio, abnormal chromatin pattern, and background cellular necrosis, the sensitivity and specificity for predicting malignancy by identifying high-grade atypia could reach 89% and 98%, respectively [36].

1.11 Micro-RNAs

These small noncoding RNAs combine with complementary sequences to modulate the expression of targeted mRNAs. Studies have shown that microRNAs can function as either oncogenes or tumor suppressors. Even at low levels, they can be detected, making them potential biomarkers. A panel consisting of miR-31-5p, miR-483-5p, miR-99a-5p, and miR-375 has been shown to differentiate serous cystadenomas from mucinous cysts with 90% sensitivity and 100% specificity [46].

1.12 Rheological Diagnosis

Cyst fluid viscosity has historically been used to identify mucinous cysts through the "string sign." This sign is measured by an endosonologist, who places a drop of fluid between the thumb and index finger and stretches it to measure the maximum length before it breaks, indirectly reflecting the fluid's viscosity. In a study, the median string length was 0 mm in benign cysts and 3.5 mm in malignant cysts (Leung et al., Ann Surg Oncol) [47].

In a recent single-center study, Khamayasi et al. measured the viscosity of cyst fluid from 22 PCF samples and analyzed the rheological behavior of the fluid in relation to the type of cyst lesion. The results revealed three distinct flow curves: types I and II were observed in nonmucinous cysts, while the third type was seen in mucinous cysts. The cutoff value of viscosity measured at a strain rate of 2000 1/s was potentially determined to distinguish between mucinous and nonmucinous cysts [48].

1.13 Novel Biomarkers

A study by Abdellah et al. involving 50 patients with pancreatic cystic lesions (PCL) demonstrated that cystic fluid interleukin-1β (IL-1β) levels could differentiate between benign and malignant cystic pancreatic lesions with a sensitivity of 84% and a specificity of 56% at a cutoff value of >150 pg/mL. However, another study indicated that IL-1β could not reliably distinguish between benign and malignant pancreatic cysts [49].

Additionally, another study assessed the role of cyst fluid chromogranin A levels in detecting cystic neuroendocrine tumors (NETs) or other pancreatic cystic lesions. The authors concluded that chromogranin A levels in cyst fluid were not useful for detecting cystic NETs or any other PCLs [50].

Cui et al. utilized mass spectrometry-based glycoproteomic analysis of pancreatic cyst fluid and identified that N-glycosylated PHKB, CEACAM5, and ATP6V0A4 could serve as potential markers for differentiating malignant from benign pancreatic cysts [51].

1.14 Algorithms

Schneider et al. conducted an intriguing study to evaluate the role of a biomarker risk score algorithm in the preoperative stratification of pancreatic cystic lesions (PCLs). The study utilized cystic fluid biomarkers such as VEGF, glucose, CEA, and amylase, combined with cytology and genetic mutations, to develop an algorithm for classifying PCLs.

The algorithm was retrospectively analyzed using a surgical cohort and prospectively validated with a surveillance cohort. In the surgical cohort, the biomarker algorithm significantly outperformed the presurgical diagnosis, with statistically significant results. In the surveillance cohort, the algorithm demonstrated a high level of confidence in predicting presurgical diagnoses [52].

1.15 Conclusion

Despite significant advances in medical technology and research, the diagnosis and management of pancreatic cystic lesions continue to pose substantial challenges. The complexity of these lesions and the limitations of current diagnostic tools often make accurate assessment and effective treatment difficult. There are currently no single blood or cyst biomarkers that can reliably predict the malignant potential or high-risk features of pancreatic cystic lesions. But, the investigation into blood and cyst markers for pancreatic cystic lesions (PCLs) has yielded valuable insights that enhance our diagnostic and prognostic capabilities. Blood-based markers such as CEA, amylase, and DNA-based biomarkers, along with microRNAs, have shown varying degrees of effectiveness in identifying and characterizing PCLs. These markers, when used in conjunction with cyst fluid biomarkers like CEA, glucose, and cyst DNA markers, provide a more comprehensive approach to differentiating between benign and malignant lesions.

The integration of these diverse biomarkers into clinical practice has the potential to significantly improve the accuracy of preoperative diagnoses. For instance, cyst fluid glucose and DNA markers have demonstrated particular promise in distinguishing malignant cysts from their benign counterparts. Similarly, the use of blood-based DNA biomarkers and microRNAs offers a noninvasive method to monitor and evaluate PCLs.

Overall, the ongoing research into blood and cyst markers continues to refine our diagnostic capabilities, paving the way for more personalized and effective management strategies for patients with PCLs. Future studies should focus on validating these markers in larger, diverse cohorts and exploring novel biomarkers to further improve diagnostic accuracy and patient outcomes. By continuing to refine and expand our biomarker toolkit, we can move closer to achieving precise, personalized care for patients with PCLs.

Conflict of Interest There are no conflicts of interest which need to be disclosed.

References

1. Körte W. Die chirurgischen krankheiten und die verletzungen des pankreas. Stuttgart: F. Enker; 1898.
2. Singhi AD, Koay EJ, Chari ST, et al. Early detection of pancreatic cancer: opportunities and challenges. Gastroenterology. 2019;156:2024–40.
3. Peller MT, Das KK. Blood-based biomarkers in the diagnosis and risk stratification of pancreatic cysts. Gastrointest Endosc Clin N Am. 2023;33:559–81.
4. Koprowski H, Brockhaus M, Blaszczyk M, et al. Lewis blood-type may affect the incidence of gastrointestinal cancer. Lancet. 1982;1:1332–3.
5. Fritz S, Hackert T, Hinz U, et al. Role of serum carbohydrate antigen 19-9 and carcinoembryonic antigen in distinguishing between benign and invasive intraductal papillary mucinous neoplasm of the pancreas. Br J Surg. 2010;98:104–10.

6. Wang W, Zhang L, Chen L, et al. Serum carcinoembryonic antigen and carbohydrate antigen 19-9 for prediction of malignancy and invasiveness in intraductal papillary mucinous neoplasms of the pancreas: a meta-analysis. Biomed Rep. 2015;3:43–50.
7. Murtaza M, Dawson S-J, Tsui DWY, et al. Non-invasive analysis of acquired resistance to cancer therapy by sequencing of plasma DNA. Nature. 2013;497:108–12.
8. Rhim AD, Thege FI, Santana SM, et al. Detection of circulating pancreas epithelial cells in patients with pancreatic cystic lesions. Gastroenterology. 2014;146:647–51.
9. Cohen JD, Li L, Wang Y, et al. Detection and localization of surgically resectable cancers with a multi-analyte blood test. Science. 2018;359:926–30.
10. Berger AW, Schwerdel D, Costa IG, et al. Detection of hot-spot mutations in circulating cell-free DNA from patients with intraductal papillary mucinous neoplasms of the pancreas. Gastroenterology. 2016;151:267–70.
11. Wu J, Matthaei H, Maitra A, et al. Recurrent GNAS mutations define an unexpected pathway for pancreatic cyst development. Sci Transl Med. 2011;3:92ra66.
12. Tan MC, Basturk O, Brannon AR, et al. GNAS and KRAS mutations define separate progression pathways in intraductal papillary mucinous neoplasm-associated carcinoma. J Am Coll Surg. 2015;220:845–854.e841.
13. Prinz C, Fehring L, Frese R. MicroRNAs as indicators of malignancy in pancreatic ductal adenocarcinoma (PDAC) and cystic pancreatic lesions. Cells. 2022;11:11.
14. Schultz NA, Dehlendorff C, Jensen BV, et al. MicroRNA biomarkers in whole blood for detection of pancreatic cancer. JAMA. 2014;311:392–404.
15. Liu J, Gao J, Du Y, et al. Combination of plasma microRNAs with serum CA19-9 for early detection of pancreatic cancer. Int J Cancer. 2012;131:683–91.
16. Yagi Y, Masuda A, Zen Y, et al. Predictive value of low serum pancreatic enzymes in invasive intraductal papillary mucinous neoplasms. Pancreatology. 2016;16(5):893–9.
17. Lee HS, Jang CY, Kim SA, et al. Combined use of CEMIP and CA 19-9 enhances diagnostic accuracy for pancreatic cancer. Sci Rep. 2018;8(1):1–7.
18. Sugimachi K, Mano Y, Matsumoto Y, et al. Neutrophil-to-lymphocyte ratio as a predictor of malignancy of intraductal papillary mucinous neoplasms. Anticancer Res. 2021;41(3):1663–9.93.
19. Arima K, Okabe H, Hashimoto D, et al. The neutrophil-to-lymphocyte ratio predicts malignant potential in intraductal papillary mucinous neoplasms. J Gastrointest Surg. 2015;19(12):2171–7.94.
20. Gemenetzis G, Bagante F, Griffin JF, et al. Neutrophil-to-lymphocyte ratio is a predictive marker for invasive malignancy in intraductal papillary mucinous neoplasms of the pancreas. Ann Surg. 2017;266(2):339–45.95.
21. Hata T, Mizuma M, Motoi F, et al. Diagnostic and prognostic impact of neutrophil to-lymphocyte ratio for intraductal papillary mucinous neoplasms of the pancreas with high-grade dysplasia and associated invasive carcinoma. Pancreas. 2019;48(1):99–106.
22. Zamir E, Zelnik Yovel D, Scapa E, Shnell M, Bar N, Bar Yishay I, et al. Pancreatic cyst fluid glucose: a rapid on-site diagnostic test for mucinous cysts. Ther Adv Gastroenterol. 2022;15:175628482211335.
23. The European Study Group on Cystic Tumours of the Pancreas. European evidence-based guidelines on pancreatic cystic neoplasms. Gut. 2018;67(5):789–804.
24. Park WG, Wu M, Bowen R, et al. Metabolomic-derived novel cyst fluid biomarkers for pancreatic cysts: glucose and kynurenine. Gastrointest Endosc. 2013;78(2):295–302.e2.
25. Ohtsuka T, Fernandez-del Castillo C, Furukawa T, et al. International evidence-based Kyoto guidelines for the management of intraductal papillary mucinous neoplasm of the pancreas. Pancreatology. 2024;24(2):255–70.
26. Park WG, Mascarenhas R, Palaez-Luna M, et al. Diagnostic performance of cyst fluid carcinoembryonic antigen and amylase in histologically confirmed pancreatic cysts. Pancreas. 2011;40(1):42–5.
27. Chiang AL, Lee LS. Clinical approach to incidental pancreatic cysts. World J Gastroenterol. 2016;22(3):1236–45.

28. Brugge WR, Lewandrowski K, Lee-Lewandrowski E, et al. Diagnosis of pancreatic cystic neoplasms: a report of the cooperative pancreatic cyst study. Gastroenterology. 2004;126(5):1330–6.
29. Ngamruengphong S, Bartel MJ, Raimondo M. Cyst carcinoembryonic antigen in differentiating pancreatic cysts: a meta-analysis. Dig Liver Dis. 2013;45(11):920–6.
30. Khan I, Baig M, Bandepalle T, et al. Utility of cyst fluid carcinoembryonic antigen in differentiating mucinous and non-mucinous pancreatic cysts: an updated meta-analysis. Dig Dis Sci. 2022;67(9):4541–8.
31. Siddappa PK, Park WG. Pancreatic cyst fluid analysis. Gastrointest Endosc Clin N Am. 2023;33(3):599–612.
32. Buerlein RCD, Shami VM. Management of pancreatic cysts and guidelines: what the gastroenterologist needs to know. Ther Adv Gastrointest Endosc. 2021;14:26317745211045769.
33. Canakis A, Lee LS. State-of-the-art update of pancreatic cysts. Dig Dis Sci. 2022;67(5):1573–87.
34. Ribeiro T, Lopes S, Moutinho-Ribeiro P, et al. Performance of intracystic glucose measurement for the characterization of pancreatic cystic lesions. J Gastrointestin Liver Dis. 2023;33(1):74–8.
35. McCarty TR, Garg R, Rustagi T. Pancreatic cyst fluid glucose in differentiating mucinous from nonmucinous pancreatic cysts: a systematic review and meta-analysis. Gastrointest Endosc. 2021;94(4):698–712.e6.
36. Gardner TB, Park WG, Allen PJ. Diagnosis and management of pancreatic cysts. Gastroenterology. 2024;167(3):454–68.
37. Singhi AD, McGrath K, Brand RE, et al. Preoperative next-generation sequencing of pancreatic cyst fluid is highly accurate in cyst classification and detection of advanced neoplasia. Gut. 2018;67(12):2131–41.
38. Whole-exome sequencing of neoplastic cysts of the pancreas reveals recurrent mutations in components of ubiquitin-dependent pathways [Internet]. [cited 2024 Aug 7]. Available from: https://www.pnas.org/doi/10.1073/pnas.1118046108.
39. Ardeshna DR, Cao T, Rodgers B, et al. Recent advances in the diagnostic evaluation of pancreatic cystic lesions. World J Gastroenterol. 2022;28(6):624–34.
40. Ren R, Krishna SG, Chen W, et al. Activation of the RAS pathway through uncommon BRAF mutations in mucinous pancreatic cysts without KRAS mutation. Mod Pathol. 2021;34(2):438–44.
41. Paniccia A, Polanco PM, Boone BA, et al. Prospective, multi-institutional, real-time next-generation sequencing of pancreatic cyst fluid reveals diverse genomic alterations that improve the clinical management of pancreatic cysts. Gastroenterology. 2023;164(1):117–133.e7.
42. Das KK. The "next generation" of pancreatic cyst fluid biomarkers? Gastroenterology. 2023;164(1):21–3.
43. Das K, Geng X, Brown J, et al. Cross validation of the monoclonal antibody Das-1 in identification of high-risk mucinous pancreatic cystic lesions. Gastroenterology. 2019;157(3):720–30.e2.
44. Das KK, Xiao H, Geng X, et al. mAb Das-1 is specific for high-risk and malignant intraductal papillary mucinous neoplasm (IPMN). Gut. 2014;63(10):1626.1–34.
45. Yang P, Han L, Zhou Z. Updates and challenges in pancreatic cytopathology. Human Pathol Rep. 2024;36:300736.
46. Prinz C, Fehring L, Frese R. MicroRNAs as indicators of malignancy in pancreatic ductal adenocarcinoma (PDAC) and cystic pancreatic lesions. Cells. 2022;11(15):2374.
47. Leung KK, Ross WA, Evans D, et al. Pancreatic cystic neoplasm: the role of cyst morphology, cyst fluid analysis, and expectant management. Ann Surg Oncol. 2009;16(10):2818–24.
48. Khamaysi I, Abu Ammar A, Vasilyev G, et al. Differentiation of pancreatic cyst types by analysis of rheological behavior of pancreatic cyst fluid. Sci Rep. 2017;7:45589.
49. Kaddah M, Okasha HH, Hasan EM, et al. The role of interleukin 1 Beta in differentiating malignant from benign pancreatic cysts. J Interf Cytokine Res. 2022;42(3):118–26.
50. Oruç N, Aydın A, Barutcuoğlu B, et al. Cystic fluid chromogranin a levels in different pancreatic cystic lesions. Turk J Gastroenterol. 2015;26(6):522–7.

51. Cui M, Hu Y, Zhang Z, et al. Cyst fluid glycoproteins accurately distinguishing malignancies of pancreatic cystic neoplasm. Signal Transduct Target Ther. 2023;8(1):406.
52. Yip-Schneider MT, Wu H, et al. Biomarker risk score algorithm and preoperative stratification of patients with pancreatic cystic lesions. J Am Coll Surg. 2021;233(3):426–34.e4.

CT and MRI of Pancreatic Cystic Lesions

2

Ujjwal Gorsi, Harsimran Bhatia, and Sonam Choudhary

Abstract

Pancreatic cystic lesions are frequently encountered in routine radiological practice. Majority of pancreatic cystic lesions are a symptomatic and detected as incidental findings in individuals. The term pancreatic cystic lesion (PCL) encompasses a large variety of lesions ranging from benign congenital cysts to frankly malignant masses with a predominant cystic appearance on imaging. Although sonography is often the screening modality, cross-sectional techniques including CT are routinely performed to diagnose these cystic lesions. MRI with its excellent soft tissue resolution is often used as a problem-solving tool to better characterize and prognosticate these lesions. In this chapter, we shall discuss in detail the role of these modalities in establishing a definitive diagnosis of PCLs. In addition, we shall also differentiate various benign and malignant pathologies based on characteristic imaging appearance. We also propose a stepwise algorithmic approach to a PCL encountered on imaging that will help radiologists and gastroenterologists alike in reaching a conclusive diagnosis.

Keywords

Pancreatic cyst · Pancreatic cystic lesion · CT · MRI · Imaging

U. Gorsi (✉) · H. Bhatia · S. Choudhary
Department of Radiodiagnosis and Imaging, Postgraduate Institute of Medical Education and Research (PGIMER), Chandigarh, India

R. K. Sharma et al. (eds.), *Differential Diagnosis and Management of Pancreatic Cystic Lesions*, https://doi.org/10.1007/978-981-92-0654-4_2

2.1 Introduction

A vast majority of cases of pancreatic cysts are incidentally detected with a prevalence as high as 4–14% in the general population. These are often detected in asymptomatic individuals or patients undergoing abdominal imaging for an unrelated etiology [1–3]. Due to the increased detection of pancreatic cystic lesions (PCLs) with the help of advanced cross-sectional imaging techniques, characterization and risk stratification of these cysts is an essential step [4, 5]. Follow-up and management guidelines have been established for all PCLs, especially the ones at risk for malignant degeneration, including IPMNs [6–9]. In addition to the available imaging tools (sonography, CT, and MRI), endoscopic ultrasound (EUS) adds essential information in cyst characterization and in determining the malignancy risk with the help of fine needle aspiration of the cyst contents, including the determination of carcino-embryonic antigen (CEA) levels.

2.1.1 Role of Sonography (USG)

Ultrasound is often used as a screening modality in symptomatic patients presenting with abdominal pain, jaundice, abdominal distention, and other symptoms. Ultrasound can clearly detect large cystic lesions with posterior acoustic enhancement in the pancreas or peri-pancreatic region. Smaller lesions are however often missed. Indirect features on sonography including biliary dilatation, ascites, and dilatation of the main pancreatic duct (MPD) are well-visualized on USG. Cases with suspected pancreatic pathologies can then undergo cross-sectional imaging with CT and/or MRI to further rule out a pancreatic lesion. Major limitations of ultrasound include its operator dependence and presence of overlying bowel gas that often obscures the sonographic window. The role of each imaging modality is discussed under a separate subheading.

2.1.2 Role of CT

Multidetector CT (MDCT) with its high spatial and temporal resolution, ease of availability, and 3D reconstruction techniques is the primary investigation of choice in detecting and characterizing pancreatic cystic lesions. CT well demonstrates the pancreatic parenchyma and in detail illustrates the intra-cystic features including calcifications, presence of septations, solid nodules, and communication with MPD. MRCP may however score over CT in delineating the latter in some cases [10–13]. A biphasic scan (arterial and venous phases) and/or a noncontrast scan helps in excellent depiction of enhancement characteristics and further classifying the lesion into aggressive and nonaggressive subtypes. Nowadays, dual-energy CT is also being increasingly used to characterize the cyst by the generation of iodine maps [14].

2.1.3 Role of MRI

Magnetic resonance imaging (MRI) due to its better soft tissue and contrast resolution is being used increasingly to characterize cystic lesions detected on CT with an accuracy as high as 90% [13]. Two-dimensional (2D) and 3D MRCP images are acquired as breath-hold or respiratory-triggered single-shot fast-spin echo sequences and excellently demonstrate the presence of communication with MPD, dilatation of MPD, and side branches. In addition, it has been proven to be superior to CT in characterizing small cysts (< 3 cm in size) and in detecting cysts not visible on CT. Another added advantage of this radiation-free modality is its utility in the follow-up of indeterminate lesions in young patients who require multiple scans for cyst surveillance [15–17].

2.2 Imaging Approach and Cyst Characterization

A PCL when identified as an incidental finding must undergo a systematic approach of characterization on imaging. The important features to be assessed include the size of the lesion, number of cysts, presence or absence of septations, presence or absence of enhancing walls or mural nodules, and relationship (or communication) to the MPD. The last is one of the key features in establishing a reliable differential diagnosis. Ductal communication may suggest a diagnosis of a pseudocyst/WON in the setting of acute pancreatitis and IPMN in the absence of such history. A small BD-IPMN, however, may not have a demonstrable ductal communication and may mimic an MCN radiologically. Lesions with a potential malignant risk must be identified by red-flag features like the presence of thick enhancing walls and/or mural nodules and solid components. MRI often shows the intra-cystic features accurately, including the type of fluid present (mucinous or hemorrhagic), and thus helps narrow down the differential diagnosis. Multiphasic CT, on the other hand, not only demonstrates the calcifications but also clearly characterizes the lesions based on enhancement characteristics [18, 19].

Table 2.1 enumerates the benign and malignant PCLs discussed further in the text.

Table 2.1 Classification of benign and malignant pancreatic cystic lesions

	Communicating with MPD	Not communicating with MPD	
Non-neoplastic	Pseudocyst	Walled off necrosis	
	Walled-off necrosis	Congenital cyst	
		Retention cyst	
Neoplastic	Intraductal papillary mucinous neoplasm (IPMN-BD/MN)	Mucinous	Non-mucinous
		MCN	SCN
			SPN
			Cystic NET
			Acinar cell neoplasm
			Ductal adenocarcinoma with cystic degeneration

2.3 Benign Lesions

These can be divided into various categories based on the origin and etiology of cyst formation and are discussed below.

(a) *Congenital Cysts*

Congenital cysts are usually multiple and often associated with a systemic syndrome affecting various organ systems as described below.

(i) *Autosomal Dominant Polycystic Kidney Disorder (ADPKD)*: While multiple renal cysts characterize the syndrome, pancreas is also a common location for the same, as are liver, spleen, thyroid, ovary, and epididymis [20, 21]. These are lined by cuboidal epithelium and are often detected incidentally as variable-sized fluid attenuation cysts in the pancreas along with the presence of cystic disease in kidneys and liver, either as a part of abdominal imaging for an unrelated purpose or as a part of syndromic evaluation [22]. The cysts may be simple or complex, and patients may be offered follow-up imaging depending on the specific guidelines.

(ii) *Cystic Fibrosis*: Though rare, cysts develop in the pancreatic parenchyma due to the obstruction of the pancreatic duct by inspissated mucin. Single or multiple cysts can be found, with the size ranging from microscopic lesions to large cysts, replacing the entire pancreas. Other associated pancreatic findings include calcifications and fatty infiltration on CT [20, 23]. MRCP may delineate the cystic lesion and dilatation of the pancreatic duct better.

(iii) *Von Hippel Lindau syndrome (VHL)*: VHL is an important autosomal dominant clinical syndrome that presents with a spectrum of pancreatic lesions including cystadenomas, hemangioblastomas, and islet cell tumors. Pancreatic cysts per se are demonstrated in only 50% of cases on imaging [20]. Familial syndromic cases must undergo active screening as pancreatic lesions are often the harbinger of lesions in other organ systems. Imaging appearance varies depending upon the type of lesion encountered in the parenchyma. CT and MRI show benign cysts (Fig. 2.1) as well as cystic tumors involving the kidneys (clear cell carcinomas), pancreas, epididymis, retinal angiomas, and posterior fossa and/or spinal hemangioblastomas. Histopathologically, congenital cysts can be either true cysts or lympho-epithelial cysts. While true cysts are epithelial-lined and unilocular or multilocular in appearance with serous fluid, the latter are rare and have a squamous lining with the keratinous material [22].

(b) *Retention Cysts*

This is another benign entity that represents a cystic dilatation of MPD occurring due to obstruction due to mucin, calculi, or a malignant cause. It is lined by mucinous epithelium and can be located anywhere in the pancreas. These are considered as indeterminate cysts with specific follow-up guidelines based on the size and age of the patient. CT and MRI often show a well-defined uni- or multilocular cystic lesion mimicking BD-IPMN or MCN. Active surveillance must be carried out to rule out the development of pancreatic cancer [24].

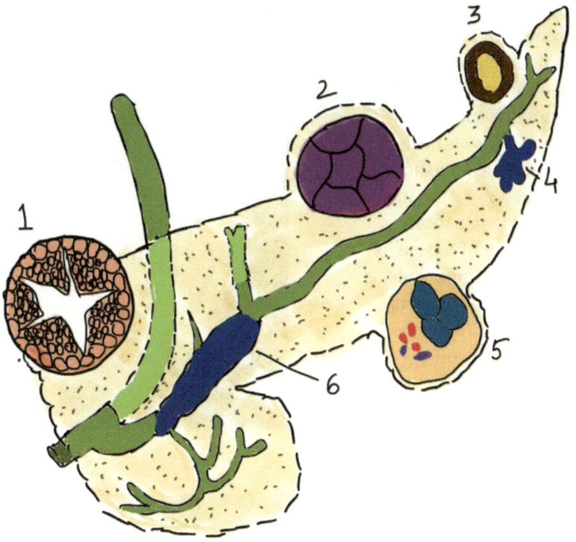

Fig. 2.1 Diagrammatic representation of pancreatic cystic lesions. 1: Serous cystadenoma; 2: Mucinous cystic neoplasm; 3: Cystic neuroendocrine tumor; 4: Branch-duct IPMN; 5: Solid pseudopapillary neoplasm; 6: Main-duct IPMN

(c) *Inflammatory or Infectious Etiology*

(i) *Abscess:* Pancreatic abscess often occurs as a morbid complication of pancreatitis developing due to infection of a pancreatic collection. Radiologically, these are often suspected due to the presence of gas in an already existing undrained fluid collection and established by the diagnostic percutaneous aspiration of the collection fluid [22]. The presence of gas in a collection on CT, however, must be treated with caution as the former can also be due to internal fistulization into the bowel or due to previous drainage of collection or secondary to a surgical procedure like pancreatico-jejunostomy. In rare scenarios, fungal and tubercular infections may present as cystic lesions on imaging [25, 26]. CT shows an ill-defined collection with intra- and peripancreatic necrosis and fat stranding and/or the presence of air. MRI often shows a heterogeneously hyperintense collection on T2 with the surrounding inflammation. Definitive diagnosis is however established only by microbiological confirmation of diagnostic aspiration of the fluid.

(ii) *Pseudocyst/Walled Off Necrosis (WON):* These are the most commonly encountered PCLs and represent encapsulated fluid collections occurring after a period of ≥4 weeks' setting of acute pancreatitis (AP) with and without necrosis. Surrounding inflammatory changes and a corroborative history of pancreatitis often clinch the diagnosis. Follow-up studies may demonstrate a decrease in the size of these lesions. CT often shows a hypodense fluid collection with the surrounding fat stranding and necrosis (in cases of WON). While pseudocysts appear uniformly hyperintense on T2WI MRI, WONs often contain internal solid debris differentiating the two radiologically (Figs. 2.2 and 2.3). These lesions, however, must be carefully assessed, as a cystic tumor may have led to the development of acute pancreatitis, and a patient with AP may have a cystic tumor on imaging.

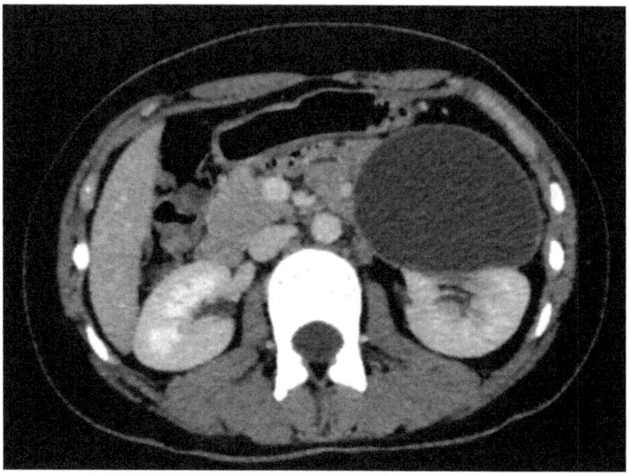

Fig. 2.2 Pancreatic pseudocyst. Axial contrast-enhanced CT of a 44-year-old man with a history of acute pancreatitis showing a well-defined, cystic attenuation lesion in the tail of the pancreas suggestive of a pseudocyst. No solid components or septations were seen

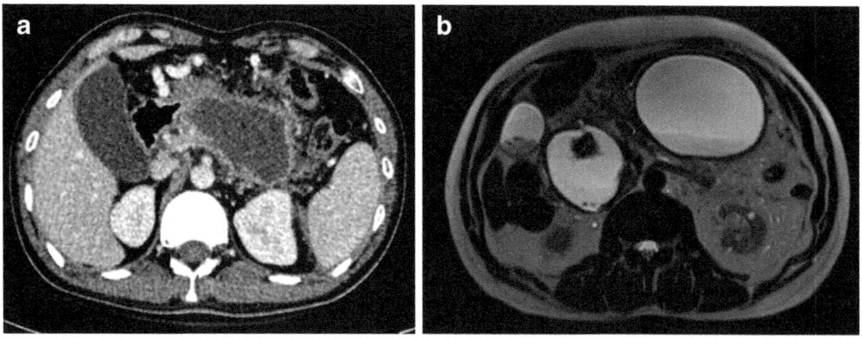

Fig. 2.3 Walled-off necrosis. Axial contrast enhanced CT image (**a**) of a young man with a history of acute necrotizing pancreatitis showing a peripherally enhancing, heterogeneous collection in the pancreatic body and tail suggestive of walled-off necrosis. Axial T2 HASTE image (**b**) of another patient showing two well-defined collections in pancreatic head and body with internal hypointense contents and fluid-debris level, respectively

2.4 Neoplastic Lesions

(a) *Serous Cystadenoma or Serous Cystic Neoplasm (SCN)*

These are benign lesions accounting for about 10–25% of all PCLs and 1–2% of pancreatic tumors. More commonly affecting old-aged females (>50 years), these lesions can be both sporadic and syndromic in nature. Up to 20% of these cases are associated with VHL, with lesions being multifocal in such cases [27]. Although this lesion can be found anywhere in the pancreas, the tumor has a specific predilection for the head region [28]. Clinically, the lesions are asymptomatic in majority of the patients; it may be symptomatic, causing abdominal pain and other pancreato-biliary symptoms [28].

Imaging wise, these lesions can be divided into three subtypes in decreasing order of prevalence: micro or polycystic pattern, macro or oligocystic pattern,

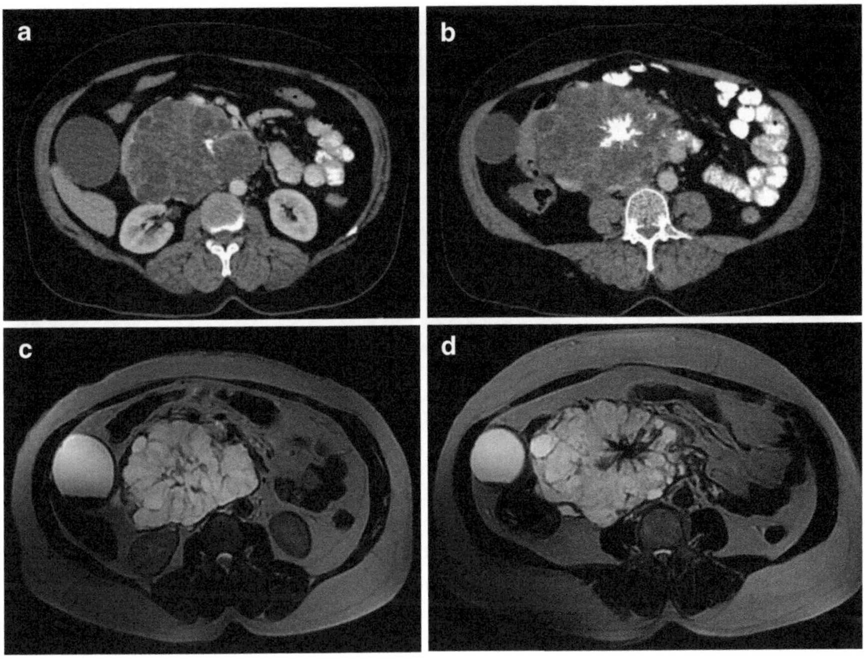

Fig. 2.4 Axial contrast enhanced CT images (**a** and **b**) of a 58-year-old woman showing multicystic lesion with microcysts in the head of the pancreas with a central scar showing stellate pattern of calcification. Axial T2 HASTE images (**c** and **d**) of the same patient show a lobulated multicystic lesion and a central T2-hypointense scar—features classical of a serous cystadenoma of the pancreas

mixed pattern, and honeycomb form which is the least common. The microcystic pattern consists of multiple (>6) cysts (< 2 cm) separated by fibrous septa forming a characteristic central stellate scar that may calcify with a lobulated contour (Fig. 2.4). The macrocystic pattern consists of small number of cysts ≥2 cm in size. Often, there is no scar within the lesion, and the lesion is often indistinguishable from other PCLs, especially MCN and BD-IPMN. Differential diagnosis is important, since SCN is a benign lesion, while MCN and IPMN have a potentially malignant behavior. In the honeycomb pattern, there are multiple tiny sub-centimetric sized closely apposed cysts that may appear solid on CT as well as MRI [29]. Mixed pattern, on the other hand, may have few larger cysts situated peripherally. Diagnosis is often established on T2-weighted MRI images and MRCP sequence where a ductal communication rules out a similar-looking lesion such as a branch duct IPMN, which may be potentially malignant. While macrocystic SCN often has a lobulated contour with septations, MCN, on the other hand, has a smooth contour [28].

(b) *Mucinous Cystadenoma or Mucinous Neoplasm (MCN)*

MCNs are potentially malignant cystic lesions often located in the body and tail region of pancreas and are almost exclusively seen in middle-aged female patients. In contrast to the glycogen lining epithelium of SCN, MCNs are lined

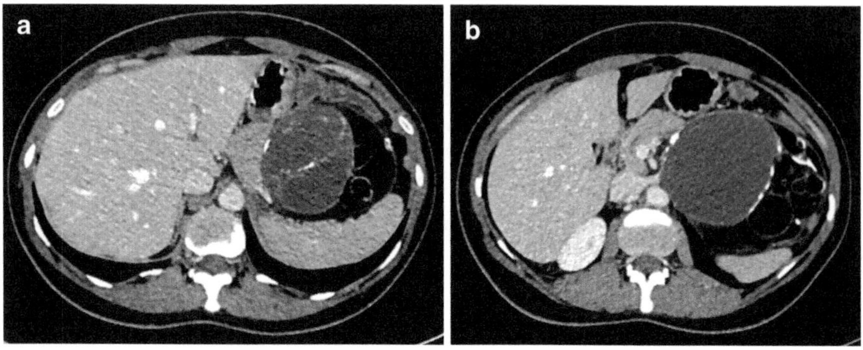

Fig. 2.5 Axial contrast enhanced CT images (**a** and **b**) of a middle-aged woman showing a large multilocular cystic lesion in the body and tail of the pancreas with thin internal septations and peripheral, curvilinear calcifications suggestive of mucinous cystadenoma of the pancreas. No obvious solid components were seen within the lesion

by mucin-producing columnar epithelium with surrounding ovarian stroma [30]. These lesions often have thickened walls and follow a spectrum from a cystic adenoma to an aggressive and invasive mucinous adenocarcinoma that is malignant. Thes lesions undergo surgical resection based on the malignancy risk and thus must be differentiated from the other more common differential diagnosis like pseudocysts based on corroborative clinical history. Characteristically, these have larger cysts (which are less in number in comparison to SCN) and have a smooth external contour. No ductal communication is demonstrated on imaging, and thus these can be differentiated from the other mucin-containing group of tumors, the IPMNs.

CT shows well-defined round fluid density hypodense lesions with cyst wall calcifications (Fig. 2.5). Thickened walls and septal nodules that enhance on contrast administration suggesting malignancy can also be seen. Distal pancreatic parenchyma may show signs of atrophy with ductal dilatation [30].

MRI: Well-defined T1 hypointense and T2 hyperintense unilocular lesions (or those with very few septae) may be seen. Enhancing septal as well as mural nodules suggesting malignancy can be seen.

Features that are considered worrisome for malignancy include the presence of thick walls, enhancing septal and mural nodularity, enhancing intra-cystic soft tissue, enlarged nodes, presence of metastases (most commonly liver), and surrounding local invasion [18].

(c) *IPMN*

This group comprises majority (about 70%) of pancreatic cystic tumors and further consists of a heterogeneous spectrum of mucin-producing tumors [28]. These mostly occur in patients over 70 years of age and are characterized by a dilated pancreatic duct (MPD or branch ducts) that histologically consist of papillary projections consisting of dysplastic mucin-producing epithelium [31]. These have a potential for malignant degeneration into adenocarcinoma and are often described to be following the adenoma–carcinoma sequence with varying grades of dysplasia. Also, it may be linked to the development of ductal adeno-

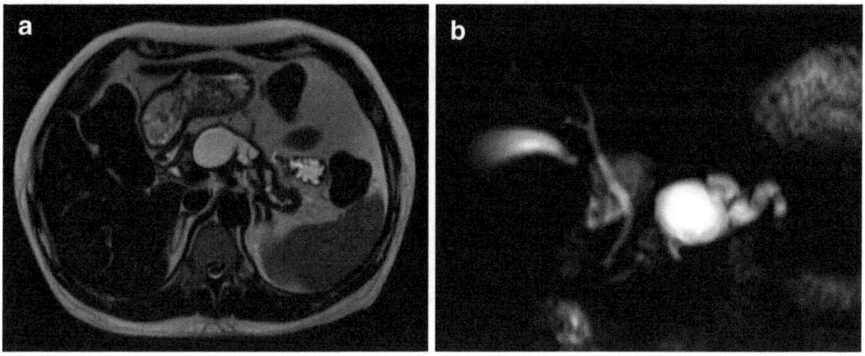

Fig. 2.6 Axial T2-HASTE (**a**) and MRCP (**b**) images of a 47-year-old man showing a cystic lesion in the body of the pancreas communicating with the main pancreatic duct. Communication with the main pancreatic duct is better depicted in the MRCP image, which suggests branch duct intraductal papillary mucinous neoplasm

carcinoma at sites not affected by the cystic tumor reflecting a diffuse pathologic process involving the entire pancreas [18]. Histologically, while these are classified into intestinal, gastric, pancreato-biliary, and oncocytic subtypes, imaging classification characterizes them into main-duct, branch-duct, or mixed-type IPMN, depending upon the type and extent of ductal involvement [32, 33].

(i) *Branch-Duct IPMN (BD-IPMN)*: This appears as a well-defined round or lobulated unilocular or multilocular lesion (grape-like appearance) communicating with the MPD. The cysts are variable in size and separated by multiple enhancing septae demonstrated on CT and/or MRI (Fig. 2.6). Location wise, this tumor is more likely to be encountered in the uncinate process [18]. Demonstration of ductal communication is essential, and thus, a definitive diagnosis is often established only on high-quality MRCP sequences that rule out or confirm suspected cystic lesions on CT. Potential differential diagnosis includes a pseudocyst, SCN, or MCN when ductal communication is difficult to establish [28]. Multiplicity of the lesion, however, favors a diagnosis of BD-IPMN over other lesions [18].

(ii) *Main-Duct IPMN (MD-IPMN)*: This represents 15–20% of the pancreatic cystic tumors and is characterized by segmental or diffuse uniform dilatation of the MPD (> 5 mm) with tumor mucin without any other cause of obstruction [34]. The duct shows cystic dilatation with a higher risk of malignancy associated with a larger MPD diameter [35].

Diffuse MD-IPMN often presents as a uniform dilatation of the MPD throughout its course without any tapering or cause of obstruction like stricture or stones. This lesion predominantly needs to be differentiated from an inflammatory dilation of MPD, as in chronic pancreatitis, where the dilatation is irregular, associated with strictures in the presence of intraductal calculi and parenchymal calcifications on CT. MD-IPMN presents as more homogeneous dilatation with a bulging ampulla. Parenchymal atrophy, however, may be seen in both the settings [28].

Segmental MD-IPMN often presents as a nonspecific segmental dilatation of MPD without obstruction or previous pancreatitis. Differentiation from chronic pancreatitis is often difficult.

Mixed-type IMPN represents dilatation of both the main and branch ducts on MRI.

2.4.1 Worrisome Features and Malignancy Risk

Risk of malignancy depends on the histological as well as ductal subtype of IPMN, with the main-duct IPMNs and pancreatico-biliary subtypes reported to have a higher risk of malignancy than the other counterparts [36]. Few features have been considered as "worrisome" for malignancy, as established by International Consensus Fukuoka Guidelines. These include an MPD dilatation of 5–9 mm {7 mm threshold by ACR [37]}, diameter of cyst >3 cm, presence of an enhancing intracystic mural nodule (< 5 mm), enhancing cyst wall, abrupt diameter change with atrophy, and presence of lymphadenopathy. All these warrant a further investigation with endoscopic ultrasound to rule out malignancy [18].

(d) *Solid Pseudo-Papillary Neoplasm (SPN)*

SPN or pseudopapillary epithelial neoplasm is a rare tumor seen almost exclusively in young females (around 35 years) with a predilection for the tail of pancreas. It accounts for about 10–12% of all exocrine pancreatic tumors and is considered to be a benign lesion or one with a low malignant potential and a favorable prognosis with a 5-year survival rate ranging from 70% to 90% [18, 30, 38]. Although rare, the lesion may be encountered as an incidental finding in asymptomatic patients. On the other hand, patients may be symptomatic due to the mass effect exerted on the surrounding structures due to the large-sized lesions.

Imaging often reveals variable-sized solid-cystic lesions in the region of tail of pancreas. While the solid component represents the tumor and is situated peripherally, the cystic nature of the tumor is attributed to tumor degeneration and is centrally located. The associated necrosis and hemorrhage often give a variable appearance to the tumor depending upon the proportion of these contents [18, 30].

CT reveals a well-encapsulated cystic lesion with enhancing solid components peripherally and central non-enhancing necrosis. Hemorrhage may be confirmed as a hyperdense fluid on noncontrast scans before the administration of intravenous contrast (Fig. 2.7).

MRI often shows a well-defined mass with hemorrhage and necrosis on T1 and T2 images. Areas of internal hemorrhage appear hyperintense on T1WI and hypointense on T2WI with the presence of a fluid debris level in a few cases. Uni- or multilocular microcystic lesions may be seen on MRI [39]. Enhancement pattern is gradual in comparison to the early enhancement of neuroendocrine tumors (Fig. 2.8).

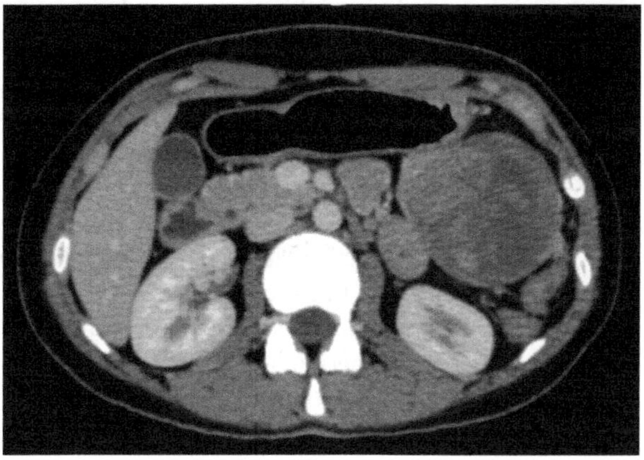

Fig. 2.7 Axial CECT image of a 21-year-old woman showing a well-defined, encapsulated soli-cystic lesion in the tail of the pancreas suggestive of solid pseudopapillary epithelial neoplasm of pancreas later confirmed on histopathology

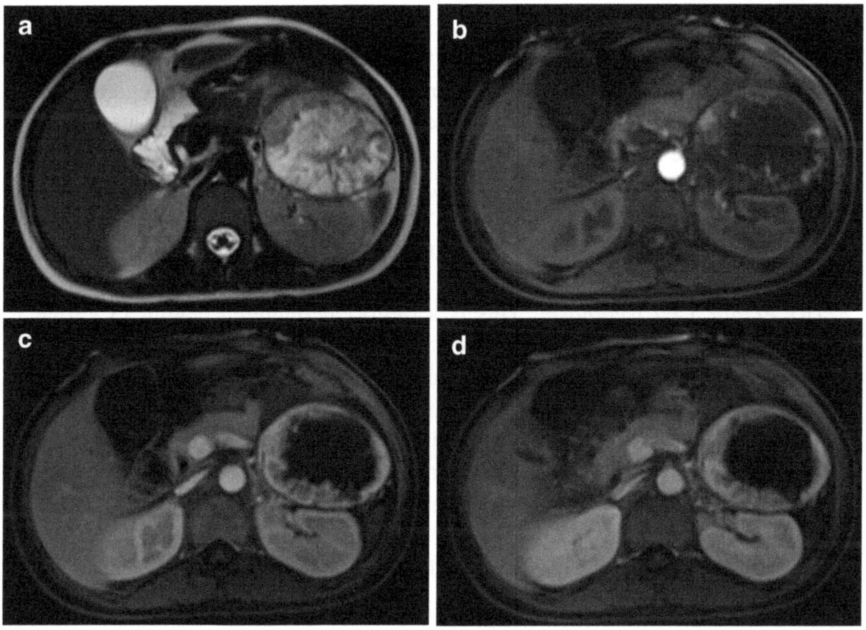

Fig. 2.8 Axial T2-HASTE image (**a**) of an 18-year-old girl showing a well-defined, encapsulated heterogeneous signal intensity lesion in the pancreatic tail. The arterial phase (**b**) image showed heterogeneous enhancement which was seen progressing in the portal venous phase (**c** and **d**). The enhancing component is seen at the periphery of the lesion while the cystic component is located at the center of the lesion. Features were suggestive of solid pseudopapillary epithelial neoplasm of the pancreas

(e) *Cystic Pancreatic Neuroendocrine Tumors (PNETs)*

NETs are rare pancreatic malignancies occurring in adult population with an equal incidence in males and females. These are often sporadic and may also occur as a part of syndromes like VHL, NF, and MEN-1 [18]. Cystic NETs comprise one subset of this tumor population, where the cystic component is attributed to tumor degeneration. PNETs can be functional and present with symptoms due to hormones they secrete or be nonfunctional in nature. The latter lesions often present due to the mass effect created by large lesions. Cystic NETs are large nonfunctional pancreatic lesions [18] that represent about 7–17% of all pancreatic NETs [18]. They often have a malignant potential and thus must be accurately differentiated from other pancreatic cystic lesions.

CT: Well-defined cystic lesion with a peripheral vascularized rim that shows avid enhancement in the arterial phase.

MRI: Shows a uni- or multilocular cystic lesion not communicating with MPD, appearing hyperintense on T2WI, with peripheral arterial enhancement that also characterizes solid NETs on imaging [18, 30].

Table 2.2 compares the imaging features among the commonly encountered pancreatic cystic tumors.

(f) *Rare Variants*

(i) *Ductal Adenocarcinoma with Cystic Degeneration*: Pancreatic ductal adenocarcinoma (PDAC) is one of the most dreaded malignant carcinomas of pancreas associated with high mortality and morbidity. Although the lesion is characteristically solid, cystic degeneration representing internal necrosis or side branch dilatation is rarely reported. The lesion is identified on cross-sectional imaging as a hypo-enhancing soft tissue (with cystic degeneration) lesion with characteristic malignant features like surrounding vascular encasement/invasion, obstruction of the MPD and/or CBD, and enlarged lymph nodes [30].

(ii) *Acinar Cell Neoplasm*: This is a rarely encountered benign PCL that is characterized histologically by acinar cell differentiation of the epithelial lining of the cyst with an ambiguous nature of origin, with theories ranging from it being a developmental anomaly to involving obstructive ductal dilatation [40]. This lesion is seen in patients of all ages with female preponderance and abdominal pain as the most common presenting symptoms. CT and MRI often show a uni- or multilocular cystic lesion with clustered cysts not communicating with the pancreatic duct and presence of cyst calcifications [41]. The final diagnosis is however established on histopathology.

Other lesions which may appear as solid-cystic on cross-sectional imaging include metastasis, lymphangioma, teratoma, paraganglioma, or rarely a sarcoma.

Flowchart 2.1 denotes a suggested imaging approach to the characterization of a PCL.

Table 2.2 Comparison among various commonly encountered pancreatic cystic tumors

	SCN	MCN	IPMN	SPN	Cystic PNET
Gender	Females > males	Females >> Males	Males = females	Females > males	Males = females
Age	5th–7th decade (grandmother lesion)	4th–5th decade (mother lesion)	6th–7th decade	2nd–4th decade (daughter lesion)	5th–6th decade
Location	Head > body and tail	Body and tail	Head, body and tail	Tail > head and body	Body and tail
Imaging appearance	Microcystic/macrocystic/ honeycomb	Large cysts ± septae	MD: Segmental or diffusely dilated MPD BD: Side branch dilated	Solid-cystic	Solid-cystic
Cyst size	<2 cm	>2 cm	Variable	Variable	Variable
Number of cysts	>6	<6	Variable	Unilocular	Unilocular
CT	Multiple cysts ± central scar ± calcifications	Few cysts ± septae ± mural nodule	Cyst communicating with MPD + dilated ducts	Heterogeneous with hyperdense hemorrhage	Cyst with peripheral hyper-vascular rim
MRI	Low T1, high T2, central scar	Low T1, high T2, thick walls and sepate	Low T1, high T2, dilated MPD	Variable with hemorrhage and necrosis	Low T1, high T2
MPD communication	No	No	Yes	No	No

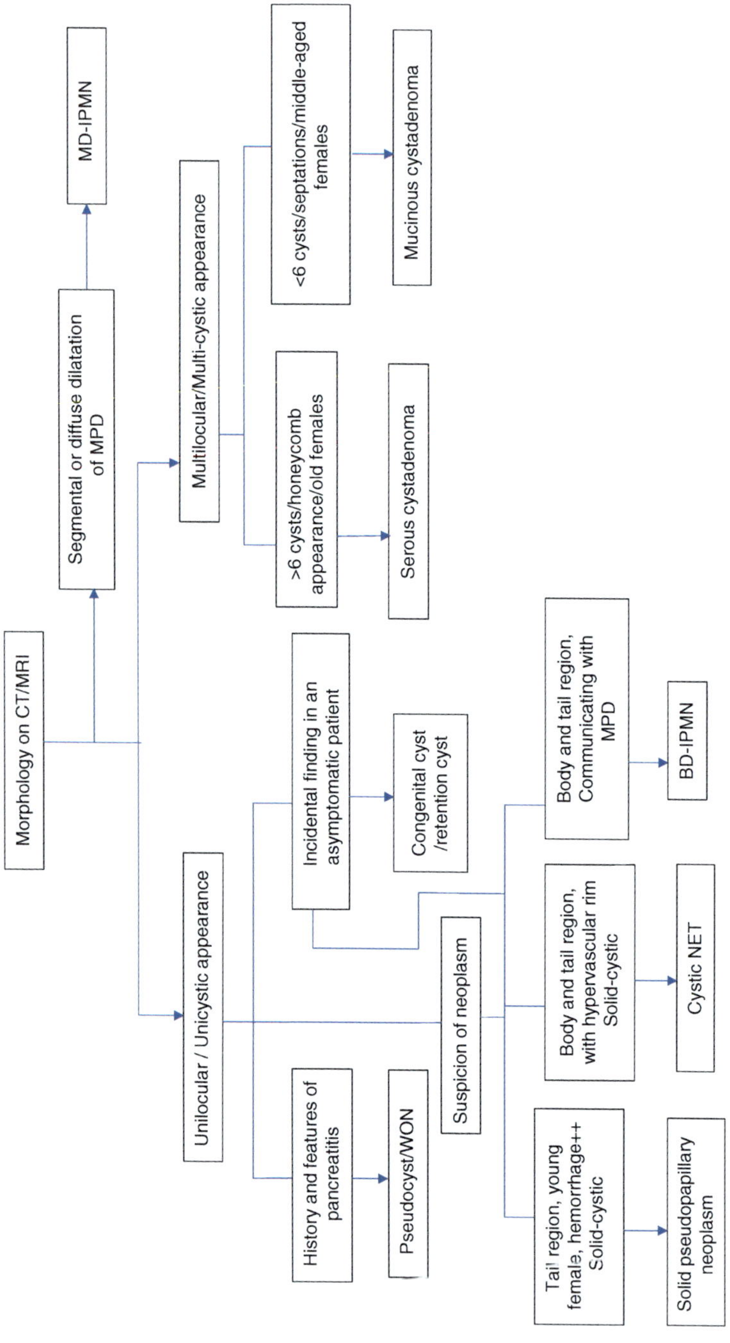

Flowchart 2.1 Imaging approach in characterizing a pancreatic cystic lesion

2.5 Role of Artificial Intelligence and Radiomics

PCLs, in particular cystic neoplasms, need to be diagnosed as early as possible in view of the associated mortality and malignancy risks. Even though cross-sectional imaging techniques well identify and characterize the lesion, the accuracy still amounts up to 50% [42].

With significant progress in the field and applications of artificial intelligence, specifically in oncology, tumor detection, classification, and characterization have become much easier and accurate [42]. Radiomics is a specific deep learning-based model that extracts quantitative features from standard input image data sets, followed by complex mathematical and computational analyses to generate specific imaging biomarkers for each tumor subtype.

Machine learning-based applications help in training of these software by using the imaging data that is available. New patient data is then processed and images analyzed based on attenuation, size, shape, enhancement characteristics, and other features. In addition, specific follow-up and surveillance protocols are also suggested for each patient [43–45].

MDCT techniques are currently in practice that use radiomics and quantitative imaging data to identify benign from malignant pancreatic cystic lesions, in particular IPMNs [28]. Although MRI-based radiomic techniques are difficult to apply, these are currently under research and being implemented along with texture analysis [28, 46].

References

1. Zaheer A, Pokharel SS, Wolfgang C, Fishman EK, Horton KM. Incidentally detected cystic lesions of the pancreas on CT: review of literature and management suggestions. Abdom Imaging. 2013;38(2):331–41.
2. Laffan TA, Horton KM, Klein AP, et al. Prevalence of unsuspected pancreatic cysts on MDCT. AJR Am J Roentgenol. 2008;191(3):802–7.
3. Lee KS, Sekhar A, Rofsky NM, Pedrosa I. Prevalence of incidental pancreatic cysts in the adult population on MR imaging. Am J Gastroenterol. 2010;105(9):2079–84.
4. Kromrey ML, Bülow R, Hübner J, et al. Prospective study on the incidence, prevalence and 5-year pancreatic-related mortality of pancreatic cysts in a population-based study. Gut. 2018;67(1):138–45.
5. Zerboni G, Signoretti M, Crippa S, Falconi M, Arcidiacono PG, Capurso G. Systematic review and meta-analysis: prevalence of incidentally detected pancreatic cystic lesions in asymptomatic individuals. Pancreatology. 2019;19(1):2–9.
6. Vege SS, Ziring B, Jain R, Moayyedi P, Clinical Guidelines Committee, American Gastroenterology Association. American gastroenterological association institute guideline on the diagnosis and management of asymptomatic neoplastic pancreatic cysts. Gastroenterology. 2015;148(4):819–22.
7. Tanaka M, Fernández-Del Castillo C, Kamisawa T, et al. Revisions of international consensus Fukuoka guidelines for the management of IPMN of the pancreas. Pancreatology. 2017;17(5):738–53.
8. Elta GH, Enestvedt BK, Sauer BG, Lennon AM. ACG clinical guideline: diagnosis and management of pancreatic cysts. Am J Gastroenterol. 2018;113(4):464–79.

9. Jeffrey RB. Imaging pancreatic cysts with CT and MRI. Dig Dis Sci. 2017;62(7):1787–95.
10. Lee HJ, Kim MJ, Choi JY, Hong HS, Kim KA. Relative accuracy of CT and MRI in the differentiation of benign from malignant pancreatic cystic lesions. Clin Radiol. 2011;66(4):315–21.
11. Sahani DV, Sainani NI, Blake MA, Crippa S, Mino-Kenudson M, del-Castillo CF. Prospective evaluation of reader performance on MDCT in characterization of cystic pancreatic lesions and prediction of cyst biologic aggressiveness. AJR Am J Roentgenol. 2011;197(1):53–61.
12. Sahani DV, Kadavigere R, Blake M, Fernandez-Del Castillo C, Lauwers GY, Hahn PF. Intraductal papillary mucinous neoplasm of pancreas: multi-detector row CT with 2D curved reformations--correlation with MRCP. Radiology. 2006;238(2):560–9.
13. Visser BC, Yeh BM, Qayyum A, Way LW, McCulloch CE, Coakley FV. Characterization of cystic pancreatic masses: relative accuracy of CT and MRI. AJR Am J Roentgenol. 2007;189(3):648–56.
14. George E, Wortman JR, Fulwadhva UP, Uyeda JW, Sodickson AD. Dual energy CT applications in pancreatic pathologies. Br J Radiol. 2017;90(1080):20170411.
15. Sainani NI, Saokar A, Deshpande V, Fernández-del Castillo C, Hahn P, Sahani DV. Comparative performance of MDCT and MRI with MR cholangiopancreatography in characterizing small pancreatic cysts. AJR Am J Roentgenol. 2009;193(3):722–31.
16. Fukukura Y, Fujiyoshi F, Sasaki M, Nakajo M. Pancreatic duct: morphologic evaluation with MR cholangiopancreatography after secretin stimulation. Radiology. 2002;222(3):674–80.
17. Sandrasegaran K, Lin C, Akisik FM, Tann M. State-of-the-art pancreatic MRI. AJR Am J Roentgenol. 2010;195(1):42–53.
18. Miller FH, Lopes Vendrami C, Recht HS, et al. Pancreatic cystic lesions and malignancy: assessment, guidelines, and the field defect. Radiographics. 2022;42(1):87–105.
19. Tamura S, Yamamoto H, Ushida S, Suzuki K. Mucinous cystic neoplasms in male patients: two cases. Rare Tumors. 2017;9(3):7096.
20. Ros PR, Hamrick-Turner JE, Chiechi MV, Ros LH, Gallego P, Burton SS. Cystic masses of the pancreas. Radiographics. 1992;12(4):673–86.
21. Nicolau C, Torra R, Bianchi L, et al. Abdominal sonographic study of autosomal dominant polycystic kidney disease. J Clin Ultrasound. 2000;28(6):277–82.
22. Demos TC, Posniak HV, Harmath C, Olson MC, Aranha G. Cystic lesions of the pancreas. AJR Am J Roentgenol. 2002;179(6):1375–88.
23. Cahill ME, Parmentier JM, Van Ruyssevelt C, Pauls CH. Pancreatic cystosis in cystic fibrosis. Abdom Imaging. 1997;22(3):313–4.
24. Ren F, Zuo C, Chen G, et al. Pancreatic retention cyst: multi-modality imaging findings and review of the literature. Abdom Imaging. 2013;38(4):818–26.
25. Robbins EG 2nd, Stollman NH, Bierman P, Grauer L, Barkin JS. Pancreatic fungal infections: a case report and review of the literature. Pancreas. 1996;12(3):308–12.
26. Pombo F, Díaz Candamio MJ, Rodriguez E, Pombo S. Pancreatic tuberculosis: CT findings. Abdom Imaging. 1998;23(4):394–7.
27. Neumann HP, Dinkel E, Brambs H, et al. Pancreatic lesions in the von Hippel-Lindau syndrome. Gastroenterology. 1991;101(2):465–71.
28. Morana G, Ciet P, Venturini S. Cystic pancreatic lesions: MR imaging findings and management. Insights Imaging. 2021;12(1):115.
29. Choi JY, Kim MJ, Lee JY, et al. Typical and atypical manifestations of serous cystadenoma of the pancreas: imaging findings with pathologic correlation. AJR Am J Roentgenol. 2009;193(1):136–42.
30. Khan A, Khosa F, Eisenberg RL. Cystic lesions of the pancreas. AJR Am J Roentgenol. 2011;196(6):W668–77.
31. Kwon JE, Jang KT, Ryu Y, et al. Subtype of intraductal papillary mucinous neoplasm of the pancreas is important to the development of metachronous high-risk lesions after pancreatectomy. Ann Hepatobiliary Pancreat Surg. 2019;23(4):365–71.
32. Fonseca AL, Kirkwood K, Kim MP, Maitra A, Koay EJ. Intraductal papillary mucinous neoplasms of the pancreas: current understanding and future directions for stratification of malignancy risk. Pancreas. 2018;47(3):272–9.

33. Procacci C, Carbognin G, Biasiutti C, Guarise A, Ghirardi C, Schenal G. Intraductal papillary mucinous tumors of the pancreas: spectrum of CT and MR findings with pathologic correlation. Eur Radiol. 2001;11(10):1939–51.
34. Levink I, Bruno MJ, Cahen DL. Management of intraductal papillary mucinous neoplasms: controversies in guidelines and future perspectives. Curr Treat Options Gastroenterol. 2018;16(3):316–32.
35. Oyama H, Tada M, Takagi K, et al. Long-term risk of malignancy in branch-duct intraductal papillary mucinous neoplasms. Gastroenterology. 2020;158(1):226–37.
36. Hecht EM, Khatri G, Morgan D, et al. Intraductal papillary mucinous neoplasm (IPMN) of the pancreas: recommendations for standardized imaging and reporting from the Society of Abdominal Radiology IPMN disease focused panel. Abdom Radiol (NY). 2021;46(4):1586–606.
37. Megibow AJ, Baker ME, Morgan DE, et al. Management of incidental pancreatic cysts: a white paper of the ACR incidental findings committee. J Am Coll Radiol. 2017;14(7):911–23.
38. Coleman KM, Doherty MC, Bigler SA. Solid-pseudopapillary tumor of the pancreas. Radiographics. 2003;23(6):1644–8.
39. Crippa S, Aleotti F, Longo E, et al. Main duct thresholds for malignancy are different in intraductal papillary mucinous neoplasms of the pancreatic head and body-tail. Clin Gastroenterol Hepatol. 2022;20(2):390–9.
40. Singhi AD, Norwood S, Liu TC, et al. Acinar cell cystadenoma of the pancreas: a benign neoplasm or non-neoplastic ballooning of acinar and ductal epithelium? Am J Surg Pathol. 2013;37(9):1329–35.
41. Delavaud C, d'Assignies G, Cros J, et al. CT and MR imaging of multilocular acinar cell cystadenoma: comparison with branch duct intraductal papillary mucinous neoplasia (IPMNs). Eur Radiol. 2014;24(9):2128–36.
42. Mao KZ, Ma C, Song B. Radiomics advances in the evaluation of pancreatic cystic neoplasms. Heliyon. 2024;10(3):e25535.
43. Lambin P, Rios-Velazquez E, Leijenaar R, et al. Radiomics: extracting more information from medical images using advanced feature analysis. Eur J Cancer. 2012;48(4):441–6.
44. Bian Y, Zhao Z, Jiang H, et al. Noncontrast radiomics approach for predicting grades of nonfunctional pancreatic neuroendocrine tumors. J Magn Reson Imaging. 2020;52(4):1124–36.
45. Li K, Yao Q, Xiao J, et al. Contrast-enhanced CT radiomics for predicting lymph node metastasis in pancreatic ductal adenocarcinoma: a pilot study. Cancer Imaging. 2020;20(1):12.
46. Tobaly D, Santinha J, Sartoris R, et al. CT-based radiomics analysis to predict malignancy in patients with Intraductal Papillary Mucinous Neoplasm (IPMN) of the pancreas. Cancers (Basel). 2020;12(11):3089.

Cytopathology of Pancreatic Cystic Lesions

3

Parikshaa Gupta, Nalini Gupta, and Radhika Srinivasan

Abstract

Pancreatic cystic lesions include both neoplastic and non-neoplastic entities with varying malignant potential and constitute significant diagnostic and management challenges. The increased use of endoscopic ultrasound-guided fine-needle aspiration (EUS-FNA) has improved the detection and characterization of these lesions. Cytologic evaluation differentiates non-neoplastic from neoplastic cysts, and also identifies mucinous from nonmucinous lesions, and dysplasia or malignancy in mucinous neoplasms. Specific diagnosis requires a unified multidisciplinary approach that combines cytomorphologic features with clinical findings, imaging characteristics, cyst fluid biochemistry, and molecular analysis. Recent advances, including standardized WHO reporting systems, immunocytochemistry, and molecular profiling, have enhanced diagnostic accuracy and risk stratification. This chapter provides a comprehensive overview of the role of cytology in pancreatic cystic lesions, detailing sampling techniques, cytomorphologic features, diagnostic pitfalls, ancillary studies, and reporting frameworks, with an emphasis on a multimodal approach to guide optimal patient management.

Keywords

Cytology · EUS-FNA · Malignant · Benign · Mucin

P. Gupta · N. Gupta · R. Srinivasan (✉)
Department of Cytology & Gynecological Pathology, Postgraduate Institute of Medical Education and Research, Chandigarh, India

R. K. Sharma et al. (eds.), *Differential Diagnosis and Management of Pancreatic Cystic Lesions*, https://doi.org/10.1007/978-981-92-0654-4_3

3.1 Introduction

Cystic lesions of the pancreas are uncommon compared to their solid counterparts. The increasing use of EUS-FNA has led to the recognition of more entities. Traditionally, a cyst is a space fully or partially filled with liquid content and lined by epithelium. However, in the pancreas, this traditional definition has expanded to include any radiolucent lesion and some lesions that may not have a true lining epithelium. Cystic lesions of the pancreas encompass diverse entities ranging from non-neoplastic cysts to benign and malignant neoplasms. The most common types include intraductal papillary mucinous neoplasms (IPMN), mucinous cystic neoplasms (MCN), serous cystadenomas (SCA), and solid pseudopapillary neoplasms (SPN) [1, 2].

Clinical diagnosis of these cystic lesions is challenging due to nonspecific and overlapping symptoms. Accurate characterization requires a multidisciplinary approach integrating clinical details, radiologic imaging, cyst fluid biochemistry, and pathologic features. Imaging modalities like MRI, MDCT, and EUS are useful in delineating cyst morphology, mural nodules, and communication with the pancreatic duct [2, 3]. EUS-guided fine-needle aspiration (FNA) allows for obtaining fluid for cytomorphologic assessment and biochemical analysis, including carcinoembryonic antigen (CEA) levels and amylase, as well as molecular testing [4–7].

In the evaluation of pancreatic cystic lesions, cytology plays a vital role, in addition to other biochemical and molecular tests [1]. However, it is pertinent here to mention that the pathologist must adopt an integrated multidisciplinary approach and interpret the cytology specimen with full knowledge of the clinical history, imaging findings, and ancillary biochemical tests, especially amylase and CEA levels [1, 7].

The primary purpose of cytologic sampling of pancreatic cystic lesions is to (i) distinguish non-neoplastic from neoplastic cysts and, if neoplastic, (ii) to distinguish nonmucinous from mucinous cysts, which may progress to malignancy. Furthermore, cytological evaluation is essential in mucinous cysts to establish if there is dysplasia and its grade and whether there is evidence of frank malignancy. A definitive diagnosis can help the surgeons and the gastroenterologists decide further course of management in these patients. A conservative approach is an option for asymptomatic patients harboring benign or low-risk lesions. In contrast, definitive surgery is the first choice for high-risk and frankly malignant lesions [8, 9]. Besides these diagnostic indications, cytologic sampling may also be employed for therapeutic aspiration in symptomatic pancreatic pseudocysts [10].

This chapter will cover the role of cytology in diagnosing various pancreatic cysts, the diagnostic approach, specific cytomorphologic features, diagnostic challenges, and the role of ancillary techniques.

3.2 EUS-FNA for Sampling of Pancreatic Cystic Lesions

In the early 1990s, Vilmann et al. used EUS-FNAC for sampling pancreatic lesions [11], which continues to be the most commonly targeted site [12]. EUS-guided FNA has become an indispensable modality in the evaluation of pancreatic lesions as it offers high-resolution imaging, precise lesion localization, and superior sensitivity, ranging from 90% to 100%, for the detection as well as characterization of various pancreatic pathologies [13, 14]. The use of linear-array echoendoscopes enables real-time fine needle aspiration through the same instrument, combining endoscopic visualization with sonographic guidance and tissue acquisition in a single procedure. EUS-FNA is now widely regarded as the standard of care for sampling solid, solid-cystic, and purely cystic pancreatic lesions [15]. It is particularly advantageous for evaluating small lesions in anatomically challenging regions, where transabdominal approaches may be less effective. The safety, reproducibility, and high diagnostic accuracy of EUS-FNA have made palpation-guided FNA unacceptable and transabdominal FNA an inferior modality for sampling pancreatic lesions in general.

The lesion is well-visualized by the endoscopist, and EUS-FNA is performed using color Doppler and a dedicated EUS FNA needle, the size ranging from 19 to 25 Gauge. A trans-duodenal approach is preferred for lesions in the head and uncinate process of the pancreas, whereas for lesions in the body and tail, a trans-gastric approach is suitable [12]. Newly designed EUS-FNA needles with back-facing bevels, larger cutting surfaces, and new techniques, including fanning, wet suction, and other techniques, have improved the diagnostic yield in general [16, 17]. FNA is performed with an occluding stylet in the needle and is guided perpendicular to puncture the cyst wall. Once within the cyst, the stylet is removed, and the cyst contents are aspirated fully with suction, leading to the cyst wall's collapse. A note is made of the quantity and nature of the cyst fluid. A representative image of cyst fluid is shown in Fig. 3.1. The aspirated cyst fluid is partitioned appropriately for

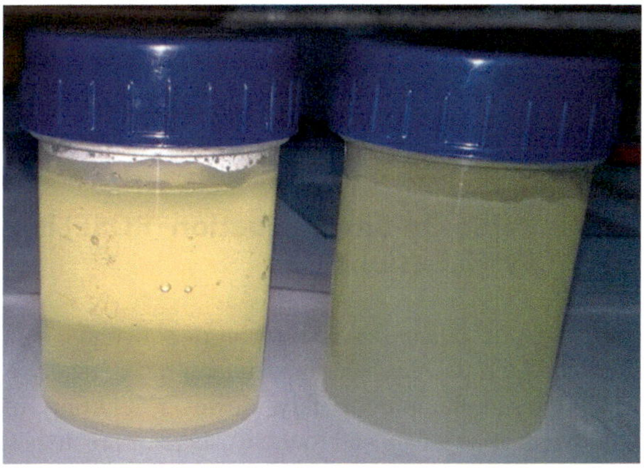

Fig. 3.1 Gross appearance of pancreatic cyst fluid. The sample on the left appears pale yellow, thin, and watery, whereas the one on the right is thicker, more opaque and darker yellow suggesting different compositions

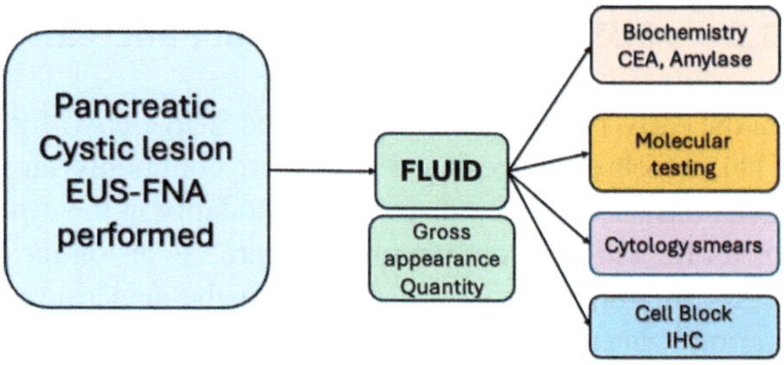

Fig. 3.2 EUS-FNA of pancreatic cystic lesions: partitioning of sample for various tests

biochemical analysis, molecular testing, and cytological evaluation (Fig. 3.2). If indicated, it may also be subjected to microbiological cultures and cell block preparation when the aspirate is sufficient. Furthermore, any residual solid areas, thick septations, or nodules in the cyst must be targeted again and subjected to FNA. Approximately 200–300 μL volume is required for performing biochemistry, 300–500 μL for molecular studies, and a minimum of 100 μL for preparing 2–3 conventional smears. If more fluid is aspirated, then more sample can be submitted to the cytopathology laboratory analysis, and no fluid should be discarded. From the larger volumes of fluid received, sediment smears following centrifugation are prepared, and a cell block may be prepared from the rest of the sediment. The supernatant can be saved for molecular analysis which will act as a "liquid biopsy" in cystic lesions.

Serous cystic neoplasms yield thin yellow/hemorrhagic fluid. On the other hand, mucinous cystic lesions yield a smaller amount of thick, viscous, or gelatinous material corresponding to mucin, which can clog the needle. In the case of a lesser volume of fluid, the allocation of cyst fluid for cytology, biochemistry, or molecular testing would depend on the major differential diagnosis [1]. For a cytological diagnosis, conventional smears are prepared. Air-dried smears are subjected to Giemsa/May-Grunwald Giemsa or Diff-Quick staining, and alcohol-fixed conventional smears are stained by Papanicolaou stain. Liquid-based cytology is not preferred for evaluating pancreatic cystic lesions as it leads to a loss of background details that are so critical in their evaluation.

Complications of pancreatic cyst FNA may include minor intracystic bleeding, which usually stops spontaneously without any sequelae. Acute pancreatitis is a rare but potentially serious complication [1].

3.3 Rapid On-Site Evaluation (ROSE) in Pancreatic Cystic Lesions

The role of ROSE in the assessment of pancreatic solid lesions is well established as it can help decrease the inadequacy rates, ensure representative sampling, and triage the sample appropriately. However, its utility in pancreatic cystic lesions is controversial as it can lead to the wastage of precious samples [9].

Key Takeaways
- EUS-FNA is the technique of choice for sampling Pancreatic cystic lesions.
- The amount of material/fluid aspirated is variable and must be partitioned appropriately for cytology, cyst fluid biochemistry, and molecular studies based on the main differential diagnosis.
- Conventional cytology smears are preferred over liquid-based cytology.

3.4 Cytopathology Reporting Format for Pancreatic Lesions

Cytology remains the primary diagnostic tool for the initial evaluation of pancreatic lesions, necessitating the use of standardized nomenclature and reporting frameworks to promote diagnostic consistency and facilitate clinical decision-making. The first reporting system for pancreaticobiliary cytology, referred to as the Papanicolaou Society Guidelines came in 2014 [18]. In 2023, the World Health Organization (WHO), in collaboration with the International Academy of Cytology and the International Agency for Research on Cancer, introduced a unified reporting system for pancreaticobiliary (PB) cytopathology [19]. This seven-tiered system aligns with the latest WHO Classification of Tumours of the Digestive System, aiming to harmonize diagnostic terminology [20]. The different reporting categories and their corresponding risk of malignancy (ROM) are shown in Table 3.1 [19]. Subsequently, there have been analyses from different parts of the world reporting on the frequency of the various categories along with their respective ROM and reiterating the superiority of the WHO system with the previous Papanicolaou society system of reporting [21–23]. Beyond standardization, the system underscores

Table 3.1 WHO reporting system for pancreaticobiliary cytopathology [19]

Diagnostic category	ROM	Recommended management
Category 1 *Insufficient/ Inadequate/Nondiagnostic*	5–25%	Repeat biopsy
Category 2 *Benign/Negative for Malignancy*	0–15%	Clinical correlation
Category 3 *Atypical*	30–40%	Repeat biopsy
Category 4 *Pancreatic Neoplasm: Low- Risk/ Low-Grade (PaN-Low)*	5–20%	Correlate clinically
Category 5 *Pancreatic Neoplasm: High Risk/ High-Grade (PaN-High):*	60–95%	Resection if surgical candidate; conservative management possible
Category 6 *Suspicious for Malignancy*	80–100%	If surgical candidate, treat as positive. Repeat biopsy before chemoradiation.
Category 7 *Malignant*	97–100%	As per the clinical stage

ROM Risk of malignancy

the critical role of clinicoradiologic correlation and the integration of ancillary studies, including biochemical and molecular assays, in accurately classifying pancreaticobiliary lesions.

Category 1: Insufficient/Inadequate/Nondiagnostic: Cystic lesions with acellular/paucicellular smears but diagnostic clinico-radiologic features should not be included in this category. The presence of any cellular atypia in the sample precludes this categorization.

Category 2: Benign/Negative for Malignancy: This category includes all benign lesions such as acute pancreatitis, chronic pancreatitis, cholangitis, autoimmune pancreatitis, pseudocyst, lymphoepithelial cyst, accessory spleen, serous cystadenoma, lymphangioma, and schwannoma.

Category 3: Atypical: This category includes samples that exhibit some features that raise the possibility of malignancy; however, overall, it is insufficient, either qualitatively or quantitatively, to diagnose a lesion as benign, premalignant, or malignant.

Category 4: Pancreatic Neoplasm: Low-Risk/Low-Grade (PaN-Low): This category includes samples with features of an intraductal and/or cystic neoplasm with low-grade atypia, including IPMN and mucinous cystic neoplasm (MCN) with low-grade atypia. Accurate grading of the epithelial atypia as low-risk/low-grade, which includes both low- and intermediate-grade dysplasia, and distinguishing it from high-risk/high-grade atypia is essential.

Category 5: Pancreatic Neoplasm: High-Risk/High-Grade (PaN-High): This category includes intraductal and/or cystic neoplasm with high-grade cytologic atypia. High-grade atypia is typically defined as a cell that (in comparison to a duodenal enterocyte measuring 12 μm) exhibits high nuclear-to-cytoplasmic ratio, nuclear membrane irregularity, abnormal chromatin (hypo- or hyperchromasia), and prominent nucleoli, with or without background necrosis.

Category 6: Suspicious for Malignancy: Samples with some cytologic features suggestive of malignancy, but these are insufficient, either qualitatively or quantitatively, for an unequivocal diagnosis of malignancy.

Category 7: Malignant: Samples demonstrating unequivocal cytologic features of malignancy. This category includes both primary and secondary malignancies (including well-differentiated PanNET and SPN) with pancreatic ductal adenocarcinoma (PDAC).

3.5 Cytology of "Contaminant" Cells

FNA from the pancreaticobiliary tract may show various cell types as "*contaminants,*" primarily due to the needle traversing via and sampling the adjacent organs [24]. These commonly include fragments of intestinal epithelium in trans-duodenal aspirates and gastric epithelium and parietal cells in trans-gastric aspirates (Fig. 3.3). The duodenal epithelium is seen as flat sheets of enterocytes interspersed with pale

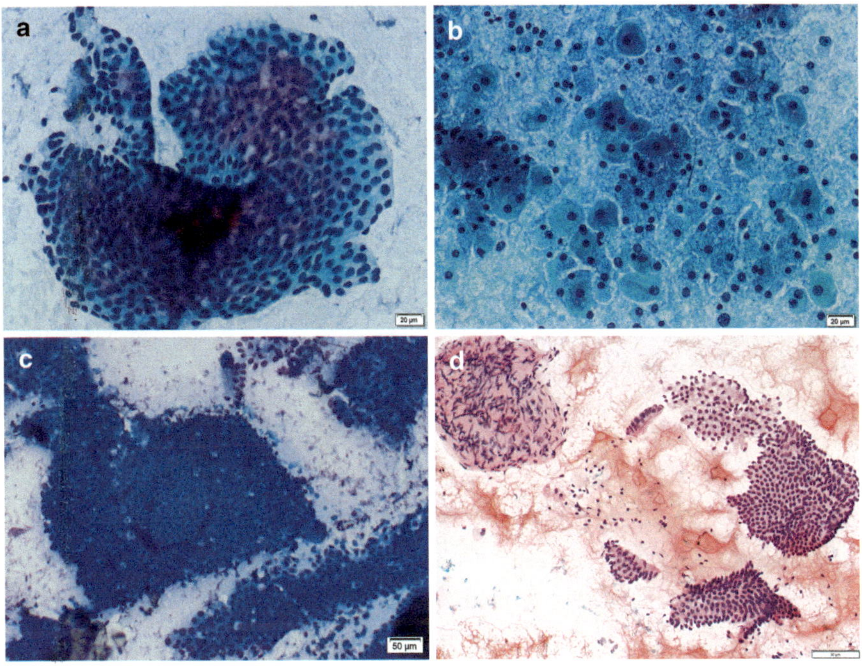

Fig. 3.3 Gastrointestinal tract contaminants in the EUS-FNA sample. (**a**) gastric epithelium; (**b**) gastric parietal cells; (**c**) duodenal epithelium showing enterocytes interspersed with pale goblet cells. (**d**) intestinal epithelium and stromal fragment (upper right side) [**a**, **b**—Papanicolaou stain. ×400; **c**—May-Grünwald Giemsa stain ×200; **d**—Hematoxylin–Eosin stain ×100]

haloed goblet cells. The gastric epithelium is also seen as flat sheets of cells or strips of columnar epithelium with basal nuclei and cup-shaped cytoplasmic vacuolation due to mucin. Parietal cells are large with abundant granular cytoplasm and small nuclei. Stromal tissue derived from the cyst wall may be seen. Knowledge of these contaminant cells is essential to avoid diagnostic misinterpretations.

3.6 Cytology of Native Pancreatic Cells

The pancreas is a mixed exocrine–endocrine gland having three anatomical parts: the head, body, and tail. Around 80–85% of the pancreas is exocrine, composed of acini, ducts, and the supporting connective tissue with blood vessels. The endocrine part is composed of the islets of Langerhans, which are concentrated in the tail of the pancreas. Needle aspirates from the normal pancreas mainly show acinar cells with few ductal epithelial cells (Fig. 3.4).

(i) *Acinar cells:* These cells are seen as cohesive aggregates or as singly scattered cells, which are small-sized, pyramidal-to-polygonal shaped, with small central

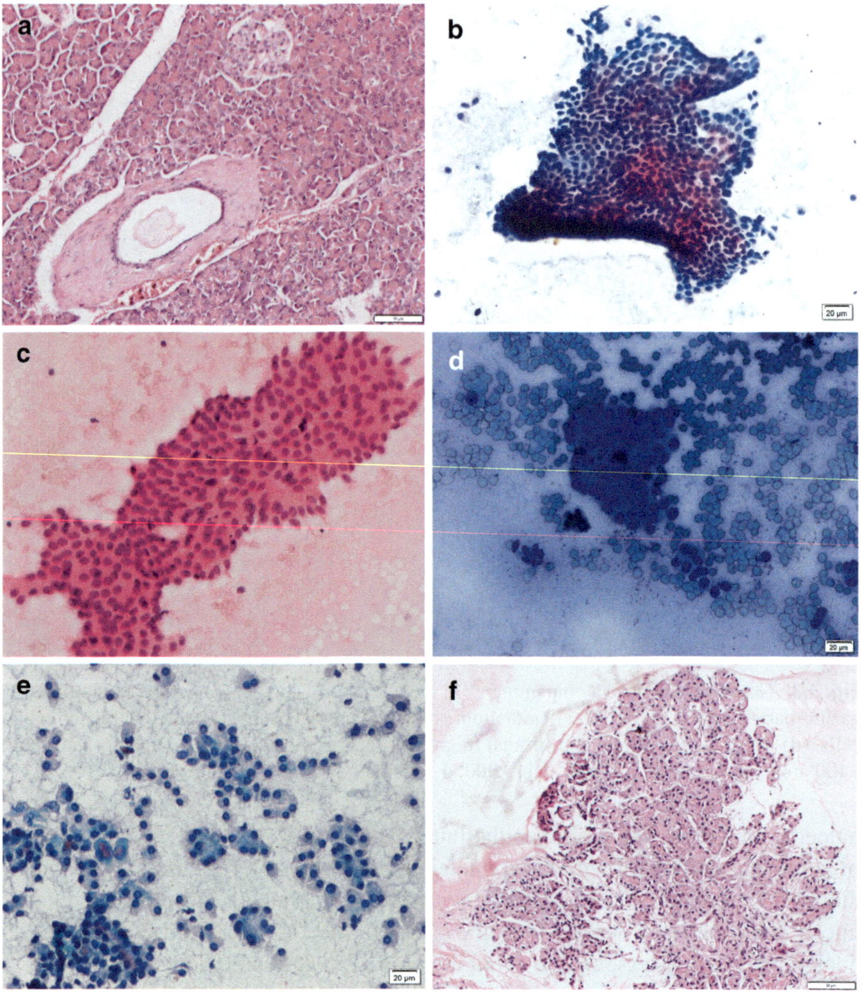

Fig. 3.4 Native cells of the pancreas. (**a**) Histology of normal pancreas showing small duct and pancreatic acini; (**b**, **c**) pancreatic ductal epithelial cluster; (**d**, **e**) different appearances of benign pancreatic acinar cells; (**f**) cell block showing normal pancreatic tissue [**a**, **c**, **f**—Hematoxylin–Eosin stain; **d**—May-Grünwald Giemsa stain; **b**, **e**—Papanicolaou stain; **a**, **f** ×200; **b**, **c**, **d**, **e** ×400]

to eccentrically placed round nuclei, fine chromatin, and inconspicuous nucleoli. They show abundant granular cytoplasm; degranulation may result in a granulo-vacuolar or a clear-vacuolated appearance.

(ii) *Ductal epithelial cells:* These cells are seen as flat, cohesive monolayered sheets of cuboidal to columnar cells with distinct cell borders, small, round, uniformly spaced nuclei, fine chromatin, inconspicuous nucleoli, and scant cytoplasm.

Pancreatic islet cells are difficult to identify on cytologic smears but may be appreciated in cell block sections.

Key Takeaways

- Cytology samples must be reported as per the current WHO system of reporting Pancreaticobiliary cytopathology which provides the risk of malignancy in each category and recommended guidelines for management
- Awareness of GI contaminants, including GI tract mucin, gastric, and duodenal epithelial cells, and knowledge of cytomorphological appearance of normal pancreatic acinar cells and ductal cells are important

3.7 Cytology of Pancreatic Cystic Lesions

Pancreatic cystic lesions encompass a vast spectrum of lesions that include both non-neoplastic and neoplastic lesions (Table 3.2).

Each of the above-listed entities will be described briefly below. The aim of this chapter is to describe the cytomorphological features. Evaluation of smears requires an algorithmic approach, as shown in Fig. 3.5. Briefly, the cellular and extracellular material should be analyzed, and once an impression is made, it has to be interpreted with knowledge of the clinical features, imaging data, and cyst fluid biochemistry. The increasing use of cell blocks has allowed for the application of immunohistochemical markers to improve diagnostic accuracy. Molecular analysis of the cyst fluid is also important and is being briefly mentioned here, and details are beyond the scope of this chapter.

Table 3.2 Cystic lesions of the pancreas

Non-Neoplastic Cystic Lesions
Pseudocyst
Lymphoepithelial cyst
Dermoid cyst
Squamoid cyst of the pancreatic ducts
Retention cyst
Enterogenous duplication cyst
Acinar cell cystadenoma (cystic acinar transformation)
Endometriotic cyst
Neoplastic Cystic Lesions
Intraductal
Intraductal papillary mucinous neoplasm (gastric/intestinal/pancreaticobiliary type)
Intraductal oncocytic papillary neoplasm
Intraductal tubulopapillary neoplasm
Nonductal/Others
Mucinous cystic neoplasm
Serous cystic neoplasm
Other neoplasms with cystic degeneration: Solid pseudopapillary neoplasm, pancreatic neuroendocrine tumor, pancreatic ductal adenocarcinoma, acinar cell carcinoma

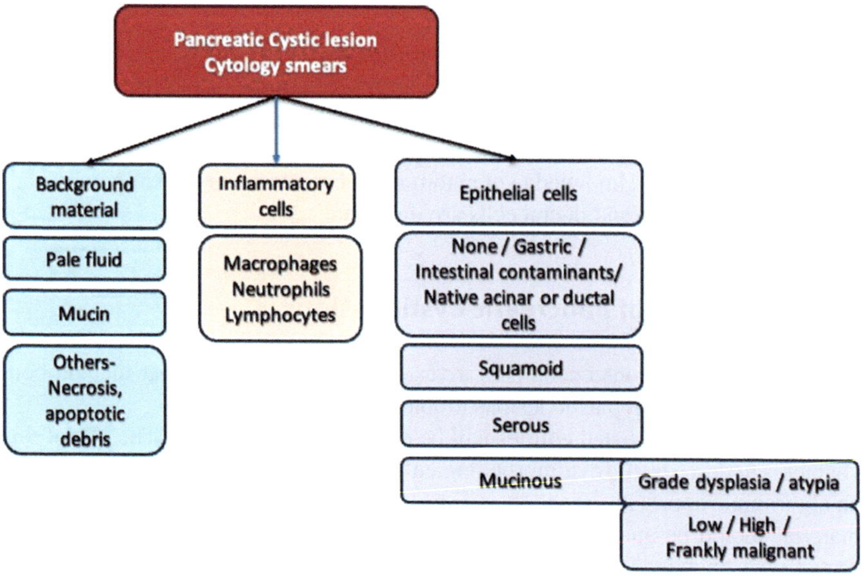

Fig. 3.5 Cytological evaluation of EUS-FNA pancreatic cystic lesions

3.8 Cytology of Non-Neoplastic Cystic Pancreatic Lesions

(a) *Pancreatic Pseudocyst*

A pseudocyst of the pancreas is a well-circumscribed, fluid-filled cavity in or near the pancreas that lacks a true epithelial lining and is lined by fibrous tissue and inflammatory cells. Etiopathogenetically, pseudocysts are formed because of enzymatic digestion and inflammation caused by leakage of pancreatic secretions consequent to pancreatitis or trauma.

The typical clinical, imaging, cyst fluid biochemistry, and cytomorphologic features are presented in Table 3.3 [25–27].

Cytomorphologic Features

- Turbid, brownish, or greenish nonmucoid fluid.
- Paucicellular smears with scattered neutrophils and macrophages in a dirty or hemorrhagic background (Fig. 3.6a and b).
- Extracellular yellow pigment (a combination of hematoidin and bile pigment) may be noted (Fig. 3.6b).
- Lack of epithelial cells.

Table 3.3 Pancreatic pseudocyst: clinical features, imaging, and cyst fluid biochemistry

Clinical features	Imaging features	Cyst fluid biochemistry
History of prior pancreatitis, alcohol-related pancreatitis	Thin-walled unilocular cyst with internal debris, with/without evidence of pancreatitis in the adjacent areas	Amylase levels: markedly elevated >250 IU/mL and usually in thousands, which is diagnostic Carcinoembryonic antigen (CEA) levels: low

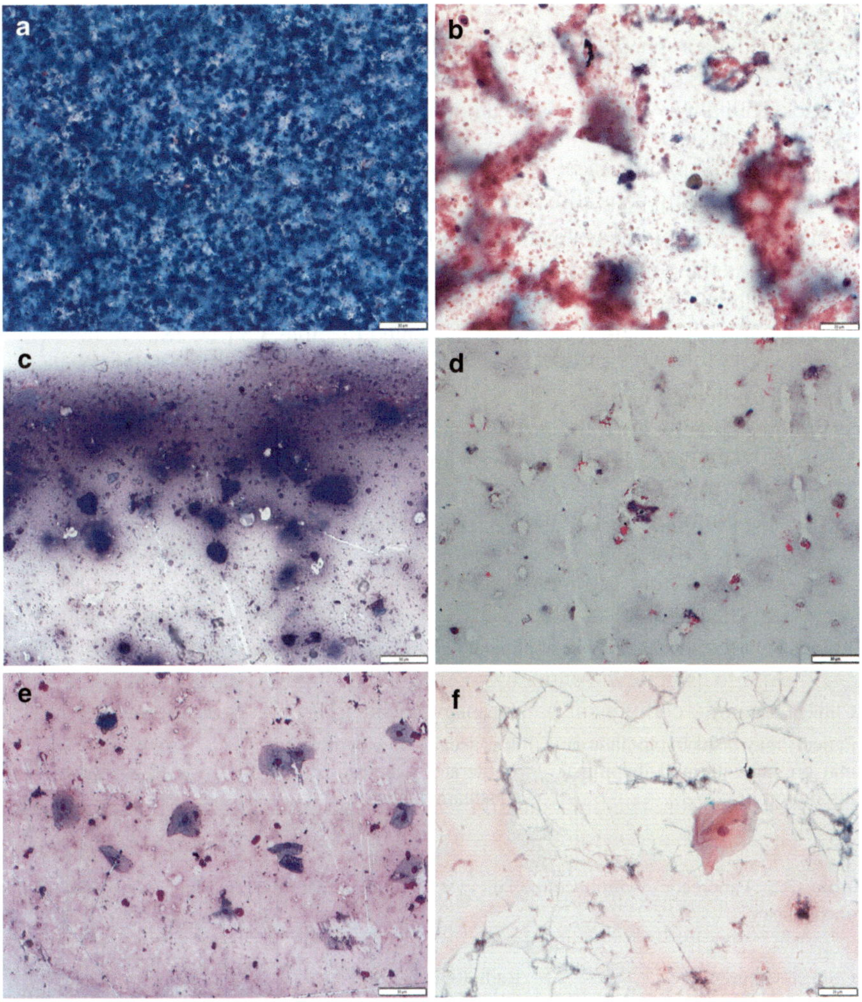

Fig. 3.6 Non-neoplastic cystic lesions of the pancreas: (**a**, **b**) Pseudocyst showing dirty hemorrhagic background and scattered macrophages with hematoidin pigment. (**c**) Retention cyst showing paucicellular smears and scattered macrophages. (**d**) Mucicarmine stain is negative. (**e**) and (**f**), Squamoid cyst with scattered benign squamous cells in a fluid background [**a**, **c**, **e**—May-Grünwald Giemsa stain; **b**, **d**, **f**—Papanicolaou stain. **a**, **c**, **d**, **e** ×200; **b**, **f** ×400]

(b) *Retention Cyst*

Retention cysts may develop because of the obstruction and fibrosis of the pancreatic duct, resulting in upstream dilatation [27]. The obstruction may be the result of chronic pancreatitis, mucus plug, stones, or neoplasm, and the retention cysts are usually small, incidentally detected cysts [27]. The typical clinical, radiologic, cyst fluid biochemistry and cytomorphologic features are presented in Table 3.4.

Cytomorphologic Features

- Paucicellular aspirate.
- Scattered macrophages and few cuboidal mucinous/nonmucinous epithelial cells (Fig. 3.6c and d).
- Background may show variable amounts of mucin.

(c) *Lymphoepithelial Cyst*

Lymphoepithelial cysts (LEC) of the pancreas are rare, benign cysts characterized by keratinizing squamous epithelium lining with surrounding lymphoid tissue. As the lymphocytes lie beneath the epithelium, they are less represented in cytology specimens. The typical clinical, radiologic, cyst fluid biochemistry and cytomorphologic features are presented in Table 3.5 [27, 28].

Cytomorphologic Features

- Viscous, creamy, or frothy gross appearance of the fluid.
- Smears show keratinous debris with anucleated and nucleated mature squamous epithelial cells.
- The background shows cholesterol crystals, macrophages, and scattered lymphocytes.

Table 3.4 Pancreatic retention cyst: clinical features, imaging, and cyst fluid biochemistry

Clinical features	Imaging features	Cyst fluid biochemistry
Patients may be asymptomatic or may present with mild abdominal discomfort	It is seen as an obstructed/ obliterated pancreatic duct with upstream dilatation	Amylase and CEA levels: variable

Table 3.5 Pancreatic lymphoepithelial cyst: clinical features, imaging, and cyst fluid biochemistry

Clinical features	Radiologic features	Cyst fluid biochemistry
Common in middle-aged men Asymptomatic or may present with abdominal pain	Seen as well-demarcated hypoattenuating uni/multiloculated cysts, which can be intrapancreatic, peripancreatic, or on the surface of the pancreas	Carcinoembryonic antigen (CEA) levels: elevated

(d) *Squamoid Cyst of the Pancreatic Ducts*

Squamoid cyst of the pancreatic ducts (SCOP) is characterized by unilocular cystic dilatation of the ducts filled with mucoproteinaceous secretions and concretions. Unlike the pseudocyst, it is not generally associated with pancreatitis. The typical clinical, radiologic, cyst fluid biochemistry and cytomorphologic features are presented in Table 3.6 [27].

Cytomorphologic Features

- Scattered squamous epithelial cells that lack keratinization in a fluidy background (Fig. 3.6e and f)
- Positive for p40, p63, and cytokeratin 5
- Columnar cells with or without mucin

(e) *Acinar Cell Cystadenoma/Cystic Acinar Transformation*

Acinar cell cystadenoma, also known as the cystic acinar transformation, is a rare, benign cystic lesion of the pancreas mainly detected incidentally. The typical clinical, radiologic, cyst fluid biochemistry and cytomorphologic features are presented in Table 3.7 [27, 29].

Cytomorphologic Features [29]

- Paucicellular aspirate.
- Scattered acinar cells with high N/C ratio and mild hyperchromasia and occasional nucleolus.
- Amorphous debris mimicking mucinous material and macrophages may also be seen.

Table 3.6 Squamoid cyst of the pancreatic ducts: clinical features, imaging, and cyst fluid biochemistry

Clinical features	Imaging features	Cyst fluid biochemistry
Patients are generally asymptomatic and rarely present with abdominal discomfort	Seen as unilocular cystically dilated ducts filled with dense contents	Amylase levels: variable CEA levels: elevated

Table 3.7 Acinar cell cystadenoma/cystic acinar transformation: clinical features, imaging, and cyst fluid biochemistry

Clinical features	Radiologic features	Cyst fluid biochemistry
Most patients are asymptomatic; rarely may present with abdominal pain	Seen as unilocular or multilocular cyst in the pancreas not connected with the main pancreatic duct	Amylase levels: elevated CEA levels: elevated

Immunocytochemistry

- Acinar cells are positive for trypsin and chymotrypsin and negative for neuroendocrine markers (synaptophysin, chromogranin, and CD56).
- Ki-67 index is low (1–2%).

Other rare cystic lesions include dermoid cyst, cystic lymphangioma, duplication, or foregut cysts.

Cytologic Differentials for Non-Neoplastic Cystic Lesions

(i) *Neoplastic mucinous cyst:* Mucin and cells derived from the gastrointestinal tract during sampling can lead to considering a mucinous neoplastic cyst. However, this mucin is thin and watery, unlike the thick, viscous mucin in true mucinous cysts. The presence of amorphous debris and inflammatory cells also favors a pancreatic origin over gastrointestinal tract contamination. The mucin of true mucinous cystic lesions is thicker, viscous, and difficult to spread and is discussed later in the chapter.

(ii) *Neoplasms with cystic change:* NET, acinar cell carcinoma, and PDAC can all show cystic change and lead to a false-negative diagnosis. Careful examination of the periphery of the smears can reveal occasional cells suggesting a neoplasm. Cyst fluid CEA and amylase levels would be low, and molecular testing would aid in excluding mucinous cysts.

3.9 Cytology of Neoplastic Cystic Pancreatic Lesions

The most common neoplastic cystic pancreatic lesions include intraductal papillary mucinous neoplasms (IPMNs), serous cystadenomas (SCAs), and mucinous cystic neoplasms (MCNs). Other neoplastic cystic pancreatic lesions have been listed in Table 3.2. The characteristic cytomorphologic, immunocytochemical, and molecular genetic features of the common lesions are presented here.

(a) *Serous Cystadenoma*

Serous cystadenomas (SCAs) are one of the most common benign cystic neoplasms of the pancreas, commonly occurring in the body and tail of the pancreas in older women [9, 27]. SCA follows a benign clinical course with negligible risk of malignant transformation. It may arise sporadically or in the context of Von Hippel Lindau's disease. Typically, they are microcystic with a sponge-like/soap-bubble appearance around a central scar. Macrocystic variants also occur. The typical clinical, radiologic, and cyst fluid biochemical features are presented in Table 3.8.

Cytomorphologic Features [9, 27, 30]

- Clear or serosanguinous fluid.
- A paucicellular smear with a few clusters of cuboidal tumor cells, which are monolayered, with round, regular nuclei with fine chromatin and a moderate amount of clear to granular, nonmucinous cytoplasm may be seen (Fig. 3.7).

Table 3.8 Serous cystadenoma of the pancreas: clinical features, imaging, and cyst fluid biochemistry

Clinical features	Imaging features	Cyst fluid biochemistry
Asymptomatic and discovered incidentally Symptomatic patients may present with abdominal pain, a palpable mass, nausea, vomiting, and weight loss	Generally seen as multicystic masses or cysts with lobulated contours with or without septations, commonly seen in the pancreatic head Lack of wall enhancement favors a radiologic diagnosis of serous cystadenoma	Carcinoembryonic antigen (CEA): low (<5 ng/mL) Amylase: low (<250 IU/L)

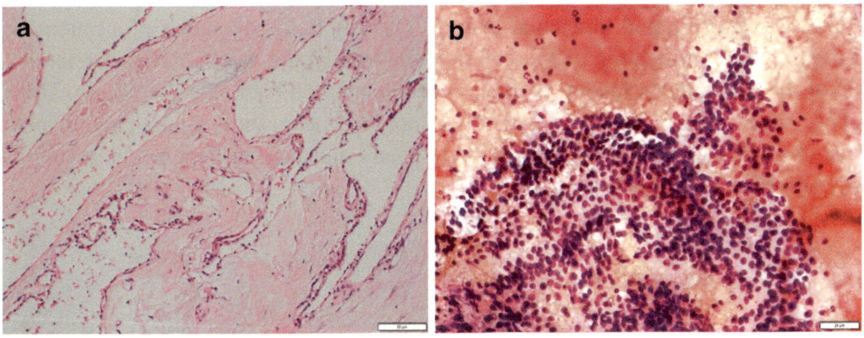

Fig. 3.7 Serous cystadenoma of the pancreas. (**a**) Histopathology showing multicystic pattern lined by cuboidal to low columnar cells. (**b**) Cytology smear showing cohesive aggregates of small cells with round, uniform nuclei, fine chromatin, inconspicuous nucleoli, and a small amount of cytoplasm, in a hemorrhagic background [Hematoxylin–Eosin stain. **a** ×200, **b** ×400]

- The background is hemorrhagic and may show hemosiderin-laden macrophages.
- In many cases, the aspirate may be completely devoid of epithelial cells, and a definite diagnosis is not possible.

Special Stains and Immunocytochemistry

- Periodic acid–Schiff (PAS) and PAS/diastase stains can help highlight the glycogen present in SCA cells [30].
- Positive for Glucose Transporter 1 (GLUT1), alpha-inhibin, cytokeratin [9, 30].

Molecular Genetics [31, 32]

- Mutations in the *VHL* gene have been identified in around two-thirds of all SCAs.

3.9.1 Differential Diagnosis

EUS-FNA has a low sensitivity for a diagnosis of serous cystadenoma. Thin or hemorrhagic fluid with some scattered macrophages and devoid of epithelial cells are seen, and a pseudocyst may be considered [27]. The cells when seen are often monotonous, and a cystic PanNET may be considered. Lastly, in aspirates with contaminating gastrointestinal epithelium and mucin, neoplastic mucinous cysts may be considered. This highlights the importance of considering the clinical, imaging, and cyst fluid biochemistry before making any conclusion.

3.9.2 Cystic Mucinous Neoplasms of the Pancreas

The two major cystic mucinous neoplasms are intraductal papillary mucinous neoplasm and mucinous cystic neoplasm. It is almost impossible to distinguish them on cytomorphology alone; however, they may be distinguished reliably using a multimodality approach by combining the clinical, radiological/imaging features, cyst fluid biochemistry, and molecular testing. The key to the diagnosis of a mucinous lesion is the identification of lesional mucin. Grossly, the mucin that is characteristic of these mucinous lesions is thick, viscous, and tends to clog the needle. Upon expressing onto the slide, it is difficult to spread. Smears show thick, magenta pink mucin in Diff-Quick or Giemsa-stained smears and pale in Papanicolaou-stained smears (Fig. 3.8a and b).

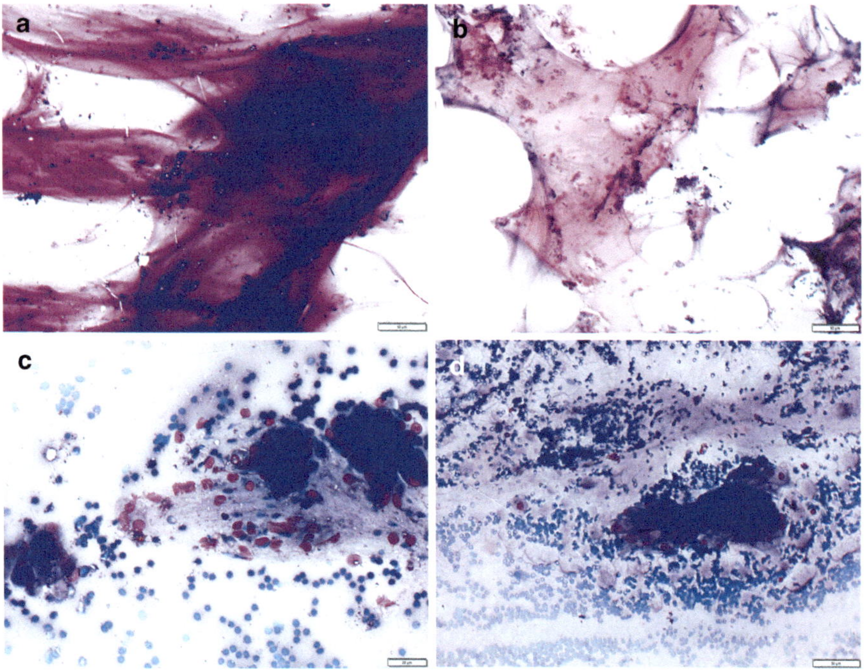

Fig. 3.8 Appearance of mucin. (**a**, **b**) Thick, difficult-to-spread mucinous material with no cells from a mucinous cystic neoplasm of the pancreas. Note the bright magenta pink color in Giemsa stain and pale appearance in the Papanicolaou stain. (**c**) Mucin from the intestinal tract, admixed with benign epithelial cells, and (**d**) thicker mucin, admixed with malignant cells from a mucinous adenocarcinoma [**a**, **c**, **d**—May-Grünwald Giemsa stain; **b**—Papanicolaou stain. **a**, **b**, **d** ×200; **c** ×400]

In both these entities, it is essential to identify and grade the dysplasia in the epithelial cells. Currently, a two-tiered grading system is used, with low and intermediate grades combined as low-grade dysplasia, with the other being high-grade dysplasia. Lesions with high-grade dysplasia are at high risk for harboring or progression to invasive carcinoma and require surgical intervention in contrast to low-grade lesions, which have a low risk for malignant transformation.

(i) *Intraductal Papillary Mucinous Neoplasm (IPMN)*

IPMNs are premalignant lesions commonly detected incidentally in elderly males. The typical clinical, radiologic [33], and cyst fluid biochemical features [34–38] are presented in Table 3.9.

Gross Pathology of IPMN [39]

- IPMNs are characterized by a grossly visible (≥1 cm) lesion in the main pancreatic duct (MD-IPMN) and/or the branch ducts (BD-IPMN).
- MD-IPMNs show diffuse or segmental dilatation of the main duct. BD-IPMNs are seen as multicystic grape-like structures.
- IPMNs associated with an invasive carcinoma may show irregular, thick cyst walls, mural nodules, or gelatinous stromal masses. In all cases, extensive sampling is essential to exclude an invasive component.

(ii) *Mucinous Cystic Neoplasm*

Mucinous cystic neoplasms (MCN) are relatively rare premalignant pancreatic tumors, almost exclusively occurring in middle-aged females. On histopathology, these are characterized by the presence of subepithelial ovarian-type stroma [40]. This stroma is often not aspirated and, hence, not

Table 3.9 Intraductal pancreatic mucinous neoplasm [IPMN]: clinical features, imaging, and cyst fluid biochemistry

Clinical features	Imaging features	Cyst fluid biochemistry
Most patients are asymptomatic; however, some may present with abdominal pain, weight loss, and jaundice Around one-third of these cases may be associated with diabetes mellitus	Upper GI endoscopy: "*fish mouth*" papilla extruding mucin Demonstration of communication with either the main pancreatic duct (MPD) or the branch duct or a combination on imaging is important (branch duct, main duct, or combined type); typical is the "*clubbed finger-like*" cystic shape [32]	Cyst fluid markers to differentiate between mucinous and nonmucinous cysts include carcinoembryonic antigen (CEA) and glucose CEA cutoff value of >192 ng/mL is widely used and has a high specificity but does not distinguish benign from malignant cysts [34] The cutoff is dependent on the assay system used and a value of 45.9 ng/mL [35] or 45 ng/mL in our experience is suggested [36] Cyst fluid glucose evaluation with a cutoff of 50 mg/dL [37, 38] is also routinely employed

Table 3.10 Mucinous cystic neoplasm of pancreas: clinical features, imaging, and cyst fluid biochemical features

Clinical features	Radiologic features	Cyst fluid biochemistry
Most cases are asymptomatic and detected incidentally on imaging; some patients may present with abdominal pain, abdominal mass, pancreatitis, or weight loss	Primarily located in the pancreatic body or tail Generally seen as smooth-contoured macrocystic lesions without any communication with the main pancreatic duct The presence of large size, thick walls, septations, calcifications, or mural nodules indicates a high-grade or invasive lesion	CEA and glucose levels in MCNs are high, similar to IPMNs Amylase levels are variable in MCNs and may not be useful in differentiation from IPMNs

reflected in cytology smears; hence, the distinction from IPMN on cytomorphology is difficult. Cell blocks with adequate material may demonstrate this stroma. Although most of these tumors are benign, they are considered premalignant as they have a predilection to develop dysplasia and invasive carcinoma. The typical clinical, radiologic, and cyst fluid biochemical features are presented in Table 3.10.

3.9.3 Cytomorphologic Features of IPMN and MCN [9, 27, 41, 42]

MCNs and IPMNs cannot be distinguished reliably based on cytologic features alone, as the subepithelial ovarian-type stroma, a diagnostic prerequisite for MCN, is not readily identifiable on smears. Hence, the cytomorphological features are being described together. The main role of the cytologic examination is to identify mucin of neoplastic origin and assess the degree of epithelial atypia. In some cases, only mucin is present in the smears, which are otherwise acellular. Neoplastic mucin is thick and viscous and difficult to spread onto the slide. Smears show thick mucin, which stains bright magenta in a Diff-Quick or Giemsa-stained smear and appears pale but thick in a Papanicolaou-stained smear (Fig. 3.8).

- Variably cellular smears
- Thick extracellular mucin is a diagnostic characteristic of a neoplastic mucinous cyst, irrespective of the presence/absence of mucinous epithelium. This, however, may be difficult to discern in liquid-based cytologic preparations.
- Papillae, micropapillae, or sheets of variably pleomorphic epithelial cells with intracytoplasmic mucin; few scattered degenerated epithelial cells within the mucin.
- The epithelial cells may be of gastric, intestinal, or pancreaticobiliary types.
- The lining epithelium may exhibit varying degrees of dysplasia; the cytology sample may or may not represent the severity of dysplasia in the lesion.

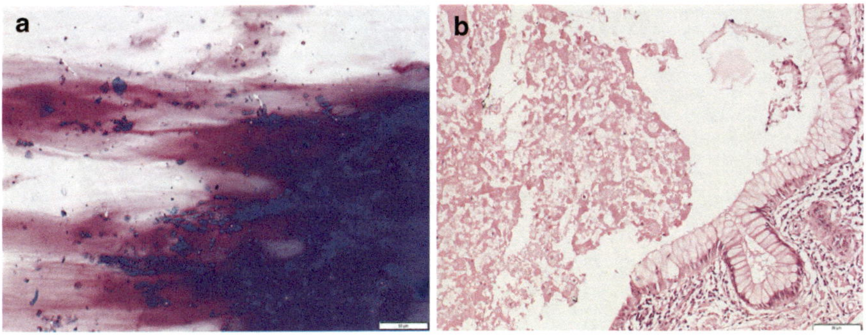

Fig. 3.9 Mucinous cystic neoplasm of pancreas. (**a**) Cytology smears showed only mucin without epithelial cells. (**b**) Histopathology showing gastric-type lining epithelium and mucin in the lumen [**a**—May-Grünwald Giemsa stain; **b**—Hematoxylin–Eosin stain. **a**, **b** ×200]

- *Low-grade epithelial atypia* on cytology includes both low-grade and intermediate-grade dysplasia cases. It is seen as mucinous cells with a low nuclear–cytoplasmic ratio, fine nuclear chromatin, and inconspicuous nucleoli. Gastric-type epithelium usually represents low-grade atypia (Figs. 3.9 and 3.10).
- *High-grade epithelial atypia* on cytology includes high-grade dysplasia and invasive mucinous carcinoma cases. Their distinction is not possible in cytology and is not clinically relevant as they are managed similarly. The epithelial cells are seen as loosely cohesive clusters with a "*drunken honeycomb*" appearance, three-dimensional and papillaroid clusters, and many singly scattered cells (Fig. 3.11). The cells show nuclear enlargement, high nucleo–cytoplasmic ratio, coarse chromatin, variably prominent nucleoli, and irregular nuclear membranes. Intracytoplasmic mucin is seen as mucinous vacuoles pushing the nucleus to the periphery. The background shows variable amounts of necrotic and apoptotic debris with inflammatory cells, all of which are clues to the high-grade lesion. A variable amount of extracellular mucin is often seen admixed with inflammatory cells.
- Cell block sections may demonstrate the characteristic subepithelial ovarian-type stroma in MCN. Alternatively, fine needle biopsy with micro-forceps, which can acquire a portion of the wall, can allow its recognition.

Immunocytochemistry [31, 40, 43]

- Gastric-type IPMN shows positivity for MUC5AC and stains variably for MUC6 and negative for MUC1 (EMA), MUC2, CDX2, and CK20.
- Pancreaticobiliary-type IPMN shows positivity for MUC1 and stains variably for MUC5AC and MUC6 and is negative for MUC2, CDX2, and CK20.
- Intestinal-type IPMN is positive for MUC2, CDX2, and CK20 and negative for MUC1 and MUC6.
- Aberrant p53, loss of p16, and loss of SMAD4 expression are common in high-grade IPMNs.

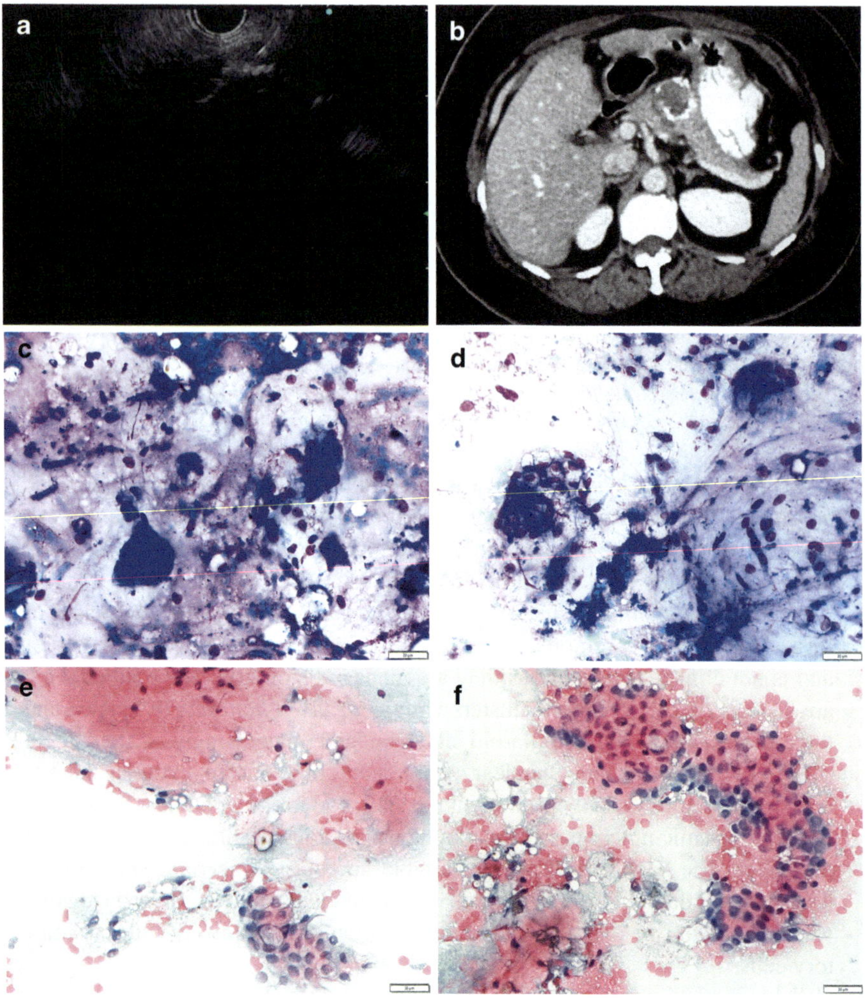

Fig. 3.10 Mucinous cystic neoplasm of the pancreas with low-grade dysplasia. (**a**) EUS-guided FNA of a cystic lesion which shows acoustic shadowing and calcification in the wall with a mural nodule. (**b**) CT scan showing cystic lesion in the neck of the pancreas. (**c**–**f**) Smears show abundant mucin admixed with cells resembling the gastric mucinous epithelium. The nuclei are relatively uniform with mild anisonucleosis. Cytoplasm shows mucinous vacuoles [**c**, **d**—May-Grünwald Giemsa stain; **e**, **f**—Papanicolaou stain. **c**–**f** ×400]

Molecular Genetics [31, 32, 44]

IPMN

- Somatic mutations of *KRAS*, *GNAS,* and *RNF43* genes are seen in 30–80% of IPMNs. A combination of *KRAS* and *GNAS* mutation testing is highly sensitive for diagnosing IPMNs.

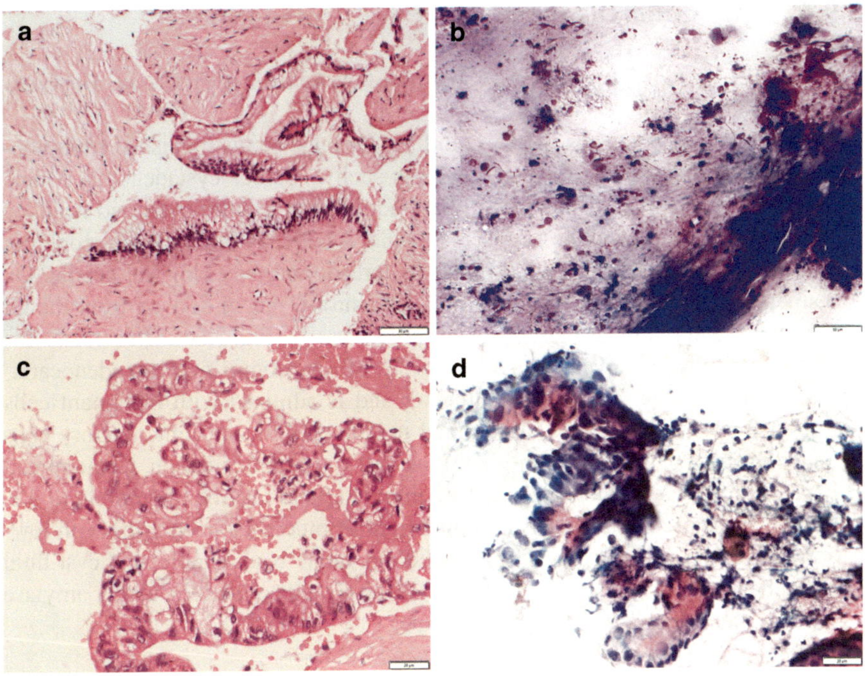

Fig. 3.11 Mucinous cystic neoplasms of the pancreas with high-grade dysplasia. (**a**, **b**) Mucinous cystic neoplasm (MCN) with high-grade dysplasia. (**c**, **d**) Intraductal pancreatic mucinous neoplasm with high-grade dysplasia. (**a**) Histopathology of mucinous cystic neoplasm with variable dysplasia; (**c**) histopathology of intraductal papillary mucinous neoplasm showing high-grade dysplasia. Corresponding smears (**b**, **d**) show abundant mucin admixed with inflammatory cells and epithelial cells, which show significant nuclear atypia with nuclear enlargement, coarse chromatin, and small nucleoli [**a**, **c**—Hematoxylin–Eosin stain; **b**—May-Grünwald Giemsa stain; **d**—Papanicolaou stain. **a**, **b** ×200; **b**, **d** ×400]

- GNAS mutations are more prevalent in intestinal-type IPMN and associated invasive carcinoma.
- *TP53, BRAF, SMAD4*, and *CDKN2A* mutations are common in cases with high-grade dysplasia.

MCN

- Mutations in the *KRAS* gene have been identified as an early event in MCNs.
- Mutations in *RNF43*, *TP53*, *SMAD4*, *PIK3CA,* and *CDKN2A* are common in MCNs with high-grade dysplasia or associated invasive carcinomas.
- Typically, *GNAS* mutations are not common in MCNs, unlike IPMNs.

3.9.4 Differential Diagnosis

(i) *Non-Neoplastic Cysts and Non-Mucinous Neoplastic Cysts from Mucinous Neoplastic Cysts*

Mucinous neoplasms, IPMNs, and MCNs must be distinguished from non-neoplastic cysts and nonmucinous cysts such as serous cystadenoma. Mucin derived from the gastrointestinal (GI) tract is often a confounder and needs to be differentiated from the neoplastic mucin. As already highlighted, neoplastic mucin is thick and viscous, difficult to spread, and may clog the needle. On smears, it stains bright magenta pink. In contrast, mucin derived from the GI tract is watery, thin, not viscous, and spreads easily (Fig. 3.6c). On smears, it is pale and thin and covers the slide entirely. Mucin from pancreatic adenocarcinoma is variable but is usually thicker and is admixed with malignant cells (Fig. 3.6d). The presence of admixed necrotic debris and inflammatory cells also favors a neoplasm (high-grade) over GI tract contamination. Contaminant gastric foveolar epithelium is a close mimicker and may be impossible to distinguish from neoplastic gastric epithelium of mucinous neoplasms with low-grade dysplasia. In such cases, morphology alone is unreliable, and cyst fluid biochemistry, which shows elevated CEA levels, glucose levels, and/or amylase levels, helps resolve the diagnostic issue.

(ii) *Mucinous Adenocarcinoma*

Invasive mucinous adenocarcinoma can arise from IPMN with high-grade dysplasia or, less commonly, from MCN. A case of mucinous adenocarcinoma that arose from an IPMN with high-grade dysplasia is illustrated in Fig. 3.12. Demonstration of invasion requires histopathological examination. On cytology, mucinous high-grade dysplasia and invasive mucinous adenocarcinoma have similar features. Colloid carcinoma shows abundant pools of extracellular mucin-trapping clusters of mucinous malignant cells.

(c) *Other Cystic Neoplastic Lesions*

(i) *Intraductal Oncocytic Papillary Neoplasm (IOPN)* [9]

Intraductal oncocytic papillary neoplasm is now regarded as a separate entity distinct from IPMN with molecular and biological association. IOPNs present as solid-cystic masses and arise from the main pancreatic duct.

Cytomorphologic Features

- Cellular smears with or without thick mucin.
- Clusters, sheets, and papillary aggregates of tumor cells. The papillae may be broad, edematous, or hyalinized.
- Oncocytic cells with well-defined borders, abundant granular cytoplasm, and large central nuclei showing vesicular chromatin and prominent nucleoli. Cells lack cytoplasmic mucin.
- IOPN is considered a tumor with high-grade dysplasia and shows mitoses, necrosis, and significant atypia.

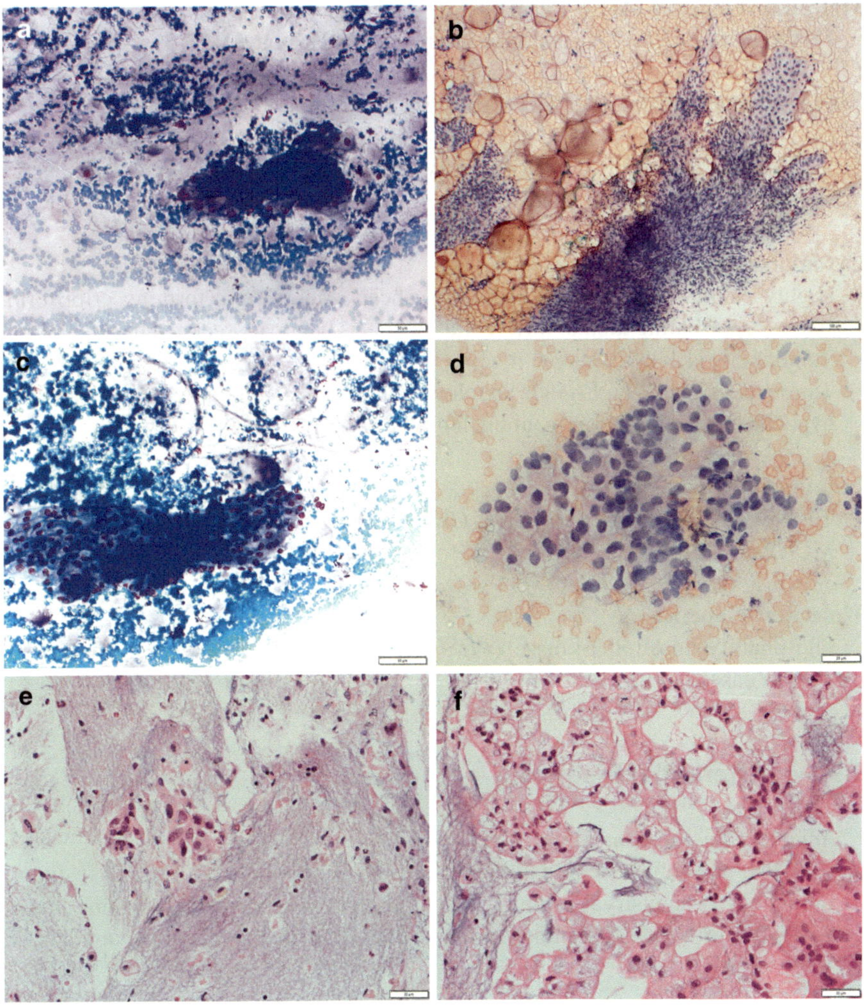

Fig. 3.12 Mucinous adenocarcinoma of the pancreas. (**a**) Pools of extracellular mucin with entrapped tumor cells; (**b**) malignant cells associated with stromal fibroblasts; (**c**, **d**) higher magnification showing tumor cells with a moderate amount of vacuolated cytoplasm, an eccentric nucleus with coarse chromatin, and a small nucleolus; (**e**) cell block showing pools of mucin with tumor cells; (**f**) cell block showing malignant cells with intracytoplasmic mucin [**a**, **c**—May-Grünwald Giemsa stain; **b**, **d**—Papanicolaou stain; **e**, **f**—Hematoxylin–Eosin stain. **a**, **b**, **c** ×200, **b**, **d**, **f**, ×400]

Immunocytochemistry

- The neoplastic cells are positive for MUC6, MUC5AC, and MUC1 and negative for intestinal markers.

Molecular Genetics [44]

- *PRKACA* and *PRKACB* gene fusions are frequently noted [45].

(ii) *Intraductal Tubular Papillary Neoplasm [ITPN]* [9, 46, 47]

ITPN is a rare, recently described entity that can present as a solid or solid-cystic mass lesion in the pancreas or biliary tree.

Cytomorphologic Features

- Highly cellular smears with branching sheets and clusters forming cribriform spaces representing tubular differentiation that is better appreciated in cell blocks.
- Tumor cells lack cytoplasmic mucin.
- Tumor cells show high-grade cytology with nuclear pleomorphism, hyper or hypochromasia, and prominent nucleoli with necrosis and apoptosis.

Immunocytochemistry

- Tumor cells are positive for CK7, CK19, MUC1, and MUC6 and negative for MUC2 and MUC5AC.

Molecular Genetics

- Phosphatidyl-inositol 3-kinase (*PIK3CA*) gene mutations are seen in around 30% of cases.

3.9.5 Differential Diagnosis

- *Acinar cell carcinoma*

  ITPN and acinar cell carcinoma share overlapping cytological features. Immunocytochemistry is useful in differentiation, as acinar cell carcinoma shows positivity for trypsin, chymotrypsin, and BCL10, which are negative in ITPN.

3.10 Cytology of Malignant Neoplastic Cystic Pancreatic Lesions

The most common pancreatic malignancies are exocrine tumors, constituting more than 95% of tumors, with pancreatic ductal adenocarcinoma (PDAC) being the most common. Other malignant neoplasms of the pancreas include neuroendocrine tumors, solid-pseudopapillary neoplasm (SPN), acinar cell carcinoma, and pancreatoblastoma (PBL). These pancreatic malignancies usually present as solid masses with variable necrosis. However, when they present as a cystic lesion, the diagnosis can be extremely challenging.

Solid pseudopapillary neoplasm is the most frequent malignancy that can present as a predominantly cystic lesion in about 12% of cases, followed by PDAC, which can be cystic in about 8% of cases [48]. In these cases, smears can be paucicellular, leading to a false-negative diagnosis [22]. Cystic change in PDAC is uncommon but can result in paucicellular aspirates, which can show occasional cells with features of malignancy in the form of moderate nuclear pleomorphism, coarse chromatin, and small to conspicuous nucleoli. Cystic change in neuroendocrine tumors can be seen in 10–17% of cases and 2% of acinar cell carcinoma [49]. Besides these tumors, other malignant tumors can show cystic degeneration and necrosis. In all these cases, careful attention to the presence of any material, such as capillary fragments with clinging tumor cells, and inspection of the edges of the smears can reveal a few cells true to their neoplastic character. Thus, SPN cells may show nuclei with grooving and vesicular chromatin and cytoplasmic fine vacuolation; PDAC can show moderate pleomorphism and atypia with prominent nucleoli; acinar cell carcinoma cells can show cytoplasm granulation and nuclei with coarse chromatin and cherry red nucleoli; and NET can show nuclei with salt and pepper chromatin. The addition of cyst fluid biochemical analysis and molecular testing of the sediment or of the cell-free liquid content can help in such cases.

Key Takeaways

- Pancreatic cystic lesions represent a wide variety of lesions, each with a distinct cytomorphology as described above.
- An accurate diagnosis requires a multimodal approach with the integration of the ultrasonographic findings, cyst fluid biochemistry, cytomorphology, and molecular abnormalities.
- Distinction of non-neoplastic from neoplastic cystic lesions and cystic change in malignant lesions is of utmost importance.
- Among neoplastic lesions, identification of mucinous cystic lesions is important. Among mucinous lesions, dysplasia must be identified and graded as low-grade or high-grade dysplasia.

3.11 Conclusion

Pancreatic cystic lesions represent a vast spectrum ranging from benign to frankly malignant, making their evaluation by the minimally invasive technique EUS-FNA a vital investigation. Appropriate partitioning of the cyst fluid sample for various biochemical and molecular testing is important by the endoscopist sampling the lesion. Accurate diagnosis on cytopathology requires knowledge of the cytomorphological features along with the nuances and caveats while interpreting smears. The recent WHO reporting system of pancreaticobiliary cytopathology is an essential step in this direction, which brought in the use of unified terminology with the risk of malignancy and management guidelines, clearly aiding good communication between the pathologist and the clinician. Needless to say, a multimodal approach combining the clinical features, imaging features, cyst fluid biochemistry, and molecular analysis is required for an accurate diagnosis that guides further patient management. Future directions include the use of cyst fluid as a liquid biopsy for discerning molecular alterations at the genetic and epigenetic levels and application of AI (artificial intelligence) in cytology for rendering an even more accurate and rapid diagnosis in pancreatic cystic lesions.

Acknowledgments We thank Dr.Ritambhra Nada, Professor, Dept of Histopathology, for providing us the histopathology images (11A, 11C, 9B, 7A).

References

1. Pitman MB, Lewandrowski K, Shen J, Sahani D, Brugge W, Fernandez-del CC. Pancreatic cysts: preoperative diagnosis and clinical management. Cancer Cytopathol. 2010;118(1):1–13. https://doi.org/10.1002/cncy.20059.
2. Hu F, Hu Y, Wang D, Ma X, Yue Y, Tang W, et al. Cystic neoplasms of the pancreas: differential diagnosis and radiology correlation. Front Oncol. 2022;12:860740. https://doi.org/10.3389/fonc.2022.860740.
3. Jang DK, Song BJ, Ryu JK, Chung KH, Lee BS, Park JK, et al. Preoperative diagnosis of pancreatic cystic lesions: the accuracy of endoscopic ultrasound and cross-sectional imaging. Pancreas. 2015;44(8):1329–33. https://doi.org/10.1097/MPA.0000000000000396.
4. Martin AK, Zhou Z. Endoscopic ultrasound-guided fine-needle aspiration for the diagnosis of pancreatic cysts by combined cytopathology and cystic content analysis. World J Gastrointest Endosc. 2015;7(15):1157–69. https://doi.org/10.4253/wjge.v7.i15.1157.
5. Pflüger MJ, Jamouss KT, Afghani E, Lim SJ, Rodriguez Franco S, Mayo H, et al. Predictive ability of pancreatic cyst fluid biomarkers: a systematic review and meta-analysis. Pancreatology. 2023;23(7):868–77. https://doi.org/10.1016/j.pan.2023.05.003.
6. Turner RC, Melnychuk JT, Chen W, Jones D, Krishna SG. Molecular analysis of pancreatic cyst fluid for the management of intraductal papillary mucinous neoplasms. Diagnostics (Basel). 2022;12(11):2573. https://doi.org/10.3390/diagnostics12112573.
7. Gillis A, Cipollone I, Cousins G, Conlon K. Does EUS-FNA molecular analysis carry additional value when compared to cytology in the diagnosis of pancreatic cystic neoplasm? A systematic review. HPB (Oxford). 2015;17(5):377–86. https://doi.org/10.1111/hpb.12364.
8. Yoon WJ, Pitman MB. Cytology specimen management, triage and standardized reporting of fine needle aspiration biopsies of the pancreas. J Pathol Transl Med. 2015;49(5):364–72. https://doi.org/10.4132/jptm.2015.07.01.
9. Reid MD. Cytologic assessment of cystic/intraductal lesions of the pancreatobiliary tract. Arch Pathol Lab Med. 2022;146(3):280–97.
10. Yoon WJ, Brugge WR. Endoscopic ultrasound and pancreatic cystic lesions—diagnostic and therapeutic applications. Endosc Ultrasound. 2012;1(2):75–9. https://doi.org/10.4103/2303-9027.105370.
11. Vilmann P, Jacobsen GK, Henriksen FW, Hancke S. Endoscopic ultrasonography with guided fine needle aspiration biopsy in pancreatic disease. Gastrointest Endosc. 1992;38:172–3. https://doi.org/10.1016/S0016-5107(92)70385-X.
12. Kumar P, Rana SS, Kundu R, Gupta P, Rohilla M, Gupta N, Srinivasan R, Dey P. Endoscopic ultrasound-guided fine-needle aspiration cytology in diagnosing intra-abdominal lesions. Cytojournal. 2022;19:56. https://doi.org/10.25259/Cytojournal_31_2021.
13. Horwhat JD, Paulson EK, McGrath K, Branch MS, Baillie J, Tyler D, et al. A randomized comparison of EUS-guided FNA versus CT or US-guided FNA for the evaluation of pancreatic mass lesions. Gastrointest Endosc. 2006;63(7):966–75. https://doi.org/10.1016/j.gie.2005.10.030.
14. Hassan GM, Laporte L, Paquin SC, Menard C, Sahai AV, Mâsse B, Trottier H. Endoscopic ultrasound guided fine needle aspiration versus endoscopic ultrasound guided fine needle

biopsy for pancreatic cancer diagnosis: a systematic review and meta-analysis. Diagnostics (Basel). 2022;12(12):2951. https://doi.org/10.3390/diagnostics12122951.
15. Banafea O, Mghanga FP, Zhao J, Zhao R, Zhu L. Endoscopic ultrasonography with fine needle aspiration for histological diagnosis of solid pancreatic masses: a meta-analysis of diagnostic accuracy studies. BMC Gastroenterol. 2016;16(1):108. https://doi.org/10.1186/s12876-016-0519-z.
16. Attam R, Arain MA, Bloechl SJ, Trikudanathan G, Munigala S, Bakman Y, et al. "Wet suction technique (WEST)": a novel way to enhance the quality of EUS-FNA aspirate. Results of a prospective, single-blind, randomized, controlled trial using a 22-gauge needle for EUS-FNA of solid lesions. Gastrointest Endosc. 2015;81(6):1401–7. https://doi.org/10.1016/j.gie.2014.11.023.
17. Bang JY, Magee SH, Ramesh J, Trevino JM, Varadarajulu S. Randomized trial comparing fanning with standard technique for endoscopic ultrasound-guided fine-needle aspiration of solid pancreatic mass lesions. Endoscopy. 2013;45(6):445–50. https://doi.org/10.1055/s-0032-1326268.
18. Pitman MB, Centeno BA, Ali SZ, Genevay M, Stelow E, MinoKenudson M, et al. Standardized terminology and nomenclature for pancreatobiliary cytology: the papanicolaou society of cytopathology guidelines. Diagn Cytopathol. 2014;42:338–50. https://doi.org/10.1002/dc.23092.
19. Pitman MB, Centeno BA, Reid MD, Siddiqui MT, Layfield LJ, Perez-Machado M, et al. The World Health Organization reporting system for pancreaticobiliary cytopathology. Acta Cytol. 2023;67(3):304–20. https://doi.org/10.1159/000527912.
20. Bosman FT, Carneiro F, Hruban RH, Theise ND, editors. WHO classification of tumours of the digestive system. 4th ed. Lyon: International Agency for Research on Cancer, WHO Press; 2010.
21. Hoda RS, Arpin RN 3rd, Rosenbaum MW, Pitman MB. Risk of malignancy associated with diagnostic categories of the proposed World Health Organization international system for reporting pancreaticobiliary cytopathology. Cancer Cytopathol. 2022;130(3):195–201. https://doi.org/10.1002/cncy.22502.
22. Kundu R, Kollabathula A, Gupta N, Rohilla M, Rana SS, Nada R, et al. The WHO system versus the Papanicolaou Society of Cytopathology system for reporting pancreaticobiliary cytology for risk stratification—which is better? Diagn Cytopathol. 2024;52(3):145–55. https://doi.org/10.1002/dc.25367.
23. Pitman MB. The World Health Organization reporting system for pancreaticobiliary cytopathology: review and comparison to the Papanicolaou Society of Cytopathology System. Arch Pathol Lab Med. 2025;149(3):e39–46. https://doi.org/10.5858/arpa.2023-0411-RA.
24. Stelow EB, Bardales RH, Stanley MW. Pitfalls in endoscopic ultrasound-guided fine-needle aspiration and how to avoid them. Adv Anat Pathol. 2005;12(2):62–73. https://doi.org/10.1097/01.pap.0000155523.41501.8e.
25. Goyal A. Pancreaticobiliary cytopathology: an update. Diagn Histopathol. 2018;24(10):397–408. https://doi.org/10.1016/j.mpdhp.2018.07.002.
26. Gonzalez Obeso E, Murphy E, Brugge W, Deshpande V. Pseudocyst of the pancreas: the role of cytology and special stains for mucin. Cancer Cytopathol. 2009;117(2):101–7. https://doi.org/10.1002/cncr.24037.
27. Abdelkader A, Hunt B, Hartley CP, Panarelli NC, Giorgadze T. Cystic lesions of the pancreas: differential diagnosis and cytologic-histologic correlation. Arch Pathol Lab Med. 2020;144(1):47–61. https://doi.org/10.5858/arpa.2019-0308-RA.
28. Raval JS, Zeh HJ, Moser AJ, Lee KK, Sanders MK, Navina S, et al. Pancreatic lymphoepithelial cysts express CEA and can contain mucous cells: potential pitfalls in the preoperative diagnosis. Mod Pathol. 2010;23(12):1467–74. https://doi.org/10.1038/modpathol.2010.134.
29. Chen AL, Misdraji J, Brugge WR, Ferrone CR, Pitman MB. Acinar cell cystadenoma: a challenging cytology diagnosis, facilitated by Moray® micro-forceps biopsy. Diagn Cytopathol. 2017;45(7):557–60. https://doi.org/10.1002/dc.23739.
30. Salomao M, Remotti H, Allendorf JD, Poneros JM, Sethi A, Gonda TA, et al. Fine-needle aspirations of pancreatic serous cystadenomas: improving diagnostic yield with cell blocks

and α-inhibin immunohistochemistry. Cancer Cytopathol. 2014;122(1):33–9. https://doi.org/10.1002/cncy.21347.
31. Reid MD, Saka B, Balci S, Goldblum AS, Adsay NV. Molecular genetics of pancreatic neoplasms and their morphologic correlates: an update on recent advances and potential diagnostic applications. Am J Clin Pathol. 2014;141(2):168–80. https://doi.org/10.1309/AJCP0FKDP7ENVKEV.
32. Matthaei H, Semaan A, Hruban RH. The genetic classification of pancreatic neoplasia. J Gastroenterol. 2015;50(5):520–32. https://doi.org/10.1007/s00535-015-1037-4.
33. Efthymiou A, Podas T, Zacharakis E. Endoscopic ultrasound in the diagnosis of pancreatic intraductal papillary mucinous neoplasms. World J Gastroenterol. 2014;20(24):7785–93. https://doi.org/10.3748/wjg.v20.i24.7785.
34. Cizginer S, Turner BG, Bilge AR, Karaca C, Pitman MB, Brugge WR. Cyst fluid carcinoembryonic antigen is an accurate diagnostic marker of pancreatic mucinous cysts. Pancreas. 2011;40(6):1024–8. https://doi.org/10.1097/MPA.0b013e31821fd360.
35. Kim D, Margolskee E, Goyal A, Siddiqui MT, Heymann JJ, Rao R, Hayden J. Optimal carcinoembryonic antigen (CEA) cutoff values in the diagnosis of neoplastic mucinous pancreatic cysts differ among assays. J Clin Pathol. 2024;77(12):848–52. https://doi.org/10.1136/jcp-2023-209136.
36. Sharma RK, Bush N, Rana SS, Srinivasan R, Nada R, Gupta R, Rana S, Singh T. Lower cyst fluid carcinoembryonic antigen cutoff is helpful in the differential diagnosis of mucinous versus non-mucinous pancreatic cysts. Indian J Gastroenterol. 2022;41(4):397–404. https://doi.org/10.1007/s12664-022-01269-w.
37. Williet N, Caillol F, Karsenti D, Abou-Ali E, Camus M, Belle A, Chaput U, Levy J, Ratone JP, Tournier Q, Grange R, Le Roy B, Becq A, Phelip JM. The level of glucose in pancreatic cyst fluid is more accurate than carcinoembryonic antigen to identify mucinous tumors: a French multicenter study. Endosc Ultrasound. 2023;12(4):377–81. https://doi.org/10.1097/eus.0000000000000024.
38. Bruni A, Eusebi LH, Lisotti A, Ricci C, Maida M, Fusaroli P, Barbara G, Sadik R, Pagano N, Hedenström P, et al. Intracystic glucose measurement for on-site differentiation between mucinous and non-mucinous pancreatic cystic lesions. Cancer. 2024;16(24):4198. https://doi.org/10.3390/cancers16244198.
39. Adsay NV, Fukushima N, Furukawa T, Hruban RH, Klimstra DS, Klöppel G, et al. Intraductal neoplasms of the pancreas. In: Bosman FT, Carneiro F, Hruban RH, Theise ND, editors. WHO classification of tumours of the digestive system. 4th ed. Lyon: IARC; 2010. p. 304–13.
40. Basturk O, Esposito I, Fukushima N, et al. Pancreatic mucinous cystic neoplasm. In: WHO Classification of Tumours Editorial Board, editor. Digestive system tumours. 5th ed. Lyon: IARC Press; 2019. p. 319–21.
41. Recine M, Kaw M, Evans DB, Krishnamurthy S. Fine-needle aspiration cytology of mucinous tumors of the pancreas. Cancer. 2004;102(2):92–9. https://doi.org/10.1002/cncr.20052.
42. Pitman MB, Centeno BA, Daglilar ES, Brugge WR, Mino-Kenudson M. Cytological criteria of high-grade epithelial atypia in the cyst fluid of pancreatic intraductal papillary mucinous neoplasms. Cancer Cytopathol. 2014;122(1):40–7. https://doi.org/10.1002/cncy.21317.
43. Lüttges J, Feyerabend B, Buchelt T, Pacena M, Klöppel G. The mucin profile of noninvasive and invasive mucinous cystic neoplasms of the pancreas. Am J Surg Pathol. 2002;26(4):466–71. https://doi.org/10.1097/00000478-200204000-00008.
44. Singhi AD, Nikiforova MN, Fasanella KE, McGrath KM, Pai RK, Ohori NP, et al. Preoperative GNAS and KRAS testing in the diagnosis of pancreatic mucinous cysts. Clin Cancer Res. 2014;20(14):4381–9. https://doi.org/10.1158/1078-0432.CCR-14-0513.
45. Singhi AD, Wood LD, Parks E, Torbenson MS, Felsenstein M, Hruban RH, et al. Recurrent rearrangements in PRKACA and PRKACB in intraductal oncocytic papillary neoplasms of the pancreas and bile duct. Gastroenterology. 2020;158(3):573–582.e2. https://doi.org/10.1053/j.gastro.2019.10.028.

46. Tajima S. Intraductal tubulopapillary neoplasm of the pancreas suspected by endoscopic ultrasonography-fine-needle aspiration cytology: report of a case confirmed by surgical specimen histology. Diagn Cytopathol. 2015;43(12):1003–6.
47. Zhao L, Hart J, Xiao SY, Antic T. Cytological features of pancreatic intraductal tubulopapillary neoplasm and an unexpected immunohistochemical profile. Pathology. 2014;46(7):662–5. https://doi.org/10.1097/PAT.0000000000000172.
48. Shah S, Mortele KJ. Uncommon solid pancreatic neoplasms: ultrasound, computed tomography, and magnetic resonance imaging features. Semin Ultrasound CT MR. 2007;28(5):357–70. https://doi.org/10.1053/j.sult.2007.08.002.
49. Yoon WJ, Daglilar ES, Pitman MB, Brugge WR. Cystic pancreatic neuroendocrine tumors: endoscopic ultrasound and fine-needle aspiration characteristics. Endoscopy. 2013;45(3):189–94. https://doi.org/10.1055/s-0032-1325990.

Role of Endoscopic Ultrasonography in the Diagnosis and Management of Pancreatic Cystic Lesions

4

Role of EUS in Pancreatic Cystic Lesion

Nikhil Sonthalia, Shivam Sethi, Rajesh Puri, and Raghavendra Puri

Abstract

Pancreatic cystic lesions are commonly detected incidentally in up to 13.5% of cross-sectional imaging studies. Broadly, a distinction needs to be made between two main groups—mucinous and nonmucinous—as mucinous cysts predominantly have malignant potential. Among mucinous cysts, a further distinction is needed between high-malignant-risk potential lesions, which require surgical intervention, and low-risk lesions which are monitored with surveillance. Endoscopic ultrasonography (EUS) has emerged as a pivotal tool in distinguishing between these types and thus influencing patient management. EUS with or without fine-needle aspiration (FNA) provides high diagnostic accuracy in differentiating mucinous from nonmucinous cysts. A panel of biochemical tests can be performed on aspirated fluid, such as amylase, glucose, carcinoembryonic antigen, molecular testing, and cytological analysis. There is an emerging role of EUS-guided confocal endomicroscopy and artificial intelligence to improve the diagnostic accuracy of EUS. Beyond diagnosis, EUS also enables therapeutic interventions such as pseudocyst drainage and ablation of selected cystic neoplasms. This chapter discusses the role of EUS in the diagnosis, characterization, and management of pancreatic cystic lesions, highlighting its advantages, limitations, and potential future directions.

N. Sonthalia
Institute of Gastrosciences and Liver Diseases, Apollo Multispecialty Hospitals, Kolkata, India

S. Sethi · R. Puri (✉)
Institute of Digestive & Hepato-biliary Sciences, Medanta, The Medicity, Gurgaon, India

R. Puri
DY Patil Medical College & Hospital, Pune, India

R. K. Sharma et al. (eds.), *Differential Diagnosis and Management of Pancreatic Cystic Lesions*, https://doi.org/10.1007/978-981-92-0654-4_4

Keywords

Endoscopic ultrasonography · Pancreatic cystic lesions · Mucinous cystadenoma Fine-needle aspiration cytology

4.1 Introduction

Pancreatic cystic lesions (PCLs) are increasingly diagnosed in day-to-day clinical practice due to the widespread use of advanced imaging technologies like computed tomography (CT) and magnetic resonance imaging (MRI). These imaging techniques have improved the ability to detect even small lesions, leading to a rise in prevalence of PCLs, many of which are asymptomatic. These cystic lesions can be broadly categorized into two major groups: nonmucinous and mucinous. Common nonmucinous cysts are pseudocysts, serous cystic neoplasms (SCN), solid pseudopapillary neoplasms (SPN), and cystic neuroendocrine tumors, whereas mucinous cysts are intraductal papillary mucinous neoplasms (IPMNs) and mucinous cystic neoplasms (MCNs). Because of the potential malignancy associated with mucinous cysts and some nonmucinous lesions (e.g., SPN, cystic neuroendocrine tumors), accurate characterization of these cysts is essential for appropriate management. This is where endoscopic ultrasonography (EUS) plays a critical role. EUS allows detailed visualization of pancreatic cysts, provides fine-needle aspiration (FNA) for cytological evaluation, and analysis of cyst fluid for biomarkers that aid in the differentiation between benign and high-risk or malignant cyst. This chapter aims to elucidate the role of EUS in the diagnosis, characterization, and management of pancreatic cystic lesions, emphasizing its advantages, limitations, and future directions.

4.1.1 Diagnostic Role of EUS in Pancreatic Cystic Lesions

While CT scans and MRIs can detect the presence of a cyst, they are less reliable in determining the cyst type, with the diagnostic accuracy for CT ranging from 39% to 40% and for MRI from 40% to 49% [1]. These imaging techniques are useful for cyst follow-up and evaluating the pancreatic duct, but they are limited in detecting mural nodules, the consistency of fluid, and mucin plugs. In contrast, EUS—with or without aspiration—plays a significant role in this regard. EUS offers high-resolution imaging of the pancreas and adjacent structures and is crucial in the management of pancreatic cysts, as treatment plans differ significantly depending on the cyst type and its malignant potential, ranging from reassurance to surveillance to surgery. For low-risk lesions, surgery might be unnecessary and overly aggressive; hence, EUS should be included in the workup for the evaluation and management of any pancreatic cyst.

Its application in the assessment of pancreatic cystic lesions is multifaceted:

- *Characterization of lesions*: EUS provides comprehensive details regarding the size, location, and morphology of cystic lesions. Key features such as wall thickness, internal echoes, and septations can suggest the nature of the cyst. For example, thickened walls or irregularities may raise suspicion for malignancy, while thin-walled, well-defined cysts are more likely to be benign.
- *Tissue sampling*: A significant advantage of EUS is its ability to facilitate fine-needle aspiration (FNA) for cytological analysis, which aids in identifying potentially malignant lesions. This real-time evaluation reduces the need for more invasive surgical interventions.

The diagnostic accuracy of EUS alone varies between 40% and 93%. However, when combined with ancillary techniques like fine-needle aspiration and contrast enhancement, its accuracy improves to 95% [2]. EUS is an invasive procedure and should be performed only after a cyst has been detected on a cross-sectional imaging.

The main goal of EUS in evaluating pancreatic cyst is to accurately differentiate between mucinous and nonmucinous cysts. This is because mucinous cysts, which include intraductal papillary mucinous neoplasms (IPMNs) and mucinous cystic neoplasms, are precursors of pancreatic adenocarcinoma. Even among them, the risk of malignant transformation can vary significantly, ranging from 10% to 70%, depending on the presence of high-risk features [3]. On the other hand, nonmucinous cysts are generally indolent and benign in nature, except SPN and cystic neuroendocrine tumors which may have malignant potential.

Key morphological features on EUS that help in differentiating benign and malignant cysts include cyst wall thickness, the presence of intracystic mural nodules, mucin plugs, septation, vascularity of lesion, adjacent lymphadenopathy, cyst number and size, as well as the relationship to the pancreatic duct and any associated background lesions.

The following table shows various high-risk stigmata and worrisome features which can be detected on EUS:

1. *Key Morphological Features of Different Pancreatic Cysts on EUS:*
   - *Pseudocysts*: These are not true cysts but rather collection of fluid and necrotic tissue that typically arise after pancreatitis. They are often managed based on their size, symptoms, and complications. On B-mode EUS, they appear as an anechoic, thick-walled lesion containing irregular debris in a background of either acute or chronic pancreatitis (Fig. 4.1a). A cystic lesion without septations or solid components and found within the pancreas having parenchymal features has sensitivity and specificity of 94 and 85%, respectively. Occasionally, communication with the main pancreatic duct is seen, and regional inflammatory nodes may be present. If symptomatic, drainage is recommended, and in cases of diagnostic uncertainty, fluid aspiration for analysis is advised.

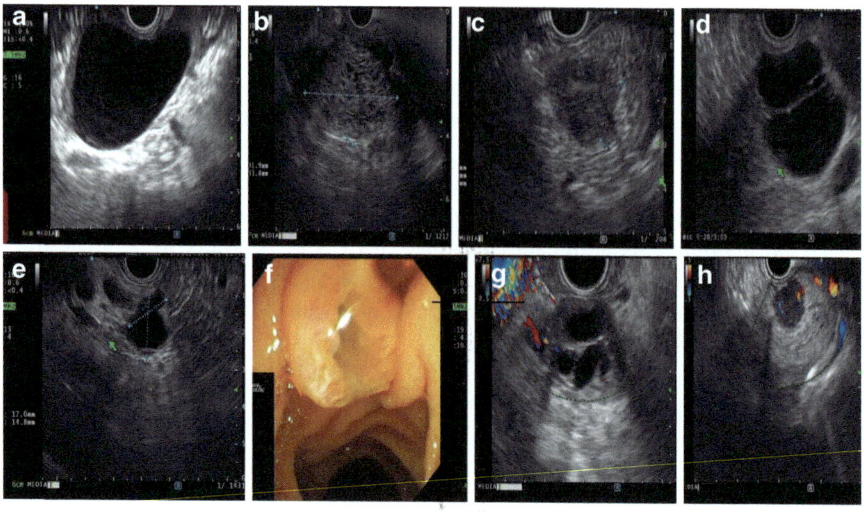

Fig. 4.1 (**a–h**) EUS appearance of various pancreatic cystic lesions: (**a**) a pseudocyst of size ~24 × 60 mm with intracystic debris; (**b**) a large (~44 × 32 mm) well-defined multiloculated microcystic lesion involving the head of pancreas, suggestive of serous cystadenoma; (**c**) a well-defined heteroechoic mass of size ~20 × 19 mm in a young female, typically seen in solid pseudopapillary epithelial neoplasm (SPEN); (**d**) a large cystic anechoic lesion of size ~45 × 40 mm with septae. Thick fluid was aspirated out, string sign was positive, and fluid analysis was suggestive of mucinous cystic neoplasm (MCN). (**e**) A thick-walled cystic lesion of size ~17 × 15 mm at the neck and body junction. MPD was dilated up to 9 mm and seen communicating with the cystic lesion s/o mixed intraductal papillary neoplasm (IPMN); (**f**) in the same case, side-view endoscopy showed characteristic fish-eyed papilla with extruding mucin, suggestive of main-duct IPMN; (**g**) multiple cystic lesions communicating with PD and MPD were nondilated, suggestive of branched duct IPMN; (**h**) a well-defined hypoechoic lesion with few cystic spaces which showed increased vascularity on Doppler application. The results of the EUS-FNA indicated a possible NET

- *Serous cystadenoma (SCA)*: These are typically benign lesions that often present as small, cystic masses filled with clear fluid. These cysts are usually located in the body or tail of the pancreas, occurring in elderly women, and are characterized by a honeycomb appearance on cross-sectional imaging. On standard B-mode EUS, they appear as microcystic lesions with a honeycomb appearance (Fig. 4.1b). Occasionally, a macrocystic component may be present, which can lead to diagnostic confusion. While central calcification is pathognomonic for SCAs, it is rarely seen. They do not communicate with the pancreatic duct, and the rest of the pancreas is usually normal, with no adjacent lymphadenopathy. On contrast-enhanced EUS, septations show hyperenhancement. In most cases, B-mode EUS is sufficient to establish the diagnosis, and FNA is generally not required.
- *Solid pseudopapillary neoplasms (SPN)*: These lesions typically occur in young women and can be located throughout the pancreas. On EUS, they appear as well-circumscribed heterogeneous mass with solid, cystic, or mixed

components, and occasionally irregular calcification can also be found (Fig. 4.1c). Internal hemorrhagic necrosis commonly occurs which results in cystic spaces.

- *Mucinous cystic neoplasm (MCN)*: These lesions predominantly occur in middle-aged women, mostly in pancreatic tail or body region, and can range from benign to malignant. On B-mode EUS, they are mostly unilocular or septated macrocysts of variable thickness that do not communicate with the main pancreatic duct (Fig. 4.1d). Sometimes, peripheral calcifications can also be seen.

  The presence of solid components within the cyst and regional lymphadenopathy raises suspicion of malignant transformation. The solid component can sometimes be confused with mucin plugs. On B-mode EUS, mucin plugs are characterized by a central hypoechoic area with a surrounding hyperechoic rim, no Doppler uptake, and may be mobile. On the other hand, mural nodules are usually isoechoic or hyperechoic with irregular margins. Contrast-enhanced EUS can also play an important role in this regard, as it reveals vascularity within mural nodules, making it helpful in distinguishing a mural nodule from a mucin ball.

  Fine-needle aspiration of fluid and sampling of solid components is recommended when MCN is suspected on B-mode EUS.

- *Intraductal Papillary Mucinous Neoplasm (IPMN)*: IPMNs are cystic neoplasms that arise within the pancreatic ductal system. They have the potential to progress to pancreatic cancer, and their management often involves careful surveillance or surgical intervention. IPMNs are classified into main-duct IPMN (M-IPMN), branched-duct IPMN (BD-IPMN), and mixed IPMN. They are more commonly found in the head of the pancreatic region than the body and tail. On B-mode EUS, IPMNs typically present as a dilated main pancreatic duct or side branches and may have septated cyst and solid components (Fig. 4.1e and g). Mucin plugs are often seen, which need to be differentiated from mural nodules. Communication with the main pancreatic duct is often seen on EUS. "Fish-eye" patulous ampulla extruding mucin during endoscopic examination is a pathognomic feature of M-IPMN (Fig. 4.1f). It is important to assess for adjacent lymphadenopathy, pancreatic atrophy, or pancreatic parenchymal mass when IPMN is suspected on B-mode EUS. FNA for fluid analysis and sampling of solid component should be done in these cases.
- *Pancreatic neuroendocrine tumors (P-NET)*: Although most P-NETs present as solid lesions, approximately 10–18% can manifest as cystic lesions. On EUS, solid NETs typically appear as well-defined, homogeneous masses with increased vascularity (Fig. 4.1h). Cystic NETs, however, can be challenging to distinguish from other pancreatic cystic lesions. P-NETs may exhibit thickened walls and septations, and they do not communicate with the pancreatic duct (PD). To establish a definitive diagnosis, EUS-guided fine-needle aspiration (FNA) should be done.

2. *EUS-Guided Fine-Needle Aspiration of Cyst Fluid for Analysis*

   EUS-FNA is a valuable technique for aspirating the contents of pancreatic cysts, aiding in the differential diagnosis of ambiguous cases, particularly in distinguishing between mucinous and nonmucinous pancreatic cystic tumors. The aspirate is often acellular or shows minimal cellularity in up to 72% of cases. Following aspiration, the fluid is generally sent for analysis, including cytology, viscosity, extracellular mucin, tumor markers (CEA, CA 19-9, CA 153, Ca 72-4, etc.), enzymes (amylase, lipase), and DNA testing. When differentiating mucinous from nonmucinous cysts, the sensitivity, specificity, and accuracy of these tests range from 12.5% to 27%, 90% to 100%, and 55%, respectively [4, 5]. The following principles should be followed during EUS-guided pancreatic cyst aspiration:

   (a) Prophylactic antibiotics: While antibiotics are commonly given prior to the procedure, recent meta-analysis have shown that prophylactic antibiotics may not significantly lower the risk of infection [6]. Therefore, the routine use of prophylactic antibiotics warrants reconsideration.
   (b) Needle choice: 19-G FNA needle is preferred due to the possibility of thick mucinous fluid in mucinous neoplasms. However, a 22-G needle may be used for small cysts, those near vascular structures, or in difficult-to-access locations.
   (c) Aim to aspirate the entire cyst content in a single pass.
   (d) If a solid component is present within the cyst, it should be sampled first, followed by aspiration of the fluid.
   (e) Post-aspiration analysis: Once fluid is aspirated, a "string sign" should be checked for. The fluid should then be sent for the analysis of glucose, amylase, CEA, and cytology.

3. *Fluid Characteristics in Different Types of Pancreatic Cysts*

   SCN: The aspirated fluid is colorless and often contain blood, typically acellular or with minimal cellularity. Cytologically, small glycogen-staining cuboidal cells may be seen against a background of acellular material. CEA is undetectable or low, amylase levels are low, and fluid glucose levels are typically >50 mg/dL.

   MCN: The aspirated fluid is colorless and thick. Cytology reveals extracellular mucin, and mucinous epithelial cells may be seen in a background of ovarian stroma. CEA levels range from moderate to very high, amylase levels are variable, and fluid glucose is <50 mg/dL. A positive string sign is observed (the fluid forms a string of ≥1 cm when stretched between fingers and lasts for ≥1 s).

   IPMN: The aspirated fluid is colorless and thick. Cytology shows extracellular mucin and mucinous epithelial cells, often with papillary projections and varying degrees of atypia. CEA levels are moderate to very high, amylase levels are elevated, and fluid glucose is typically <50 mg/dL. A positive string sign is also present.

Pseudocyst: The aspirated fluid is yellow to brown and thin. Cytologically, macrophages and mixed inflammatory infiltrate are observed, with no mucin present. CEA levels are low, while amylase levels are elevated.

Cystic NET: The aspirated fluid typically has low cellularity, and amylase and CEA levels are also low.

4. *Ancillary Tests for Enhancing the Diagnostic Accuracy of EUS*

   Several studies have reported the diagnostic accuracy of EUS in evaluating pancreatic cystic lesions. A meta-analysis reported that EUS-FNA has a sensitivity of approximately 85% for detecting malignancy in cystic lesions [5]. The diagnostic accuracy of EUS can be further enhanced by analyzing the cyst fluid, including cytology and biochemical markers. Cyst fluid glycoprotein markers, such as, CEA, CA 19-9, CA 125, CA 15-3, and CA 72-4, which are secreted by the epithelial lining, can provide valuable insights. Among these, CEA is currently considered the most reliable for identifying mucinous cystic pancreatic lesions, with values >192 ng/mL suggesting mucinous neoplasms [7]. In addition to fluid analysis, DNA and mutational analysis of the cystic fluid aspirated can assist in predicting malignancy. The presence of loss of heterozygosity (LOH) associated with tumor suppressor genes serves as a surrogate marker for gene inactivation and mutation [8]. In IPMNs, there is a transformation process where hyperplastic lesions progress to dysplastic and carcinoma cells. The oncogene GNAS has been linked to IPMN tissue, with some studies suggesting that GNAS mutations are associated with more aggressive and invasive forms of IPMN. Additionally, mutations in K-*ras*, *p*16, and *p*53 have been associated with the progression of cystic pancreatic lesions from nondysplastic to dysplastic stages.

High-risk stigmata	Worrisome features
MPD dilated to >10 mm	MPD diameter 5–10 mm
Solid enhancing mural nodule ≥ 5 mm in size	Solid enhancing mural nodule <5 mm in size
Biliary obstruction by cyst	Cyst diameter > 3 cm
	Enhancing or thickened cyst wall
	Thickened septations
	Lymphadenopathy
	Change in caliber of MPD with distal pancreatic atrophy
	Increase in cyst size >20% in diameter per year

The use of Moray micro-forceps through the EUS needle enables tissue sampling from the cyst wall, septum, or mural nodules. Studies have shown that cyst fluid analysis and Moray forceps-guided biopsy offer similar performance in distinguishing mucinous from nonmucinous cysts and in identifying high-risk cysts. However, tissue sampling using Moray forceps has been found to be superior for diagnosing specific cyst subtypes, providing valuable information for preoperative patient management.

4.1.2 Therapeutic Role of EUS in Pancreatic Cystic Lesions

The management of PCLs varies significantly based on their characteristics, clinical presentation, and potential for malignancy. For benign lesions, such as serous cystadenomas and low-risk cysts, regular surveillance using cross-sectional imaging or EUS allows monitoring of any changes in size or morphology and helps identify any worrisome features that may suggest malignancy. In contrast, lesions suspected to be malignant or exhibiting high-risk features warrant surgical intervention [9]. The therapeutic role of EUS is limited to the management of symptomatic pseudocysts and ablation of certain PCLs.

1. *Endoscopic drainage*: For symptomatic pseudocysts, EUS-guided drainage is commonly the treatment of choice. This minimally invasive technique provides symptom relief and prevents complications like infection, bleeding, or rupture.
2. *EUS-guided ablation*: It has emerged as an innovative, minimally invasive technique in the treatment of certain PCLs. Below is an overview of the indications, procedure, and outcomes associated with EUS-guided ablation.
   (a) *Indications for EUS-Guided Ablation*
   EUS-guided ablation is particularly beneficial for lesions that are not amenable to surgical resection, providing a less invasive alternative. The main indications for EUS-guided ablation of PCLs include:
   - Symptomatic lesions
   - Cysts with worrisome features for malignancy
   - Lesions that require intervention due to the size or growth rate

   (b) *Techniques of Ablation*
   Several techniques are used in EUS-guided ablation of pancreatic cystic lesions, each with its own mechanism of action and clinical indications:
   (i) *Ethanol ablation*: It is one of the most established methods which involve the injection of absolute ethanol into the cyst cavity, leading to dehydration and necrosis of the cyst lining. The effectiveness of this approach has been documented in various studies, showing significant reduction in cyst size and resolution of symptoms [10].
   (ii) *Radiofrequency ablation (RFA)*: RFA uses high-frequency electromagnetic waves to generate heat and cause coagulative necrosis of the target tissue. This technique has become popular due to its efficacy and safety profile. Studies have demonstrated the successful reduction of cyst size and the low incidence of complications [11].
   (iii) *Cryoablation*: This emerging technique involves the application of extreme cold to induce cellular destruction. Although still in the experimental stages, preliminary results suggest it may be a viable option for managing certain types of PCLs.

(c) Procedure Overview

The success of EUS-guided ablation hinges on proper patient selection and a well- executed procedure. Below is an outline of the typical steps involved:

(i) *Patient selection and preparation*: Proper patient selection is critical for the success of EUS-guided ablation. Pre-procedural assessment includes imaging studies along with cytological analysis to characterize the cyst. Pre-procedural counseling should inform patients about the risks, benefits, and alternative management options.

(ii) *Technical aspects of EUS-guided ablation*: The procedure is typically performed under sedation. A linear echoendoscope is advanced into the duodenum or stomach to visualize the pancreas and the target cyst. A fine-needle aspiration needle is then advanced into the cyst under ultrasound guidance.

- For ethanol injection, the absolute ethanol is slowly injected into the cyst in small, incremental doses, ensuring the entire cavity is treated. Care must be taken to avoid extravasation into surrounding structures.
- For radiofrequency ablation, EUS needle is inserted within the cyst, followed by placement of an RFA probe. The probe is then activated, delivering energy that induces thermal damage to the cyst wall.

(iii) *Post-ablation care*: After the procedure, patients are monitored for potential complications, such as abdominal pain or pancreatitis. Follow-up imaging is essential to assess the efficacy of the procedure and to monitor for any recurrence.

(d) *Efficacy and Outcomes*

Multiple studies have evaluated the efficacy of EUS-guided ablation therapies. In a systematic review, RFA showed a successful reduction in cyst size in over 80% of patients with a low complication rate [12]. Ethanol injection has also demonstrated therapeutic success, especially in mucinous cystic neoplasms.

(e) *Complications and Safety*

EUS-guided ablation is generally well-tolerated; however, complications can occur. These include:

- Pancreatitis: The most common complication, occurring in a small percentage of cases.
- Infection: Both the cyst and surrounding tissues are at risk of infection, especially with ethanol injections.
- Bleeding: Although rare, bleeding can occur, particularly if major vessels are inadvertently damaged during the procedure.

Patient selection, meticulous technique, and appropriate post-procedural monitoring can mitigate these risks.

4.2 Advantages of EUS in Evaluating Pancreatic Cysts

EUS offers several advantages compared to other imaging modalities:

- *High sensitivity and specificity*: EUS is superior in differentiating between various cystic lesions, especially when combined with FNA.
- *Minimally invasive*: EUS is less invasive than surgical exploration, reducing patient risk and recovery time. The procedure can often be performed on an outpatient basis.
- *Real-time imaging*: The ability to visualize structures in real time allows for immediate intervention if necessary. For instance, if a suspicious lesion is identified, FNA can be performed during the same session.

4.3 Limitations of EUS

Despite its advantages, EUS has certain limitations:

- *Operator dependence*: The success of EUS is highly dependent on the operator's skill and experience. Accurate interpretation of EUS findings requires extensive training and expertise.
- *Limited accessibility*: EUS may not be available in all medical facilities, and its use can be restricted in certain regions due to limited access to the necessary equipment or trained personnel.
- *Potential complications*: Although rare, complications such as pancreatitis, bleeding, or infection can occur. The risk of these complications must be weighed against the potential benefits of the procedure.

4.4 Future Directions

The landscape of EUS in pancreatic cystic lesions continues to evolve, driven by advancements in technology and a growing understanding of pancreatic pathology. Some promising developments include:

- *Enhanced imaging techniques*: The use of contrast-enhanced EUS may improve the characterization of lesions, allowing for better differentiation between benign and malignant entities [13]. This technique enhances the visualization of vascularity and tissue perfusion.
- *Artificial intelligence*: AI applications in EUS image analysis are under investigation, potentially increasing diagnostic accuracy and efficiency. Machine learning algorithms may assist in the interpretation of complex EUS images, which might help in standardizing assessment and thus reducing variability [14].

- *Longitudinal studies*: Large-scale, multicenter studies are needed to establish clear guidelines for the management of PCLs based on EUS findings and defining appropriate follow-up intervals and intervention thresholds.
- *Integration with other modalities*: Combining EUS with other imaging modalities, such as MRI, offers a more comprehensive assessment, enhancing the overall diagnostic yield.

4.5 Conclusion

EUS plays a central role in the diagnosis and management of PCLs. Its ability to offer high-resolution imaging and tissue sampling makes it an indispensable tool in distinguishing benign from malignant lesions. With continued advancements in EUS technology and ablation techniques, it is likely that the role of EUS in manging PCLs will continue to grow, improving patient outcomes and offering new, minimally invasive options for treatment.

Author's Contribution's NS, RP, SS, RP did the literature search; NS and RP wrote the manuscript; RP, SS, RP did critical review; NS and RP did final editing and approval of the manuscript.

Conflict of Interest No conflict of interest to declare.

References

1. Kwon RS, Scheiman JM. EUS and pancreatic cyst fluid analysis: is the juice worth the aqueeze? J Gastrointest Oncol. 2011;2(4):199.
2. Ahmad NA, Kochman ML, Brensinger C, Brugge WR, Faigel DO, Gress FG, Kimmey MB, Nickl NJ, Savides TJ, Wallace MB, Wiersema MJ. Interobserver agreement among endosonographers for the diagnosis of neoplastic versus non-neoplastic pancreatic cystic lesions. Gastrointest Endosc. 2003;58(1):59–64.
3. Fritz S, Schirren M, Klauss M, Bergmann F, Hackert T, Hartwig W, Strobel O, Grenacher L, Büchler MW, Werner J. Clinicopathologic characteristics of patients with resected multifocal intraductal papillary mucinous neoplasm of the pancreas. Surgery. 2012;152(3):S74–80.
4. Kelvin YM, Park JS, Seo DW. Role of endosonography in the management of incidental pancreatic cystic lesions. Gastrointest Intervent. 2014;3(1):40–5.
5. Thornton GD, McPhail MJ, Nayagam S, Hewitt MJ, Vlavianos P, Monahan KJ. Endoscopic ultrasound guided fine needle aspiration for the diagnosis of pancreatic cystic neoplasms: a meta-analysis. Pancreatology. 2013;13(1):48–57.
6. Facciorusso A, Mohan BP, Tacelli M, Crinò SF, Antonini F, Fantin A, Barresi L. Use of antibiotic prophylaxis is not needed for endoscopic ultrasound-guided fine-needle aspiration of pancreatic cysts: a meta-analysis. Expert Rev Gastroenterol Hepatol. 2020;14(10):999–1005.
7. Cizginer S, Turner B, Bilge AR, Karaca C, Pitman MB, Brugge WR. Cyst fluid carcinoembryonic antigen is an accurate diagnostic marker of pancreatic mucinous cysts. Pancreas. 2011;40(7):1024–8.
8. Bhutani MS, Gupta V, Guha S, Ionuţ Gheonea D, Săftoiu A. Pancreatic cyst fluid analysis–a review. J Gastrointestin Liver Dis. 2011;20(2):175–80.

9. Elta GH, Enestvedt BK, Sauer BG, Lennon AM. ACG clinical guideline: diagnosis and management of pancreatic cysts. Am J Gastroenterol. 2018;113(4):464–79.
10. Zhang WY, Li ZS, Jin ZD. Endoscopic ultrasound-guided ethanol ablation therapy for tumors. World J Gastroenterol: WJG. 2013;19(22):3397.
11. Pai M, Habib N, Senturk H, Lakhtakia S, Reddy N, Cicinnati VR, Kaba I, Beckebaum S, Drymousis P, Kahaleh M, Brugge W. Endoscopic ultrasound guided radiofrequency ablation, for pancreatic cystic neoplasms and neuroendocrine tumors. World J Gastrointestinal Surg. 2015;7(4):52.
12. Fahmawi Y, Mehta A, Abdalhadi H, Merritt L, Mizrahi M. Efficacy and safety of endoscopic ultrasound-guided radiofrequency ablation for management of pancreatic lesions: a systematic review and meta-analysis. Transl Gastroenterol Hepatol. 2022;7:7.
13. Reddy NK, Ioncică AM, Săftoiu A, Vilmann P, Bhutani MS. Contrast-enhanced endoscopic ultrasonography. World J Gastroenterol: WJG. 2011;17(1):42.
14. Park JS, Jeong S. Endoscopic ultrasound-based artificial intelligence diagnosis of pancreatic cystic neoplasms. Korean J Pancreas Biliary Tract. 2023;28(3):53–8.

Pancreatic Cysts: Risk Stratification and Follow-Up

5

Amit Kumar, Nimesh Kumar Tarway, A. S. Prasad, and Ravi Kumar Sharma

Abstract

Pancreatic cysts are increasingly identified due to the widespread use of advanced imaging techniques. While most cysts are benign, a subset can progress to malignancy, necessitating robust risk stratification and follow-up protocols. This chapter outlines the current approaches to evaluating pancreatic cysts, emphasizing risk stratification based on size, morphology, and the presence of high-risk features such as main duct involvement, mural nodules, or solid components. Guidelines from leading organizations, including the American Gastroenterological Association (AGA), the International Association of Pancreatology (IAP), and the European Evidence-Based Consensus, are summarized to provide clarity on diagnostic and surveillance strategies. Patients with low-risk cysts, such as those under 3 cm without worrisome features, are often managed conservatively, with periodic imaging recommended to monitor for changes. High-risk cysts, defined by specific imaging findings or concerning clinical symptoms, require further evaluation with endoscopic ultrasound (EUS) and, in some cases, surgical consultation. The chapter highlights the balance between avoiding overtreatment of benign cysts and ensuring timely intervention for malignancy-prone lesions. Recent advances in biomarkers and genetic testing, along with imaging modalities, are discussed as emerging tools for refining risk stratification. Surveillance strategies and intervals vary depending on cyst

A. Kumar (✉) · A. S. Prasad
Department of Gastroenterology, Command Hospital (Southern Command), Pune, Maharashtra, India

N. K. Tarway
Department of Gastroenterology, Army Hospital R&R, New Delhi, Delhi, India

R. K. Sharma
Department of Biotechnology, Chandigarh University, Mohali, Punjab, India

R. K. Sharma et al. (eds.), *Differential Diagnosis and Management of Pancreatic Cystic Lesions*, https://doi.org/10.1007/978-981-92-0654-4_5

stability and risk profile, with many guidelines recommending discontinuation of surveillance after 5 years for stable, low-risk cysts. This comprehensive chapter underscores the importance of individualized patient care, multidisciplinary decision-making, and adherence to evidence-based guidelines in optimizing outcomes for patients with pancreatic cysts.

Keywords

Pancreatic cysts · Risk stratification · Surveillance · Malignancy · High-risk features · Endoscopic ultrasound · Biomarkers · Cyst management

5.1 Introduction

Pancreatic cysts are fluid-filled lesions within the pancreas, often discovered incidentally during imaging for unrelated conditions. While many pancreatic cysts are benign, some carry a significant risk of malignant transformation, making their management a critical component of patient care. Accurate risk stratification is essential to guide appropriate follow-up and determine the need for surgical intervention. This chapter focuses on the methods and guidelines for risk stratification and the strategies for monitoring pancreatic cysts over time.

5.2 Types of Pancreatic Cysts Relevant to Risk Stratification

Pancreatic cysts can be broadly classified into several categories, each with distinct implications for malignancy risk (Fig. 5.1):

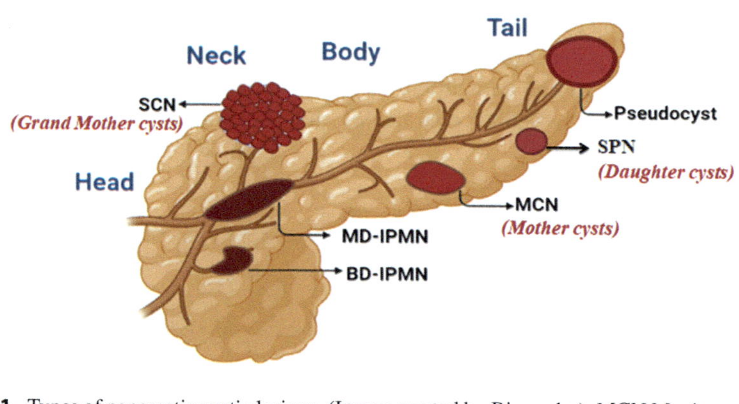

Fig. 5.1 Types of pancreatic cystic lesions. (Image created by Biorender). MCN Mucinous Cystic Neoplasm, IPMN Intraductal Papillary Mucinous Neoplasm, SCN Serous Cystic Neoplasm, SPN Solid Pseudopapillary Neoplasm

Serous cystadenomas (SCAs): These are generally benign and have a very low risk of malignancy. They often require minimal surveillance and rarely necessitate surgical intervention unless symptomatic [1].

Mucinous cystic neoplasms (MCNs): These cysts have a higher risk of malignancy, particularly in cases with certain high-risk features. They are typically found in the body or tail of the pancreas and occur predominantly in women [2].

Intraductal papillary mucinous neoplasms (IPMNs): These cysts are divided into main-duct and branch-duct types. Main-duct IPMNs carry a significant risk of malignancy, while branch-duct IPMNs have a variable risk depending on specific imaging and clinical features [3, 4].

Solid pseudopapillary neoplasms (SPNs): Although rare, SPNs are typically low-grade malignant tumors that require surgical resection [5].

Pseudocysts: These are associated with pancreatitis and do not have malignant potential, but differentiation from neoplastic cysts is crucial [6].

5.3 Diagnostic Approaches for Risk Stratification

Accurate diagnosis and risk stratification of pancreatic cysts involve a combination of clinical evaluation, imaging studies, and sometimes cyst fluid analysis.

5.3.1 Clinical Presentation

Many pancreatic cysts are asymptomatic and found incidentally. However, symptoms such as abdominal pain, jaundice, or weight loss may indicate a higher risk of malignancy, particularly in cysts with associated ductal obstruction or when presenting with rapid growth [7].

5.3.2 Imaging Techniques

Imaging is central to the initial assessment and ongoing surveillance of pancreatic cysts. The following modalities are most commonly used:

Ultrasound (US): Often the first imaging modality used, particularly for abdominal pain evaluation. However, its sensitivity in detecting and characterizing pancreatic cysts is limited compared to other techniques [8].

Computed tomography (CT): Provides detailed anatomical information and is useful for identifying cyst characteristics such as size, presence of calcifications, and the relationship to surrounding structures. CT is particularly valuable in identifying solid components or nodules within cysts, which may indicate a higher risk of malignancy [9, 10].

Magnetic resonance imaging (MRI) and magnetic resonance cholangiopancreatography (MRCP): MRI/MRCP is the preferred modality for evaluating pancreatic

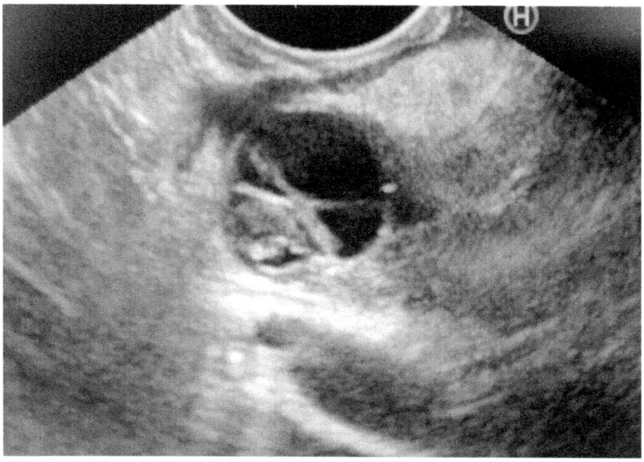

Fig. 5.2 BD-IPMN

cysts due to its superior soft tissue contrast, allowing for better characterization of cystic lesions. MRCP is particularly useful in assessing ductal communication, a critical factor in the evaluation of IPMNs [11].

Endoscopic ultrasound (EUS): EUS allows for high-resolution imaging of the pancreas and the opportunity to perform fine-needle aspiration (FNA) of cystic fluid for further analysis. EUS is invaluable in assessing cyst wall thickness, septations (Fig. 5.2), and the presence of mural nodules (Fig. 5.3) [12].

5.3.3 Cyst Fluid Analysis

For cysts that are indeterminate on imaging, cyst fluid analysis can provide additional diagnostic information:

Naked eye examination: Aspirated fluid bed-side examination yields important information about whether the fluid is serous or viscous (as also tested by string sign, Fig. 5.4).

Cytology: Examination of cyst fluid for malignant cells is important but has limitations due to low sensitivity [13].

5.3.3.1 Biochemical Markers

Carcinoembryonic antigen (CEA): High levels (>192 ng/mL) are suggestive of mucinous cysts, which have a higher risk of malignancy [14].

Amylase and lipase: Elevated levels suggest communication with the pancreatic duct, often seen in pseudocysts or IPMNs [15].

Molecular analysis: Genetic mutations such as KRAS, GNAS, and VHL can provide insights into the neoplastic nature of the cyst and its potential for malig-

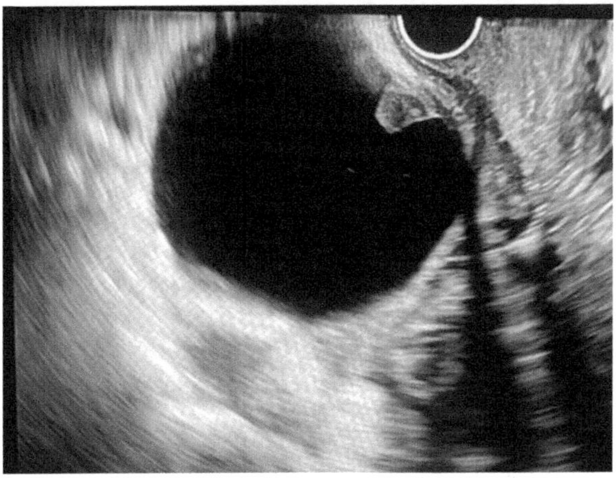

Fig. 5.3 Mural nodule in pancreatic cystic lesion

nancy. Emerging techniques in molecular analysis are increasingly being integrated into routine clinical practice [16, 17].

5.4 Risk Stratification

Risk stratification is the process of assessing the potential for a pancreatic cyst to develop into malignancy. It involves evaluating several factors, including cyst size, growth rate, the presence of solid components, and patient characteristics.

5.4.1 Key Risk Factors for Malignancy

Several factors are critical in determining the risk of malignancy in pancreatic cysts.

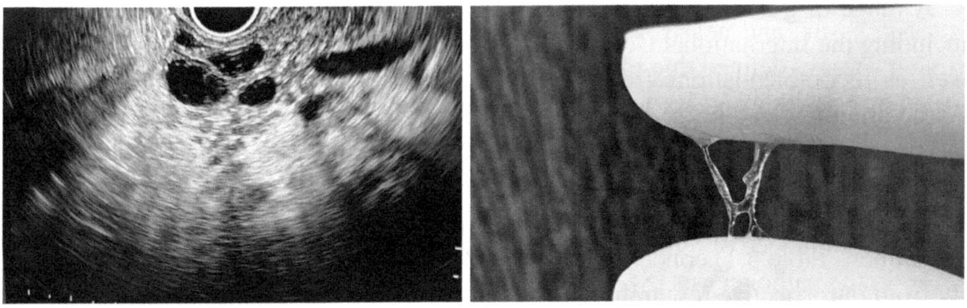

Fig. 5.4 BD-IPMN (bile duct IPMN) with dilated main pancreatic duct and string sign from aspirated mucinous material

5.4.1.1 Size of the Cyst

Larger cysts (particularly those >3 cm) are more likely to harbor malignancy or high-grade dysplasia. Cyst size is one of the most significant risk factors considered in guidelines [18, 19].

5.4.1.2 Cyst Growth Rate

An increase in cyst size over time suggests a higher risk of malignancy. Guidelines often recommend closer follow-up for cysts demonstrating growth, typically defined as an increase of more than 5 mm over 1 year [17].

5.4.1.3 Presence of Solid Components or Mural Nodules

Solid components or mural nodules seen on imaging are associated with a higher risk of malignancy. EUS can be particularly useful in evaluating these features [20].

5.4.1.4 Ductal Dilatation

Involvement of the main pancreatic duct, particularly ductal dilatation (>5 mm), is a concerning feature, especially in IPMNs. Main-duct IPMNs carry a significantly higher risk of malignancy compared to branch-duct IPMNs [21, 22].

5.4.1.5 Patient Age and Sex

Older age is associated with an increased risk of malignancy. Additionally, certain cyst types, like MCNs, are more common in women, which can influence management decisions [23].

5.4.1.6 Symptomatic Presentation

Symptomatic cysts, particularly those causing jaundice, abdominal pain, or weight loss, are more likely to be malignant and often warrant a more aggressive approach to management [24].

5.4.2 Stratification Systems

Several stratification systems and guidelines have been developed to assist clinicians in managing pancreatic cysts based on their risk of malignancy.

A range of guidelines exists to direct the diagnosis and management of PCLs, including the International Consensus Guidelines (such as Sendai and Fukuoka), as well as recommendations from organizations like the American Gastrointestinal Association (AGA), American College of Radiology (ACR), American College of Gastroenterology (ACG), and European societies. The recommendations vary in terms of imaging techniques, endoscopic ultrasound (EUS) evaluations, analysis of cyst fluid, criteria for surgical intervention, and follow-up schedules. Many of these guidelines (Table 5.1) concentrate on IPMNs and MCNs, deriving insights primarily from retrospective research, which tends to have lower-quality evidence.

Table 5.1 Guidelines for pancreatic cystic neoplasms

Year	Guidelines
2006	Consensus (Sendai)
2010	Radiology
2012	Consensus (Fukuoka)
2013	European
2014	Italian
2015	AGA Institute
2016	ASGE
2017	Revised Fukuoka
2018	European, ACG

5.4.2.1 Fukuoka Guidelines (2017)

- These guidelines are among the most widely used for managing IPMNs and MCNs. They categorize cysts into low-risk, moderate-risk, and high-risk, based on features such as cyst size, mural nodules, and main duct involvement [25].
- High-risk stigmata: These include obstructive jaundice with a cystic lesion in the head of the pancreas, enhancing solid component within the cyst, and main duct size ≥10 mm.
- Worrisome features: These include cyst size ≥3 cm, thickened/enhancing cyst walls, and main duct size 5–9 mm, among others. The presence of worrisome features typically prompts EUS evaluation.

5.4.2.2 American Gastroenterological Association (AGA) Guidelines (2015)

- The AGA provides a more conservative approach, recommending less frequent surveillance for cysts without high-risk features and suggesting surgery for those with concerning features [26].
- Surveillance intervals are based on cyst size, with less frequent monitoring for smaller, stable cysts.

5.4.2.3 European Evidence-Based Guidelines (2018)

- These guidelines emphasize a risk-based approach similar to the Fukuoka Guidelines but incorporate a broader range of evidence from recent studies. They recommend a tailored approach based on cyst type, size, and patient characteristics [27].

Various guidelines and the surveillance protocols are summarized in Table 5.2.

5.4.3 Role of Cyst Fluid Analysis, Cytology and Molecular Testing

5.4.3.1 Carcinoembryonic Antigen (CEA) and Molecular Testing

Fukuoka and AGA Guidelines:

- Recognize cyst fluid CEA as a marker for identifying mucinous cysts.

Table 5.2 Guidelines and surveillance protocols

Guideline	Target population	Preferred imaging method	EUS and FNA recommendations	Surgical Indications	Surveillance Protocols
American Gastroenterological Association (AGA) (2015)	Asymptomatic pancreatic cysts; does not cover solid pseudopapillary neoplasms or cystic neuroendocrine tumors	MRI	Performed when two high-risk features are present (e.g., size ≥3 cm, main pancreatic duct (MPD) dilation, or solid component)	Requires two criteria: presence of solid component and MPD dilation	*Based on cyst size*: 1–4 cm: MRI annually *Discontinuation of surveillance*: If no change in cyst size for 5 years or patient no longer surgery candidate *Postsurgery*: MRI every 2 years
Fukuoka Guidelines (2017)	Focus on main duct and branched duct intraductal papillary mucinous neoplasms (MD-IPMNs and BD-IPMNs)	Combine pancreatic protocol CT or MRI with MRCP	Assess presence of any "worrisome features" or "high-risk stigmata"	High-risk features include obstructive jaundice, mural nodules ≥5 mm, MPD > 10 mm	*Based on cyst size*: 1–2 cm: MRI/CT yearly 2–3 cm: EUS 3–6 monthly 3–4 cm: EUS or MRI 3–6 monthly *Discontinuation of surveillance*: Data not available *Postsurgery*: indefinite monitoring for MD-IPMN

Guideline	Target population	Preferred imaging method	EUS and FNA recommendations	Surgical Indications	Surveillance Protocols
American College of Radiology (ACR) (2017)	Incidentally discovered asymptomatic lesions	Both MRI and CT are acceptable	Recommend for lesions with "worrisome features" or "high-risk stigmata"	Referral for surgical consultation if worrisome features noted	Based on cyst size (i.e., <1.5 cm, 1.5–2.5 cm, >2.5 cm), patient age, interval growth, and presence of risk factors *Discontinuation of surveillance*: 9- to 10-year follow-up for most patients, terminating at the age of 80 years *Postsurgery*: no recommendations

(continued)

Table 5.2 (continued)

Guideline	Target population	Preferred imaging method	EUS and FNA recommendations	Surgical Indications	Surveillance Protocols
American College of Gastroenterology (ACG) (2018)	Newly diagnosed pancreatic cysts without known genetic predisposition	MRI-MRCP is preferred	Similar indications to Fukuoka guidelines for EUS	Surgical decisions recommended following multidisciplinary discussion of high-risk cases	*Based on cyst size*: 1–2 cm: MRI yearly 2–4 cm: EUS/MRI 6 –12 monthly *Discontinuation of surveillance*: Lifelong surveillance unless patient is a surgery candidate *Postsurgery*: *IPMN*—every 2 years if no remnant cyst. IPMN in remnant pancreas—surveillance based on the largest IPMN *MCNs* without cancer—no surveillance *Solid pseudopapillary neoplasm*—yearly surveillance for at least 5 years*SCAs, pseudocyst, other benign cysts*—no surveillance

Guideline	Target population	Preferred imaging method	EUS and FNA recommendations	Surgical Indications	Surveillance Protocols
European Guidelines (2018)	Includes various cyst types in management recommendations	MRI-MRCP preferred; CT for specific cases	EUS should be considered for uncertain diagnoses and when expected to impact treatment	Recommends surgery for cysts with characteristics such as size ≥4 cm or high-risk features	*Screening*: Clinical setting with Ca 19-9 and MRI/EUS 6 monthly *Duration*: Lifetime surveillance is required *Postsurgery*: *IPMN with high-grade dysplasia or MD-IPMN*—every 6 months for the first 2 years, followed by yearly surveillance. *IPMN with low-grade dysplasia*—as nonresected IPMN *IPMN in the remnant pancreas, no high-grade dysplasia or MD-IPMN*—followed same manner as nonresected BD-IPMN

- Do not specify definitive thresholds for CEA levels.
- Consider molecular analysis investigational, and do not recommend it routinely.

ACG, European, and ASGE Guidelines:

- Recommend measuring cyst fluid CEA and performing cytology if there is adequate fluid available.
- Cyst fluid CEA levels >192 ng/mL are often used in practice as a threshold for identifying mucinous cysts, though this is not explicitly endorsed in all guidelines.
- Suggest molecular and genetic testing in cases where the diagnosis is uncertain and results could significantly impact management decisions.
- Examples include KRAS, GNAS, and TP53 mutations for mucinous differentiation or malignancy risk.

5.5 Management and Follow-Up

The management of pancreatic cysts hinges on their risk stratification. Follow-up strategies are designed to monitor cysts for changes that might indicate a progression toward malignancy, with the goal of intervening before malignancy develops.

5.5.1 Surveillance Strategies

Surveillance is crucial for pancreatic cysts that do not warrant immediate surgery but have a potential risk of malignancy. The frequency and duration of surveillance depend on the cyst's characteristics:

5.5.1.1 Frequency of Imaging

- For low-risk cysts (<2 cm, no worrisome features), imaging may be performed every 1–2 years [28].
- For cysts with worrisome features or those larger than 2 cm, more frequent imaging, typically every 6–12 months, is recommended [8].

5.5.1.2 Duration of Follow-Up

- Lifelong surveillance may be necessary for cysts with potential for malignant transformation, particularly in younger patients or those with worrisome features [4].
- For older patients with small, stable cysts, the duration of follow-up may be more limited, balancing the risks of repeated imaging with the likelihood of clinical benefit [29].

5.5.2 Indications for Surgical Intervention

Surgical intervention is indicated for pancreatic cysts that have a high risk of malignancy or those that become symptomatic:

5.5.2.1 High-Risk Features

Cysts with high-risk stigmata (e.g., obstructive jaundice, enhancing mural nodules, main duct involvement) are typically referred for surgical resection, as the likelihood of malignancy is significant [30].

5.5.2.2 Types of Surgery

Enucleation: A limited resection for small, benign-appearing cysts that are symptomatic [31].

Distal pancreatectomy: Commonly performed for cysts located in the body or tail of the pancreas, often with splenectomy [32].

Total pancreatectomy: Reserved for extensive disease involving the entire pancreas but carries significant morbidity [33].

5.5.3 Nonsurgical Management

For cysts that do not meet criteria for surgery, nonsurgical management options include:

5.5.3.1 Observation

- Most appropriate for small, asymptomatic cysts without high-risk features. Regular imaging is used to monitor for changes that might prompt surgery [34].

5.5.3.2 Minimally Invasive Techniques

Ablative therapies: EUS-guided ethanol ablation or radiofrequency ablation is being explored for certain cystic lesions, though these techniques are still largely experimental [35].

Drainage: Indicated primarily for pseudocysts, particularly those that are symptomatic or infected [36].

5.6 Emerging Technologies and Future Directions

As the understanding of pancreatic cysts continues to evolve, new technologies and methods are being developed to improve risk stratification and management.

5.6.1 Advances in Imaging

Advances in imaging, particularly the integration of artificial intelligence (AI) and machine learning, offer the potential for more accurate and individualized risk assessment. AI-driven tools could enhance the ability to detect subtle changes in cysts over time, improving early detection of malignancy [37].

5.6.2 Molecular and Genetic Markers

The role of molecular and genetic markers in pancreatic cysts is expanding, with research focusing on the identification of specific mutations that correlate with malignancy. The future of pancreatic cyst management may involve personalized medicine approaches, where the genetic profile of a cyst guides treatment decisions [38, 39].

5.6.3 Role of Endoscopic Techniques

Endoscopic techniques, particularly EUS-guided interventions, are becoming increasingly important in the management of pancreatic cysts. Innovations such as confocal laser endomicroscopy (CLE) allow for real-time microscopic examination of cyst walls, potentially improving the accuracy of risk stratification [40].

5.7 Conclusion

Pancreatic cystic neoplasms (PCLs) are being identified more frequently, largely due to advancements in imaging techniques and an aging demographic. Diagnosing and assessing the risk associated with PCLs is challenging because of the diverse types of cysts and their varying potential for cancerous transformation. Risk stratification and follow-up of pancreatic cysts are essential components of managing this increasingly recognized clinical entity. The goal is to balance the need for early detection and treatment of malignancy with the risks of overtreatment and unnecessary surgery. Current guidelines provide a framework for decision-making, but ongoing research and technological advancements promise to refine these strategies further. Clinicians must remain vigilant in monitoring patients with pancreatic cysts, adapting their management approach as new evidence emerges.

References

1. Valsangkar NP, Morales-Oyarvide V, Thayer SP, Ferrone CR, Wargo JA, Warshaw AL, et al. 25-year experience of pancreatic serous cystadenomas. J Gastrointest Surg. 2012;16(12):2175–80.
2. Zamboni G, Scarpa A, Bogina G, Iacono C, Bassi C, Cavallini G, et al. Mucinous cystic tumors of the pancreas. Am J Surg Pathol. 1999;23(4):410–22.
3. Salvia R, Crippa S, Falconi M, Butturini G, Landoni L, Bassi C, et al. Branch-duct intraductal papillary mucinous neoplasms of the pancreas: to operate or not to operate? Gut. 2007;56(8):1086–90.
4. Tanaka M, Chari S, Adsay V, Fernandez-del Castillo C, Falconi M, Shimizu M, et al. International consensus guidelines 2012 for the management of IPMN and MCN of the pancreas. Pancreatology. 2012;12(3):183–97.
5. Papavramidis T, Papavramidis S. Solid pseudopapillary tumors of the pancreas: review of 718 patients reported in English literature. J Am Coll Surg. 2005;200(6):965–72.

6. Tandon A, Bensoussan V, Berger F, Mitchell A, Hammel P, Couvelard A, et al. Pseudocysts of the pancreas are not always innocent. J Gastrointest Surg. 2012;16(8):1629–37.
7. Goh BK, Tan YM, Cheow PC, Chung YF, Chow PK, Wong WK, et al. Cystic neoplasms of the pancreas with mucin production: an appraisal of their clinicopathological features and outcome after surgery. Ann Surg. 2006;244(2):256–61.
8. Brugge WR, Lewandrowski K, Lee-Lewandrowski E, Centeno BA, Szydlo T, Regan S, et al. Diagnosis of pancreatic cystic neoplasms: a report of the cooperative pancreatic cyst study. Gastroenterology. 2004;126(5):1330–6.
9. Sahani DV, Kadavigere R, Saokar A, Fernandez-del Castillo C, Brugge WR, Hahn PF. Cystic pancreatic lesions: a simple imaging-based classification system for guiding management. Radiographics. 2005;25(6):1471–84.
10. Wu BU, Sampath K, Berberian CE, Kwok KK, Lim BS, Shah JN. Prediction of malignant high-grade dysplasia in branch-duct intraductal papillary mucinous neoplasms of the pancreas: a multi-institutional review. Pancreas. 2011;40(3):270–5.
11. Takeshita K, Shiratori K, Kamisawa T, Nakagomi K, Takayanagi R. Differential diagnosis of pancreatic cystic lesions by MRC and MRI. Eur J Radiol. 2008;65(2):274–82.
12. Bhutani MS, Gupta V, Guha S. Pancreatic cyst fluid analysis. Gastrointest Endosc Clin N Am. 2002;12(4):741–8.
13. Pitman MB, Lewandrowski K, Shen J, Sahani D, Brugge WR. Pancreatic cysts: preoperative diagnosis and clinical management. Cancer Cytopathol. 2010;118(1):1–13.
14. Brugge WR, Lewandrowski K, Lee-Lewandrowski E, Centeno BA, Szydlo T, Regan S, et al. Cyst fluid analysis in the differential diagnosis of pancreatic cysts: a report of the cooperative pancreatic cyst study. Gastroenterology. 2004;126(5):1330–6.
15. van der Waaij LA, van Dullemen HM, Porte RJ. Cyst fluid analysis in the differential diagnosis of pancreatic cystic lesions: a pooled analysis. Gastrointest Endosc. 2005;62(3):383–9.
16. Khalid A, Brugge W, Aabakken L. Role of cyst fluid analysis in the diagnosis of pancreatic cystic lesions. Acta Gastroenterol Belg. 2004;67(4):384–7.
17. Matthaei H, Norris AL, Tsiatis AC, Olino K, Hong S-M, Dal Molin M, et al. Clinicopathological characteristics and molecular analyses of multifocal intraductal papillary mucinous neoplasms of the pancreas. Ann Surg. 2012;255(3):442–9.
18. Crippa S, Fernandez-del Castillo C, Salvia R, Finkelstein D, Mino-Kenudson M, Pergolini I, et al. Risk of pancreatic malignancy in branch-duct IPMNs increases with cyst size. Gut. 2019;68(4):780–8.
19. Yoon WJ, Brugge WR. Pancreatic cysts: what you need to know. J Clin Gastroenterol. 2013;47(8):667–75.
20. Schmidt CM, White PB, Waters JA, Yiannoutsos C, Cummings OW, Baker M, et al. Intraductal papillary mucinous neoplasms: predictors of malignant and invasive pathology. Ann Surg. 2007;246(4):644–51.
21. Rodriguez JR, Salvia R, Crippa S, Warshaw AL, Bassi C, Falconi M, et al. Branch-duct intraductal papillary mucinous neoplasms: observational management versus resection. A systematic review and meta-analysis. Ann Surg. 2007;246(5):741–9.
22. Sahani DV, Kambadakone A, Macari M, Cho A, Thiim M, Ros PR, et al. Diagnosis and management of cystic pancreatic neoplasms: CT and MRI imaging paradigms. Radiology. 2013;266(1):62–71.
23. Kosmahl M, Pauser U, Peters K, Sipos B, Lüttges J, Kremer B, et al. Cystic neoplasms of the pancreas and tumor-like lesions with cystic features: a review of 418 cases and a classification proposal. Virchows Arch. 2004;445(2):168.
24. Del Chiaro M, Segersvärd R, Lohr M, Verbeke C. Early detection and prevention of pancreatic cancer: is it really possible today? World J Gastroenterol. 2014;20(34):12118–31.
25. Vege SS, Ziring B, Jain R, Moayyedi P. American Gastroenterological Association Institute guideline on the diagnosis and management of asymptomatic neoplastic pancreatic cysts. Gastroenterology. 2015;148(4):819–22.

26. Tanaka M, Fernández-del Castillo C, Kamisawa T, Jang JY, Levy P, Ohtsuka T, et al. Revisions of international consensus Fukuoka guidelines for the management of IPMN of the pancreas. Pancreatology. 2017;17(5):738–53.
27. Correa-Gallego C, Ferrone CR, Thayer SP, Wargo JA, Warshaw AL, Fernández-del CC. Incidental pancreatic cysts: do we really know what we are watching? Pancreatology. 2010;10(2–3):144–50.
28. European Study Group on Cystic Tumours of the Pancreas. European evidence-based guidelines on pancreatic cystic neoplasms. Gut. 2018;67(5):789–804.
29. Allen PJ, D'Angelica M, Gonen M, Jaques DP, Brennan MF, Conlon KC. A selective approach to the resection of cystic lesions of the pancreas: results from 539 consecutive patients. Ann Surg. 2006;244(4):572–82.
30. Sahora K, Mino-Kenudson M, Brugge W, Thayer SP, Ferrone CR, Sahani D, et al. Branch duct intraductal papillary mucinous neoplasms with main duct involvement: an intermediate-risk category. Ann Surg. 2013;258(3):502–10.
31. Sahani DV, Saokar A, Hahn PF, Brugge WR, Fernandez-Del Castillo C, Fernández-del Castillo C, et al. Pancreatic cysts: imaging evaluation and diagnostic accuracy. Radiology. 2006;240(1):130–8.
32. Lennon AM, Wolfgang CL, Canto MI, Klein AP, Herman JM, Goggins M, et al. The early detection of pancreatic cancer: what will it take to diagnose and treat curable pancreatic neoplasia? Cancer Res. 2014;74(13):3381–9.
33. Correa-Gallego C, D'Angelica M, Gonen M, Muzikansky A, Allen PJ, DeMatteo RP, et al. Comparison of preoperative imaging and histopathology in the assessment of patients with cystic pancreatic lesions: implications for surgical management. Ann Surg. 2011;254(6):977–83.
34. Megibow AJ, Baker ME, Morgan DE, Kamel IR, Sahani DV, Lachman MF, et al. Management of incidental pancreatic cysts: a white paper of the ACR incidental findings committee. J Am Coll Radiol. 2017;14(7):911–23.
35. Sarr MG, Murr M, Smyrk TC, Yeo CJ, Fernández-del Castillo C, Hawes RH, et al. Primary cystic neoplasms of the pancreas: neoplastic disorders of emerging importance—current state-of-the-art and unanswered questions. J Gastrointest Surg. 2003;7(3):417–28.
36. Chari ST, Yadav D, Smyrk TC, DiMagno EP, Miller LJ, Raimondo M, et al. Study of recurrence after surgical resection of intraductal papillary mucinous neoplasm of the pancreas. Gastroenterology. 2002;123(5):1500–7.
37. Pergolini I, Sahora K, Ferrone CR, Morales-Oyarvide V, Wolpin BM, Mucci LA, et al. Long-term risk of pancreatic malignancy in patients with branch-duct intraductal papillary mucinous neoplasm in a referral center. Gastroenterology. 2017;153(5):1284–94.
38. Winter JM, Brennan MF, Tang LH, D'Angelica MI, Dematteo RP, Fong Y, et al. Survival after resection of pancreatic adenocarcinoma: results from a single institution over three decades. Ann Surg Oncol. 2012;19(1):169–75.
39. Reddy S, Wolfgang CL. The role of surgery in pancreatic cancer: a review. Clin Adv Hematol Oncol. 2009;7(5):399–407.
40. Hackert T, Hinz U, Fritz S, Strobel O, Schneider L, Hartwig W, et al. Enucleation in pancreatic surgery: indications, technique, and outcome compared to standard pancreatic resections. Langenbeck's Arch Surg. 2011;396(8):1197–203.

PET in Pancreatic Cystic Neoplasm

6

Rajender Kumar, Vinisha Gunasekaran,
and Bhagwant Rai Mittal

Abstract

Pancreatic cystic lesions (PCLs) are often found due to increased usage of cross-sectional imaging. The prevalence of PCLs rises significantly with age. These lesions comprise a diverse group that may occur from benign cyst, premalignant as well as malignant neoplasms, making diagnosis and treatment extremely difficult. Their detailed morphological information is provided by conventional imaging modalities. But their significant similarities in imaging features often restrict accurate lesions characterization and risk stratification.

Positron emission tomography (PET), especially with 18F-fluorodeoxyglucose (18F-FDG), provides functional and metabolic evaluation for cystic lesions. The utilization of FDG differs among cyst subtypes and represents tumor metabolic activity. While mucinous cysts exhibit enhanced uptake in the presence of high-grade dysplasia or invasive carcinoma, benign lesions such as serous cyst adenomas typically show minimal uptake. FDG PET/CT shows better specificity, positive predictive value, and overall diagnostic accuracy, especially in uncertain cystic lesions with high-risk morphological characteristics. Therefore, accurate evaluation of localized diseases, distant metastases, and synchronous cancers is made possible by whole-body PET/CT, which has the potential to significantly alter therapy.

Rajender Kumar and Vinisha Gunasekaran contributed equally with all other contributors.

R. Kumar (✉) · V. Gunasekaran · B. R. Mittal
Department of Nuclear Medicine, Postgraduate Institute of Medical Education and Research, Chandigarh, India

R. K. Sharma et al. (eds.), *Differential Diagnosis and Management of Pancreatic Cystic Lesions*, https://doi.org/10.1007/978-981-92-0654-4_6

In addition to FDG, new radiotracers that target tumor neovasculature, somatostatin receptor expression, cellular proliferation, and tumor stroma, respectively, include 68Ga-PSMA, 68Ga-DOTATATE, 18F-fluorothymidine, and 68Ga-FAPI. By integrating enhanced soft-tissue contrast with metabolic data, hybrid PET/MRI significantly improves diagnostic performance. This chapter overall includes the changing role of PET imaging in PCLs and its potential to enhance personalized risk assessment and treatment.

Keywords

FDG · Tumor · PET CT · Imaging · 18F-fluorothymidine · 68Ga-FAPI

6.1 Introduction

Pancreatic cystic lesions encompass a wide range of pathologies, ranging from simple benign cysts to highly malignant ones. With the advancement in the imaging techniques and its widespread application, the detection of incidental pancreatic cystic lesions has increased significantly. Hence, it is important to know the exact nature of the lesions for accurate diagnosis and management. Since pancreatic surgeries hold high morbidity and mortality, it is essential to differentiate benign lesions from malignant ones, where surgery can be safely avoided [1]. Molecular imaging plays a crucial role in characterization and risk stratification of lesions which guide accurate management. This chapter aims to explore the various types of pancreatic cystic lesions and diagnostic utility of PET/CT in their management.

6.2 Pancreatic Cystic Lesions

The global prevalence of pancreatic cysts, using only magnetic resonance imaging (MRI) as the imaging modality, ranges from 10% to 20% [2]. Prevalence varies with the imaging modality used and the age of population. It can be as high as 30% to 40% in patients above 80 years of age [2, 3]. These lesions may be asymptomatic or present with abdominal pain, jaundice, and features of pancreatitis depending on their location. The World Health Organization (WHO) classification broadly classifies pancreatic cystic neoplasms into four major histological subtypes which are serous cystic neoplasms (SCN), mucinous cystic neoplasms (MCN), intraductal papillary mucinous neoplasm (IPMN), and solid pseudopapillary epithelial neoplasm (SPEN). Other non-neoplastic cystic lesions like congenital cysts, lymphoepithelial, retention cysts, and pseudocysts encompass a separate group. Various solid neoplasms like adenocarcinoma and neuroendocrine tumors of pancreas can also undergo cystic degeneration and present like cystic lesions.

6.3 Imaging Modalities

Contrast-enhanced computerized tomography (CECT), magnetic resonance imaging (MRI) abdomen, and transabdominal or endoscopic ultrasound (EUS) are the initial imaging modalities available for evaluation. Ultrasound remains the first non-invasive imaging for pancreatic evaluation despite being limited by body habitus and bowel gas obscuring pancreas. EUS is highly sensitive than a transabdominal US for detecting small pancreatic tumors, particularly less than 2 cm [4]. Contrast-enhanced US is another cost-effective method in evaluating enhancement in the lesion which helps in differentiating malignancy from chronic pancreatitis. However, individually, it is not sufficient for the characterization of tumor, and it should be complemented by the CT or MRI findings. Multidetector row computed tomography (MDCT) gives additional information about the vascular involvement and also has high accuracy of 85–95% for tumor detection. Double duct sign, the traditional sign of malignancy, even though not specific, is easily identified in the CT [5]. One major disadvantage is high radiation exposure. Techniques like "split-bolus CT" optimizes the pancreatic enhancement and reduces radiation exposure [6]. Magnetic resonance imaging (MRI) and MR cholangiopancreatography (MRCP) are the imaging modalities of choice and problem-solving tools. It has high soft tissue contrast resolution and aids in precise evaluation of lesion characteristics and ductal system. It identifies the communication between duct and the cystic lesions [7, 8]. The radiological features of all these cystic lesions exhibit a significant overlap, creating challenges in the accurate diagnosis. Another major drawback in conventional imaging is failure to provide the functional significance of lesion. Over the past decade, molecular imaging has gained interest and has been explored in identifying the lesion and guiding management. ^{18}F-Fluorodeoxyglucose (FDG) positron emission tomography (PET) is effective in detecting malignancy in cystic neoplasms. Co-registered imaging with CT and MRI enhances the diagnostic performance of PET/CT and PET/MRI.

6.4 Role of ^{18}F-FDG PET/CT in Pancreatic Cystic Neoplasms

^{18}F-FDG PET/CT imaging is based on the principle that the malignant cells exhibit high metabolic activity, leading to increased glucose uptake. This enhanced FDG uptake serves as a marker for detecting malignancy. The uptake pattern differs with the different types and components of cysts. Benign cysts such as serous cystadenomas typically do not show FDG uptake, whereas MCN and IPMN are premalignant lesions and have high risk for malignant transformation and show higher FDG uptake (Fig. 6.1).

Sperti et al. initially evaluated the utility of ^{18}F-FDG PET/CT in differentiating benign and malignant pancreatic cysts in a group of 50 patients. A total of 17 patients had malignancy which was proven with histopathology. CT features were

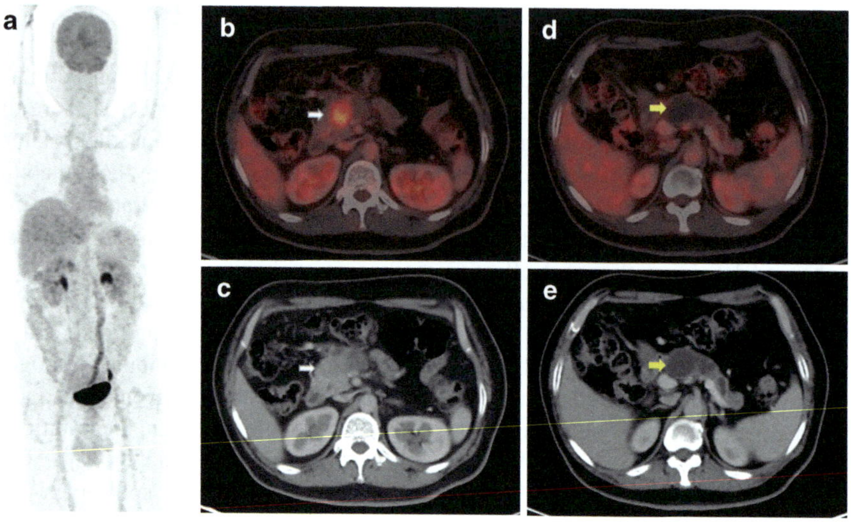

Fig. 6.1 ^{18}F-FDG PET/CT (**a**) done in an elderly female patient with complaints of abdominal pain for 1 year, for characterization of pancreatic lesion found in CT. Trans-axial fused PET/CT and CT images show isodense FDG avid suspicious malignant mass in the head of pancreas (white arrows, **b** and **c**) with SUV of 5.0 and MPD dilatation secondary to it (yellow arrows, **d** and **e**)

suggestive of malignancy only in 65% patients, whereas FDG PET/CT detected malignancy in 16/17 (94%) patients, with the standardized uptake value ranging from 2.5 to 7. ^{18}F-FDG PET/CT detected liver metastasis in additional two patients than CT. In the same study, rest 33 patients had benign lesions. CT showed high-risk features like internal septations and MPD dilatation in 10 and 8 patients, respectively, which were proved as benign lesions in histopathology later. However, in ^{18}F-FDG PET/CT, again 94% of patients (31/33), no FDG uptake was seen. So, the presence of high-risk features in conventional imaging alone can be misleading and cannot help characterizing the nature of lesion. It emphasizes the need for combining molecular imaging in preoperative evaluation [9].

In a network meta-analysis by Lee SW et al., aiming to compare the preoperative imaging modalities for assessing the malignant potential of pancreatic cystic lesions showed that ^{18}F-FDG PET/CT has significantly higher PPV and accuracy than CT. Other preoperative imaging modalities did not show significant differences in diagnosis when compared with each other [10].

When an indeterminate cystic lesion with high-risk CT features such as presence of septations, MPD communication, and solid component were found in CT or MRI, clinical dilemma occurs whether the cyst should be resected or safe for observation. The role of ^{18}F-FDG PET/CT was explored in indeterminate lesions and found to have an accuracy of 94% in differentiating benign from malignant cysts [11]. So, PET-positive lesions strongly suggest malignancy and warrant surgical resection. PET-negative lesions can be followed up safely.

In few studies, it was found that ^{18}F-FDG PET/CT has sensitivity comparable to that of CT (89% vs 93%), whereas the specificity of PET/CT is higher in the diagnosis of pancreatic malignancy (69% vs 21%) [12]. And PET/CT shows superior diagnostic accuracy over PET alone [13, 14]. Also, in the evaluation of the locoregional spread and distant metastases, PET/CT has huge advantage of whole-body imaging which aids in analyzing the whole body for distant lesions which will upstage the disease. In patients with distant metastasis and locoregionally advanced disease in the whole-body scan, clinical management varies drastically from surgery to others. PET/CT enables the identification of distant tumors, especially in liver, which might be missed in conventional imaging. It was observed that ^{18}F-FDG PET/CT influenced the management strategy and upstaged the disease in around 16% of patients [12, 15]. It also has an advantage of identifying the presence of any synchronous malignancy in the whole body. Sensitivity and specificity of PET/CT for the detection of distant metastasis are up to 80% and 95%, respectively [15].

6.4.1 Intraductal Papillary Mucinous Neoplasm (IPMN)

IPMNs are the most clinically significant mucinous neoplasm of the pancreas due to a higher risk of malignant transformation to pancreatic ductal adenocarcinoma. They are predominantly asymptomatic, hence detected more incidentally. They are classified based on the involvement of the pancreatic duct. Main-duct IPMN carries a high risk of malignancy, whereas the branch-duct IPMN has a lower risk. Many researches focused on IPMN since the risk of malignancy in IPMN is higher up to 35% [16, 17]. The Sendai and Fukuoka guidelines have been used for the management of IPMN. Revised Fukuoka guidelines highlighted "high-risk" and "worrisome features" based on morphological features such as main-duct dilatation, presence of enhancing mural nodules, cyst size, growth rate, and biochemical values of the carbohydrate antigen 19-9 (CA19-9) to guide surgery [18]. However, these guidelines often led to high false-positive rates, resulting in a high rate of unwarranted surgeries. A meta-analysis showed that the chances of progression of low-risk IPMN without the abovementioned features into invasive malignancy in 10 years is around 8% [19]. This highlights the necessity for early detection and characterization of mucinous neoplasm. ^{18}F-FDG PET/CT has proven highly effective in detecting malignant changes in IPMN, making it useful in preoperative assessment. Studies have also proven that ^{18}F-FDG PET/CT is a better investigation modality not only for IMPN but also for other pancreatic cystic neoplasms than the traditional guidelines [18]. A recent meta-analysis by Serafini et al. found that ^{18}F-FDG PET/CT is more sensitive (80% vs 67%), specific (95% vs 58%), and has superior PPV (94.4% vs 66.1%) and NPV (82.2% vs 59.3%) values compared to International Consensus Guidelines [20]. Low-grade dysplasia or benign IPMNs have low or negligible FDG uptake. Invasive carcinoma or high-grade dysplasia exhibits a higher FDG uptake due to increased metabolism and hence SUV. Studies have indicated that a SUV cutoff of 3.6 can effectively differentiate between benign and malignant lesions [8]. Kim et al. investigated the diagnostic performance of ^{18}F-FDG PET/CT in the subgroup of IPMN, which showed the pooled sensitivity, specificity, and diagnostic odd's ratio of 0.84, 0.95, and 101, respectively, to determine malignancy in IPMN [21].

Although PET/CT can serve as a complementary diagnostic tool, additional studies are required to establish its role. Current guidelines do not recommend PET/CT in the management of cystic neoplasms. More randomized controlled studies and clinical trials are required to establish its role.

6.4.2 Mucinous Neoplasms (MCNs)

MCNs are large loculated mucin-producing cystic lesions occurring commonly in middle-aged women. They are commonly seen in the distal pancreas. The lesions vary from benign cystic adenomas to aggressive invasive cystadenocarcinomas. Communication with MPD is not seen often. Risk for malignant transformation ranges from 18% to 27%. ^{18}F-FDG PET/CT helps identifying the malignant lesions. Few false-negative results are also noted in PET/CT in MCN due to sparse cellularity in MCN [22].

6.4.3 Serous Cystadenoma (SCA)

Serous cystadenoma of pancreas are rare and benign cystic lesions. It occurs mostly in elderly female and often presents as clusters of cysts and central calcified scar [23]. However, it has a wide range of overlapping imaging features with other cystic lesions, raising suspicion of malignancy. Multiple cystic lesions throughout the pancreas can be seen in patients with von Hippel–Lindau syndrome, resembling serous cystadenomas. SCAs can be classified into micro- and macrocystic variants depending upon the cyst size. Macrocystic SCAs are difficult to differentiate from MCN. ^{18}F-FDG PET/CT has limited role in the evaluation of SCAs.

6.4.4 SPEN

SPENs are cystic tumors with low malignant potential. They typically involve the distal part of the pancreas in young female patients. Lesions are characterized by large encapsulated mass with solid, cystic components and calcification. The cystic component is the result of tumor degeneration and internal hemorrhage [24]. Even though less malignant, presurgical evaluation for aggressive malignancy is necessary. Focal or multifocal FDG uptake in the periphery of lesion is predictive of highly aggressive tumor [25, 26].

6.4.5 Other Forms of Cystic Neoplasms

Sometimes, pancreatic ductal adenocarcinoma, because of the central necrosis, may undergo cystic degeneration and appear as cystic neoplasm. Often in conventional imaging, it mimics other benign cystic neoplasms. ^{18}F-FDG PET/CT is highly useful in this scenario, differentiating it from other benign lesions with high FDG uptake along with the additional CT features [23].

6.5 Benign Cysts

6.5.1 Pseudocysts

The most common benign cystic lesions of pancreas are pseudocysts. Pseudocysts of pancreas are non-neoplastic cysts accounting for 30–50% of cystic lesions of pancreas. The diagnosis is made easily from the history of an episode of pancreatitis. Pseudocysts complicated by acute pancreatitis may present with a large mass and false-positive FDG uptake which mimic a MCN [23]. Detailed history and follow-up imaging will be useful to rule out malignancy. MRCP is the most accurate and sensitive investigation with high sensitivity for the visualization of duct and guide drainage.

6.5.2 Limitations

Although ^{18}F-FDG PET/CT has a high diagnostic accuracy, it is not specific for malignancy. False-positive FDG uptake is seen in the inflammatory cystic lesions such as some pseudocysts and in the inflammatory component of a non-neoplastic cyst and can misdirect the management [27]. And mucinous neoplasms accumulate very less FDG. Clinical correlation and other imaging findings are crucial to avoid misdiagnosis. Newer radiotracers like ^{68}Ga-PSMA and somatostatin receptor imaging also help overcome the limitations of FDG PET/CT and help in establishing diagnosis.

6.6 New PET Tracers

6.6.1 PSMA

Prostate-specific membrane antigen (PSMA) expression is seen in the neovasculature of the tumor cells [28]. PSMA uptake is established in many nonprostatic malignancies with high tumor-to-background ratio. Studies have also shown that

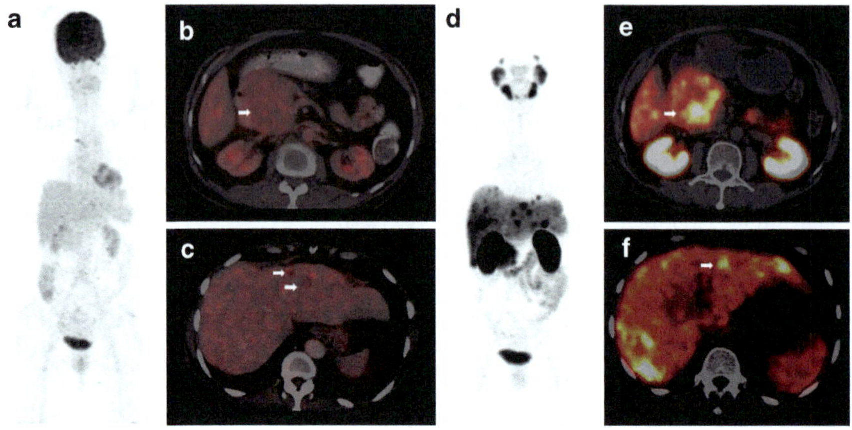

Fig. 6.2 Fifty-year-old female patient with complaints of abdominal pain underwent ^{18}F-FDG PET/CT (**a**). Trans-axial fused FDG PET/CT images show a large mass in the head of the pancreas with mild FDG uptake (white arrows, **b**) and mild FDG uptake in the hypodense liver lesions (**c**). ^{68}Ga-PSMA PET/CT (**d**) done in the same patient showed intense PSMA uptake in both the pancreatic mass (**e**) and liver lesions (**f**). Histopathology revealed pancreatic adenocarcinoma

^{68}Ga-PSMA PET/CT has a very high negative predictive value and a high degree of accuracy than ^{18}F-FDG PET/CT in pancreatic malignancies [29]. Figure 6.2 shows intense PMSA-expressing pancreatic mass (Fig. 6.2e) and liver lesions (Fig. 6.2f) in a case of pancreatic adenocarcinoma and low FDG uptake (Fig. 6.2a–c).

6.6.2 Somatostatin Receptor Imaging

Cystic pancreatic neuroendocrine tumors (NET) account for 17% of all pancreatic NETs [30]. They are mostly nonfunctional and asymptomatic. These are most commonly located in the body and tail of pancreas. They are usually less aggressive than solid NETs with less ki-67 index and low-grade tumors [31, 32]. ^{68}Ga-DOTATATE PET/CT targeting somatostatin receptor (SSTR) expression has high sensitivity and specificity for well-differentiated NET (Fig. 6.3). In poorly differentiated NETs, ^{18}F-FDG PET/CT has increased sensitivity owing to the high-grade nature and lack of SSTR expression. High SUV values are noted in ^{18}F-FDG PET/CT than SSTR imaging in poorly differentiated NET [33, 34].

6.6.3 Fluorothymidine PET

^{18}F-Fluorothymidine (FLT) is a radiolabeled thymidine analogue which is used to assess the cellular proliferation. Malignant cells have high rate of metabolism and DNA replication, leading to increased FLT uptake. Herrmann et al. demonstrated

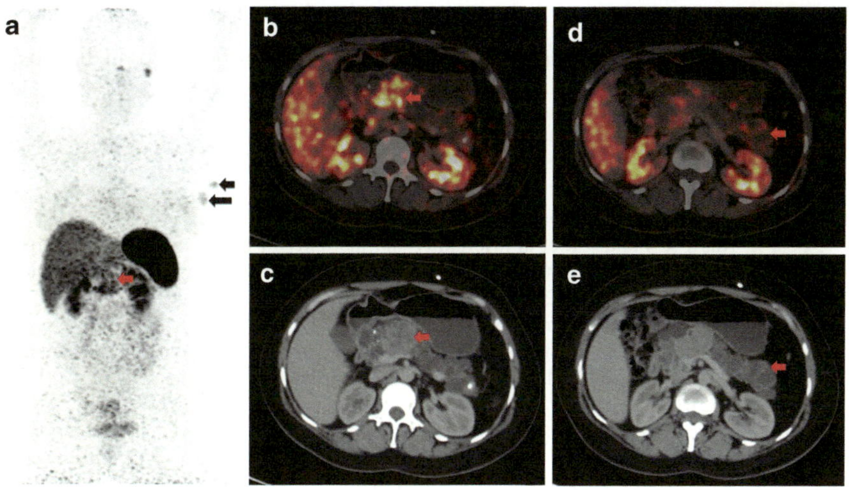

Fig. 6.3 ^{68}Ga-DOTATATE PET/CT (**a**) done in a 30-year-old female patient, who is a known case of VHL syndrome. Trans-axial fused PET/CT and CT images show intense SSTR expressing NET in the proximal body of the pancreas (red arrows, **b** and **c**), with the SUV value of 20.8. Rest of the pancreas is replaced by multiple nontracer avid cysts (**d** and **e**). Black arrows in the maximum intensity projection image (**a**) is the contamination of radiotracer on the patient's body surface

focal FLT uptake in the malignant pancreatic lesions opening up a new radiotracer for future exploration [35]. Mean SUV cutoff of 1.8 was found to be 81% sensitive and 100% specific for differentiating benign from malignant lesions.

6.6.4 ^{68}Ga-FAPI

Fibroblast activation protein (FAP) inhibitor (FAPI) imaging targets the FAP which is highly expressed in stromal cells that are cancer-associated fibroblasts. FAPI-based imaging is being explored in different malignancies [36]. Higher FAP expression is noted in the high-grade IPMN and pancreatic adenocarcinoma [37]. Few case reports have also shown mild FAPI uptake in the serous cystadenoma, extending the role of FAPI imaging in both benign and malignant lesions [38].

6.6.5 PET/MRI in Pancreatic Cystic Neoplasms

Hybrid PET/ MR imaging is available clinically since 2011. Since then, the utility of PET/MR is also explored in a wide range of oncological and non-oncological conditions. ^{18}F-FDG PET/MR imaging can efficiently diagnose pancreatic lesion, whether it is benign or malignant [39]. Also, in differentiating solid and cystic neoplasms, PET/MRI has high accuracy then PET/CT (100% vs 87%). PET/MRI has better performance than CT when imaging small cystic lesions. Overall, PET/MRI and PET/CT were found to have comparable diagnostic performances in diagnosing pancreatic neoplasms [40].

Bibliography

1. Zeni L, Russi R, Fialho A, et al. Morbidity and mortality of pancreatic tumors undergoing surgical treatment. Arq Bras Cir Dig ABCD Braz Arch Dig Surg. 2014;27(4):275–9. https://doi.org/10.1590/S0102-67202014000400011.
2. Vilela A, Quingalahua E, Vargas A, et al. Global prevalence of pancreatic cystic lesions in the general population on magnetic resonance imaging: a systematic review and meta-analysis. Clin Gastroenterol Hepatol. 2024;22(9):1798–809.e6. https://doi.org/10.1016/j.cgh.2024.02.018.
3. Farrell JJ. Prevalence, diagnosis and management of pancreatic cystic neoplasms: current status and future directions. Gut Liver. 2015;9(5):571–89. https://doi.org/10.5009/gnl15063.
4. Yousaf MN, Chaudhary FS, Ehsan A, et al. Endoscopic ultrasound (EUS) and the management of pancreatic cancer. BMJ Open Gastroenterol. 2020;7(1):e000408. https://doi.org/10.1136/bmjgast-2020-000408.
5. Menges M, Lerch MM, Zeitz M. The double duct sign in patients with malignant and benign pancreatic lesions. Gastrointest Endosc. 2000;52(1):74–7. https://doi.org/10.1067/mge.2000.105775.
6. Scialpi M, Pierotti L, Gravante S, et al. Split-bolus multidetector-row computed tomography technique for characterization of focal liver lesions in oncologic patients. Iran J Radiol. 2016;13(2):e20143. https://doi.org/10.5812/iranjradiol.20143.
7. Ozaki K, Ikeno H, Kaizaki Y, et al. Pearls and pitfalls of imaging features of pancreatic cystic lesions: a case-based approach with imaging-pathologic correlation. Jpn J Radiol. 2021;39(2):118–42. https://doi.org/10.1007/s11604-020-01032-1.
8. Kauhanen S, Rinta-Kiikka I, Kemppainen J, et al. Accuracy of 18F-FDG PET/CT, multidetector CT, and MR imaging in the diagnosis of pancreatic cysts: a prospective single-center study. J Nucl Med. 2015;56(8):1163–8. https://doi.org/10.2967/jnumed.114.148940.
9. Sperti C, Pasquali C, Decet G, Chierichetti F, Liessi G, Pedrazzoli S. F-18-fluorodeoxyglucose positron emission tomography in differentiating malignant from benign pancreatic cysts: a prospective study. J Gastrointest Surg. 2005;9(1):22–8; discussion 28–9. https://doi.org/10.1016/j.gassur.2004.10.002. PMID: 15623441.
10. Lee SW, Shim SR, Jeong SY, Kim SJ. Comparison of preoperative imaging modalities for the assessment of malignant potential of pancreatic cystic lesions: a network meta-analysis. Clin Nucl Med. 2022;47(10):849. https://doi.org/10.1097/RLU.0000000000004323.
11. Jones MJ, Buchanan AS, Neal CP, Dennison AR, Metcalfe MS, Garcea G. Imaging of indeterminate pancreatic cystic lesions: a systematic review. Pancreatology. 2013;13(4):436–42. https://doi.org/10.1016/j.pan.2013.05.007.
12. Heinrich S, Goerres GW, Schäfer M, et al. Positron emission tomography/computed tomography influences on the management of resectable pancreatic cancer and its cost-effectiveness. Ann Surg. 2005;242(2):235–43. https://doi.org/10.1097/01.sla.0000172095.97787.84.
13. Casneuf V, Delrue L, Kelles A, et al. Is combined 18F-fluorodeoxyglucose-positron emission tomography/computed tomography superior to positron emission tomography or computed tomography alone for diagnosis, staging and restaging of pancreatic lesions? Acta Gastro-Enterol Belg. 2007;70(4):331–8.
14. Saif MW, Cornfeld D, Modarresifar H, Ojha B. 18F-FDG positron emission tomography CT (FDG PET-CT) in the management of pancreatic cancer: initial experience in 12 patients. J Gastrointest Liver Dis JGLD. 2008;17(2):173–8.

15. Pery C, Meurette G, Ansquer C, Frampas E, Regenet N. Role and limitations of 18F-FDG positron emission tomography (PET) in the management of patients with pancreatic lesions. Gastroenterol Clin Biol. 2010;34(8–9):465–74. https://doi.org/10.1016/j.gcb.2009.04.014.
16. Nilsson LN, Keane MG, Shamali A, et al. Nature and management of pancreatic mucinous cystic neoplasm (MCN): a systematic review of the literature. Pancreatology. 2016;16(6):1028–36. https://doi.org/10.1016/j.pan.2016.09.011.
17. Kim SC, Park KT, Lee YJ, et al. Intraductal papillary mucinous neoplasm of the pancreas: clinical characteristics and treatment outcomes of 118 consecutive patients from a single center. J Hepato-Biliary-Pancreat Surg. 2008;15(2):183–8. https://doi.org/10.1007/s00534-007-1231-8.
18. Takaori K. "Revisions of the international consensus Fukuoka guidelines for the management of IPMN of the pancreas": progress for twelve years. Pancreatology. 2017;17(5):645–6. https://doi.org/10.1016/j.pan.2017.08.008.
19. Choi SH, Park SH, Kim KW, Lee JY, Lee SS. Progression of Unresected Intraductal papillary mucinous neoplasms of the pancreas to cancer: a systematic review and meta-analysis. Clin Gastroenterol Hepatol. 2017;15(10):1509–20.e4. https://doi.org/10.1016/j.cgh.2017.03.020.
20. Serafini S, Sperti C, Brazzale AR, et al. The role of positron emission tomography in clinical management of intraductal papillary mucinous neoplasms of the pancreas. Cancer. 2020;12(4):807. https://doi.org/10.3390/cancers12040807.
21. Diagnostic Role of F-18 Fluorodeoxyglucose Positron Emission Tomography/Computed Tomography for Characterization of Intraductal Papillary Mucinous Neoplasms: an Updated Systematic Review and Meta-analysis – PubMed. https://pubmed.ncbi.nlm.nih.gov/33835966/. Accessed 2 Oct 2024.
22. Sperti C, Pasquali C, Decet G, Chierichetti F, Liessi G, Pedrazzoli S. F-18-fluorodeoxyglucose positron emission tomography in differentiating malignant from benign pancreatic cysts: a prospective study. J Gastrointest Surg. 2005;9(1):22–8; discussion 28–29. https://doi.org/10.1016/j.gassur.2004.10.002.
23. Cystic Lesions of the Pancreas | AJR. https://ajronline.org/doi/full/10.2214/AJR.10.4378. Accessed 4 Oct 2024.
24. Zhang W, Qiu J, Bian W, et al. Clinical characteristics, surgical strategies, and outcome of solid pseudopapillary tumor of the pancreas: retrospective analysis in a single center. Wideochirurgia Inne Tech Maloinwazyjne Videosurgery Miniinvasive Tech. 2022;17(1):163–9. https://doi.org/10.5114/wiitm.2021.108804.
25. Kurihara K, Hanada K, Serikawa M, et al. Investigation of Fluorodeoxyglucose positron emission tomography for the diagnosis of solid pseudopapillary neoplasm of the pancreas: a study associated with a national survey of solid pseudopapillary neoplasms. Pancreas. 2019;48(10):1312. https://doi.org/10.1097/MPA.0000000000001424.
26. Kim JS, Hao EIU, Rho SY, et al. Clinical pattern of preoperative positron emission tomography/computed tomography (PET/CT) can predict the aggressive behavior of resected solid Pseudopapillary neoplasm of the pancreas. Cancer. 2021;13(9):2119. https://doi.org/10.3390/cancers13092119.
27. Mbakaza O, Vangu MDTW. 18F-FDG PET/CT imaging: normal variants, pitfalls, and artifacts musculoskeletal, infection, and inflammation. Front Nucl Med. 2022:2. https://doi.org/10.3389/fnume.2022.847810.
28. Prostate-specific Membrane Antigen Is Produced in Tumor-associated Neovasculature1 | Clinical Cancer Research | American Association for Cancer Research. https://aacrjournals.org/clincancerres/article/5/10/2674/288237/Prostate-specific-Membrane-Antigen-Is-Produced-in. Accessed 30 Sept 2024.
29. Krishnaraju VS, Kumar R, Mittal B, et al. Utility of prostate specific membrane antigen expression in pancreatic lesions to differentiating inflammatory and malignant masses by using Ga-68 PSMA PET/CT: exploring a new diagnostic avenue. Published online November 15, 2019. https://doi.org/10.2139/ssrn.3487796.
30. Carr RA, Bletsis P, Roch AM, et al. Cystic pancreatic neuroendocrine tumors: a more favorable lesion? Pancreatology. 2019;19(2):372–6. https://doi.org/10.1016/j.pan.2019.01.017.

31. Koh YX, Chok AY, Zheng HL, Tan CS, Goh BKP. A systematic review and meta-analysis of the clinicopathologic characteristics of cystic versus solid pancreatic neuroendocrine neoplasms. Surg US. 2014;156(1):83–96.e2. https://doi.org/10.1016/j.surg.2014.03.026.
32. Ilhan H, Fendler WP, Cyran CC, et al. Impact of 68Ga-DOTATATE PET/CT on the surgical management of primary neuroendocrine tumors of the pancreas or ileum. Ann Surg Oncol. 2015;22(1):164–71. https://doi.org/10.1245/s10434-014-3981-2.
33. Hindié E. The NETPET score: combining FDG and somatostatin receptor imaging for optimal management of patients with metastatic well-differentiated neuroendocrine tumors. Theranostics. 2017;7(5):1159–63. https://doi.org/10.7150/thno.19588.
34. Panagiotidis E, Alshammari A, Michopoulou S, et al. Comparison of the impact of 68Ga-DOTATATE and 18F-FDG PET/CT on clinical management in patients with neuroendocrine tumors. J Nucl Med. 2017;58(1):91–6. https://doi.org/10.2967/jnumed.116.178095.
35. Herrmann K, Eckel F, Schmidt S, et al. In vivo characterization of proliferation for discriminating cancer from pancreatic pseudotumors. J Nucl Med. 2008;49(9):1437–44. https://doi.org/10.2967/jnumed.108.052027.
36. FAPI PET/CT imaging—an updated review. https://www.mdpi.com/2075-4418/13/12/2018. Accessed 4 Oct 2024.
37. Spektor AM, Gutjahr E, Lang M, et al. Immunohistochemical FAP expression reflects 68Ga-FAPI PET imaging properties of low- and high-grade intraductal papillary mucinous neoplasms and pancreatic ductal adenocarcinoma. J Nucl Med. 2024;65(1):52–8. https://doi.org/10.2967/jnumed.123.266393.
38. Xu W, Zhao L, Meng T, Shang Q, Chen H. Serous cystadenoma of the pancreas showing increased uptake on 68 Ga-FAPI PET/CT. Clin Nucl Med. 2022;47(12):1095–8. https://doi.org/10.1097/RLU.0000000000004348.
39. Haodan D, Ruimin W, Jiajin L, Mu L, Xiang F, Baixuan X. Positron emission tomography/magnetic resonance imaging for the diagnosis and differentiation of pancreatic tumors. Nucl Med Commun. 2020;41(2):155. https://doi.org/10.1097/MNM.0000000000001125.
40. Xing H, Ding H, Hou B, Hao Z, Hu Y, Zhu W, Liang S, Feng F, Li F, Zhao Y, Huo L. The performance comparison of ^{18}F-FDG PET/MRI and ^{18}F-FDG PET/CT for the identification of pancreatic neoplasms. Mol Imaging Biol. 2022;24(3):489–97. https://doi.org/10.1007/s11307-021-01687-w. Epub 2022 Mar 24. PMID: 35332447.

Management of Solid Pseudopapillary Neoplasm of the Pancreas

7

Nirmaljeet Singh Malhi, Rajiv Grover, and Jasmeet Singh Dhingra

Abstract

Solid pseudopapillary neoplasm (SPN) of the pancreas is a rare, low-grade malignant tumor that predominantly affects young women in the second to fourth decades of life.

It accounts for 1–2% of all pancreatic neoplasms and has very different clinical, radiological, and pathological features, which differentiate it from other cystic pancreatic lesions. SPN is mainly composed of a large, well-encapsulated mass with mixed solid and cystic components and is frequently an incidental finding or presents with symptoms like abdominal pain, indigestion, and a palpable mass. Radiologically, the tumor has an irregular enhancement pattern with areas of hemorrhage and necrosis, while histopathologically, it shows pseudopapillary structures consisting of uniform epithelial cells with nuclear grooves and cytoplasmic vacuolation. The immunohistochemical staining for β-catenin (nuclear and cytoplasmic) and vimentin is positive in majority of cells and helps in confirming the diagnosis. Complete surgical removal of the tumor is the standard of care and is associated with an almost complete cure, the 5-year survival rates exceeding 95%. This chapter on SPN elucidates its characteristics, diagnostic work-up, imaging features, along with histopathological profile and management strategies.

Keywords

Pancreatic cystic lesions · Pancreatic tumors · Solid pseudopapillary neoplasm Endoscopic ultrasound · EUS-guided biopsy

N. S. Malhi (✉) · R. Grover · J. S. Dhingra
Department of Gastroenterology, Advanced Gastroenterology Institute (AGI)-The Gastrociti, Ludhiana, India

R. K. Sharma et al. (eds.), *Differential Diagnosis and Management of Pancreatic Cystic Lesions*, https://doi.org/10.1007/978-981-92-0654-4_7

7.1 Introduction

Solid pseudopapillary neoplasm (SPN) of the pancreas represents a rare, indolent type of cystic pancreatic neoplasm (CPN) with a potential for malignant transformation. First described in 1959 by Virginia Frantz, the tumor over the years has been known by various names such as Frantz's tumor, Hamoudi's neoplasm, papillary cystic tumor of pancreas, and solid pseudopapillary epithelial neoplasm (SPEN), till it was officially classified as the solid pseudopapillary tumor of pancreas (SPTP) by World Health Organization (WHO) in 1996 and later renamed as solid pseudopapillary neoplasm (SPN) in 2010 [1–3].

SPN typically presents as a mass lesion comprising of both solid and cystic areas, commonly involving the body and tail of pancreas and seen frequently among young females in their third and fourth decades. Although the incidence rates of SPN are low, there is a sevenfold rise in detection of SPN cases since the year 2000, possibly due to better understanding and awareness about the disease and refined imaging modalities [4].

Despite their rarity, SPN poses significant diagnostic and therapeutic challenges. This chapter aims to provide a comprehensive overview of SPNs, including their epidemiology, clinical presentation, diagnostic approach, management strategies, and recent advances in research.

7.2 Epidemiology

SPNs are rare pancreatic tumors, accounting for approximately 1–2% of all pancreatic neoplasms and nearly 3–5% of all CPNs [5, 6]. The epidemiology of SPNs remains poorly defined due to lack of large epidemiological studies. The estimated prevalence is likely to be less than one in a million per year with no definitive regional or racial predilection [7]. They predominantly affect young women, with a peak incidence in the third to fourth decades of life. The female-to-male ratio is approximately 9:1, highlighting the tumor's strong predilection for females possibly due to the influence of female sex hormones like progesterone and estrogen being a factor in the pathogenesis [8].

7.3 Pathophysiology

The exact etiology of SPN remains largely unknown. However, several genetic mutations and molecular pathways have been implicated in its pathogenesis. The commonest and most plausible pathogenetic mechanism of SPN is genetic alterations in the WNT/β-catenin signaling pathway, which plays a crucial role in cellular proliferation, differentiation, and adhesion. In SPN, Exon 3 mutation of CTNNB1 gene (which encodes the β-catenin protein) is seen in 85–90% cases, which leads to abnormal accumulation of mutated β-catenin in the cytoplasm that later translocates to the nucleus. Here, it acts as a transcriptional activator of oncogenic genes involved in cellular proliferation and tumorigenesis [9, 10].

In normal cells, β-catenin at the level of cell membrane is also a part of the E-cadherin complex and is responsible for maintaining intracellular adhesions. In SPN, due to the accumulation of mutated β-catenin, there is loss of E-cadherin expression that leads to disruption of cell adhesions causing loosely cohesive tumor cells giving rise to pseudopapillary structures with cystic degeneration of the tumor [11, 12].

Hormonal influences may also contribute to the tumor's development, as SPN predominantly affects young women. Immunohistochemical studies frequently demonstrate progesterone receptor (PR) positivity and less commonly estrogen receptor (ER) positivity. These findings suggest a possible role of sex hormones, particularly progesterone, in SPN pathogenesis, although the exact mechanisms remain unclear [13].

7.4 Clinical Presentation

SPN often presents with nonspecific symptoms, making its diagnosis challenging. Common symptoms include abdominal pain and discomfort, palpable abdominal mass, and nonspecific gastrointestinal complaints like nausea, vomiting, bloating, early satiety, and back pain. The uncommon manifestations include obstructive jaundice, pancreatitis, and portal hypertension seen in less than 5% cases [14, 15]. In more than 40% cases, SPN is discovered incidentally during imaging studies conducted for other reasons, with patients being completely asymptomatic [16]. SPN is generally considered a low-grade tumor having favorable prognosis, with the 5-year survival rate exceeding 97% and 10-year survival rate of 94% [17, 18]. There is variability in the clinical behavior and outcomes based on certain important factors which include tumor size, histological features, and the presence of extra-pancreatic spread. Metastatic spread is uncommon but can occur particularly in cases with aggressive histological features.

The common differential diagnosis for SPN includes cystic pancreatic neuroendocrine tumor (cPNET) and other cystic neoplasms of pancreas, the differences of which have been enumerated in Table 7.1.

Table 7.1 Characteristic features of different cystic lesions of pancreas

Feature	SPN	cPNET	SCN	MCN	IPMN	Pseudocyst
Epidemiology						
Age	20–40 years	Any age, often in adults	50–70 years	40–60 years	50–70 years	Any age, often in adults
Gender predilection	Strong female predominance (9:1)	Slight female predominance	Female predominance (3:1)	Strong female predominance (9:1)	Equal gender distribution	None
Location	Pancreatic tail or body	Variable, can be anywhere	Pancreas head	Pancreas tail or body	Pancreas head and body	Variable, can be anywhere
Clinical behavior	Generally indolent, low-grade, favorable prognosis	Malignant potential, varies based on grade	Benign, indolent, rarely malignant	Potentially malignant, particularly if invasive	Variable behavior, can progress to invasive cancer	Benign, no malignant potential
Malignant potential	10–15%	5–10%	0%	10–34%	BD-IPMN: 1–3% MD-IPMN: 33–85%	0%
Imaging appearance	Well-defined, solid and cystic components, often with hemorrhage	Well-defined cystic mass with variable solid components	Well-defined, microcystic, often central scar	Well-defined, unilocular or multilocular, often with mucinous fluid	Dilated pancreatic duct with papillary projections, mucin-rich fluid	Well-defined cystic with minimal solid necrotic components
Histology	Solid and cystic areas with pseudopapillary structures; low mitotic activity	Neuroendocrine tumor features, often with cystic and solid components	Microcystic spaces with a central stellate scar; cuboidal epithelium	Cystic spaces lined by mucin-secreting columnar epithelium, often with ovarian-type stroma	Cystic areas lined by mucin-secreting epithelial cells with or without papillary projections	Inflammatory exudates and necrotic parenchyma
Treatment	Surgical resection, often curative	Surgical resection; possible chemotherapy/radiation	Surgical resection if symptomatic	Surgical resection, especially if invasive	Surgical resection; surveillance for noninvasive types	Watchful observation or drainage, if symptomatic
Prognosis	Excellent with complete resection; low recurrence	Variable; generally less favorable due to potential malignancy	Excellent with complete resection, low recurrence	Variable; good with complete resection but depends on invasive nature	Variable; good for noninvasive types, worse for invasive	Excellent

SPN Solid pseudopapillary neoplasm, *cPNET* Cystic pancreatic neuroendocrine tumor, *SCN* Serous cystic neoplasm, *MCN* Mucinous cystic neoplasm, *IPMN* Intraductal papillary mucinous neoplasm, *BD-IPMN* Branch-duct intraductal papillary mucinous neoplasm, *MD-IPMN* Main-duct intraductal papillary mucinous neoplasm

7.5 Diagnostic Approach

The diagnosis of SPN involves a combination of imaging studies, histopathological examination, and immunohistochemical analysis.

7.5.1 Imaging Techniques

Imaging studies, including abdominal ultrasound, computerized tomography (CT), magnetic resonance imaging (MRI), and endoscopic ultrasound (EUS), are essential for initial tumor evaluation and assessment of local extent and metastasis.

Ultrasonography (USG) is generally the first investigation for symptomatic patients and for screening. SPN on USG reveals a variabl-sized, heterogeneous, hypoechoic mass surrounded by a hyperechoic rim. Contrast-enhanced ultrasound (CEUS) further highlights this feature, showing hyperenhancement of the rim and capsular boundaries during the arterial phase with a nonenhanced central region, thus improving the diagnostic accuracy [19].

Computerized tomography (CT) scan is the most widely used and sensitive method for the diagnosis and staging of SPN. CT imaging of SPN typically reveals an encapsulated mass with both solid and cystic components, often resulting from hemorrhagic degeneration. Calcifications and solid areas can be found at the periphery of the mass, resulting in egg shell pattern of calcification [20]. On multiphasic CT scan, during the pancreatic phase, there is mild enhancement compared to the surrounding pancreatic parenchyma, with a gradual increase in enhancement during the delayed venous phase, more so in small lesions. A fibrous pseudo-capsule often shows peripheral enhancement, and the fibrous components within cystic areas give a characteristic "floating cloud" pattern [21]. Atypical SPNs lack a surrounding capsule, may be entirely solid or cystic, show hyperattenuation during the pancreatic phase, and often have dense internal calcifications with poorly defined margins [22].

Li et al. classified SPNs into five types based on the solid-to-cystic component ratio, with types III, IV, and V being more common in females. The most prevalent type, type III (29.4%), presented as a well-circumscribed mass with mixed solid and cystic components and no clear boundary between these regions [23]. Interestingly, as SPNs grow, the ratio of solid to cystic components may shift, with smaller tumors (less than 3 cm) tending to be predominantly solid, while larger ones (greater than 3 cm) have more cystic areas [24].

MRI is better than CT to correlate the clinicopathological and radiological findings of SPN and is advantageous for patients with contrast allergies or renal insufficiency. MRI findings of SPN are an aseptate encapsulated lesion with both solid and cystic components along with hemorrhage. It typically presents with T2 hyperintensity, T1 hypointensity, and heterogeneous enhancement on contrast-enhanced T1-weighted images. Yu et al. proposed three MRI subtypes based on solid and cystic contents (Type 1, Type 2, and Type 3) that correlated well with the clinicopathological features of SPN [25].

Positron emission tomography/CT (PET/CT) serves as a valuable complement to routine imaging for assessing the histopathological composition and staging of SPN. As higher FDG uptake indicates increased metabolic activity, SPNs with predominantly solid components tend to be more FDG-avid compared to lesions with cystic or hemorrhagic components. Additionally, the standard uptake value (SUV), which measures FDG uptake, has been found to correlate strongly with the pathological features such as tumor cellularity and proliferative index [26]. In cases of SPN, where FDG uptake is negative, a potential alternative option is the use of a fibroblast activation protein inhibitor (FAPI) radiotracer, as suggested by some of the recent reports [27]. Although less commonly used, PET/MRI offers a combined advantage of anatomical and functional imaging, providing detailed insights in a single session. However, despite their clinical benefits, the high cost of these technologies may limit their widespread use.

Endoscopic ultrasound (EUS) plays a crucial role in the preoperative pathological diagnosis of SPN. Similar to abdominal ultrasound, SPN appears as a well-circumscribed, heterogeneously hypoechoic mass with mixed solid and cystic components and/or calcifications at the periphery, with no characteristic findings seen either on EUS elastography or Doppler assessment. Overall, SPN remains a difficult diagnosis to confirm through EUS imaging only, as it lacks distinctive pathognomonic features. Along with imaging for morphological characteristics, EUS has an additional advantage over other modalities for sampling of the lesion via aspiration (FNA) and /or biopsy (FNB) for histological confirmation, with the sensitivity and specificity rates exceeding 90% [28].

EUS-FNA enables sampling both from the solid part of the lesion and the collection of the cyst fluid that helps it to differentiate from other CPNs, as summarized in Table 7.2 [29, 30].

However, due to the predominant solid component in SPN and the limited accuracy of cyst fluid analysis, EUS-guided fine-needle biopsy (EUS-FNB) is often a more effective diagnostic tool, providing larger tissue samples for both histopathological and immunohistochemical analyses. A recent multicenter retrospective study reported an impressive 97.2% (103/106 patients) preoperative diagnostic accuracy for SPN using EUS-guided biopsy. The needle type used (19G v/s 22G) did not appear to have a significant impact on the diagnostic yield. Thus, EUS-guided biopsy from SPN, currently, is the gold standard in establishing the diagnosis [31].

Another promising diagnostic technique is EUS-guided needle-based confocal laser endomicroscopy (EUS-nCLE), which has demonstrated high diagnostic accuracy. On EUS-nCLE, typical features of solid pseudopapillary tumors (SPT) include small, round, dark cellular clusters interspersed with white stroma bands. Furthermore, advancements in artificial intelligence, particularly deep learning analysis of EUS images, hold the potential to significantly improve the diagnostic accuracy of endoscopic methods [32, 33].

Table 7.2 Characteristic features of fluid analysis in different cystic lesions of pancreas

Feature	SPN	cPNET	SCN	MCN	IPMN	Pseudocyst
Viscosity	Low	Low	Low	High	High	Low
Amylase level	Low	Low	Low	Variable, low	Variable, high	High
CEA level	Low	Low	Low	High	High	Low
Cytology	Hemorrhagic debris, monomorphic discohesive small cells, hyaline globules, grooved nuclei	Uniform cells in loosely cohesive clusters, coarse granular chromatin containing nuclei	Protienaceous debris and blood glycogen containing cuboid cell	Thick mucinous fluid mucinous epithelial cells Ovarian-type stroma	Thick mucinous fluid Mucinous epithelial cells papillary structures	Dirty macrophages, inflammatory cells, debris
NGS	*CTNNB1*	Mostly sporadic	*vHL*	*KRAS* *RNF43*	*KRAS*, *GNAS* *RNF43* *CTNNB1*	No sequence variation

7.5.2 Histopathological Examination

Macroscopically, majority of SPNs are typically well-circumscribed masses ranging from a few centimeters to more than 20 cm in size, with a fine fibrous capsule having cystic and solid areas. The solid areas consist of sheets of tumor cells, while cystic areas result from hemorrhagic degeneration [5].

On microscopic examination, the characteristic features are pseudopapillary structures which are formed due to loosely cohesive clusters of tumor cells around delicate fibrovascular cores or stalks. Foamy macrophages with hyalinized stroma and hyaline globules are commonly observed in these tumors. There may be hemorrhage and necrosis leading on to cystic degeneration within the tumor. There is generally a low mitotic index with minimal cellular atypia [34, 35].

7.5.3 Cytopathological Examination

The cytology smears are generally cellular with delicate papillary fronds. There are monomorphic tumor cells which are relatively uniform with round, oval or reniform nuclei, occasional nuclear grooves with eosinophilic cytoplasm. Another characteristic feature is the presence of single cells with a cytoplasmic tail described as "cercariform" cells [34, 35].

7.5.4 Immunohistochemical (IHC) Staining

IHC is critical in confirming the diagnosis of SPN and distinguishing it from other pancreatic neoplasms (e.g., pancreatic neuroendocrine tumor, acinar cell carcinoma, and adenocarcinoma). The following markers are typically used.

1. *Positive Markers*
   - β-catenin (98%): SPNs show nuclear and cytoplasmic staining for β-catenin, a hallmark of the tumor due to mutations in the Wnt/β-catenin signaling pathway.
   - Vimentin (88%): This mesenchymal marker is strongly positive in SPNs.
   - CD10 (63%): Shows diffuse positivity in most SPN cases.
   - Progesterone receptor (PR) (63%): PR positivity is common, which aligns with the tumor's prevalence in young women.
   - Neuron-specific enolase (NSE) (70%): Typically positive, although it is a less specific marker.
   - Synaptophysin (55%): Shows focal positivity, although widespread expression is rare (important in differentiating from neuroendocrine tumors).
   - CD56 (96%): Frequently positive, further complicating differentiation from neuroendocrine tumors.

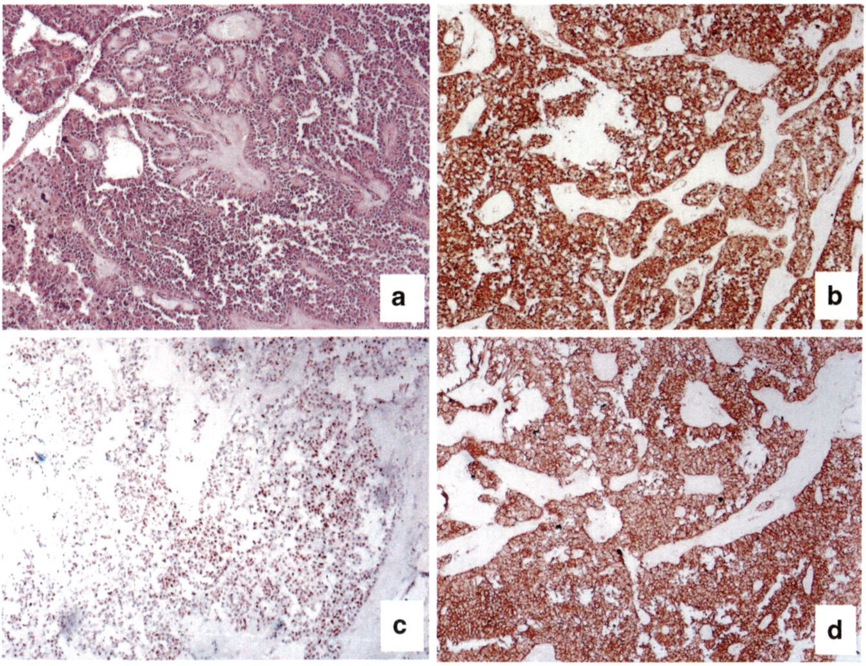

Fig. 7.1 Histopathological and IHC staining in SPNs. (**a**) H&E stain showing variable admixture of solid and pseudo-papillary areas. Solid areas are comprised of uniform cells admixed with capillary-sized blood vessels. Stroma shows focal hyalinization and cystic degeneration. Tumor cells have moderate amount of eosinophilic cytoplasm and uniform nuclei with finely textured chromatin. (**b**) IHC showing strong positivity for β-catenin stain. (**c**) IHC showing strong positivity for PR stain. (**d**) IHC showing strong positivity for CD56 stain

2. *Negative Markers*
   - Chromogranin-A: SPN is typically negative for chromogranin-A, which helps in differentiating it from pancreatic neuroendocrine tumors, which are chromogranin-A positive.
   - CA19–9 and CEA: Typically negative, ruling out pancreatic adenocarcinoma [12, 36–38] (Fig. 7.1).

7.6 Management Strategies

Surgical resection is the preferred treatment for SPN, with a focus on organ preservation, if feasible. The majority of patients with SPN are candidates for surgical intervention due to the tumor's typically low-grade behavior and localized presentation. The surgical approach depends on the tumor's size, location, and involvement of surrounding structures. Pancreaticoduodenectomy (PD), both conventional

Whipple's procedure and pylorus-preserving Pancreaticoduodenectomy (PPD), central pancreatectomy (CP), distal pancreatectomy (DP) with or without splenectomy, and enucleation can be performed [29, 39, 40].

Enucleation should be attempted for SPN less than 5 cm in size and distant from MPD, although the risk of postoperative pancreatic fistula stays high. For SPN, where enucleation is not feasible, surgical approach should be aimed to perform complete resection (R0) with the maximum preservation of pancreatic parenchyma [41]. For lesions in the distal body and tail, distal pancreatectomy with the preservation of spleen is the recommended treatment option. However, spleen preservation is not contemplated in cases of splenomegaly, involvement of splenic hilum, and vascular encasement (splenic artery and vein) [41, 42].

In cases where the tumor is in the neck or proximal body of the pancreas, central pancreatectomy (CP) with distal pancreatojejunostomy or pancreaticogastrostomy is preferred. However, due to the potential for leaks at both the proximal pancreatic stump and the distal pancreatico-enteric anastomotic site, it should only be performed at specialized centers [31, 43].

For tumors located in the head of the pancreas, pylorus-preserving pancreaticoduodenectomy (PPD) and duodenum-preserving pancreatic head resection (DPPHR) are recommended to minimize postoperative complications such as dumping syndrome, diarrhea, delayed gastric emptying, and marginal ulcers [29, 44].

The surgical treatment for SPN is summarized in an algorithmic approach in Fig. 7.2.

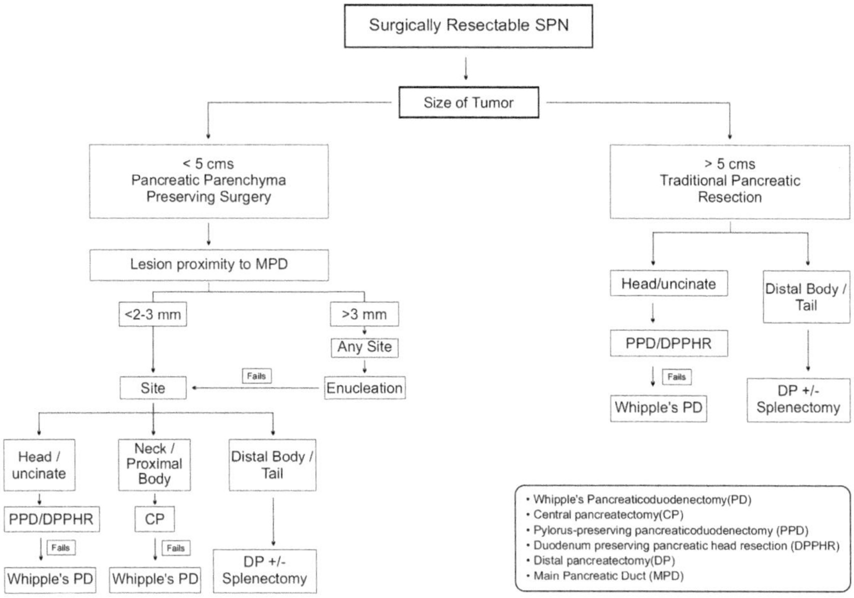

Fig. 7.2 Algorithmic approach of surgical treatment for SPN

As lymph node metastasis is extremely uncommon (1.0%–7.9% cases) in SPN, routine lymph node dissection is not required [24, 29]. However, in cases where the SPN involves surrounding structures like the portal vein, superior mesenteric vein or artery, spleen, or duodenum, an attempt for en bloc resection with clear margins is advised [16, 42].

Lately, with advancements in technology, EUS RFA has emerged as an important minimally invasive treatment option for small SPN patients who are unfit for surgical intervention. It can achieve localized tumor necrosis and potentially prevent further tumor progression. EUS-RFA is particularly useful for targeting lesions in challenging anatomical locations, such as those near major blood vessels or bile ducts, where traditional surgical resection might carry higher risks [45, 46].

Adjuvant therapy is not routinely indicated for SPNs due to their generally indolent nature and localization. However, in cases with high-risk features such as large tumor size, vascular invasion, or aggressive histology, additional treatment modalities, including chemotherapy or radiation therapy, may be considered.

Follow-up after surgical resection typically involves regular imaging studies and clinical evaluations to monitor for potential recurrence or metastasis. The overall prognosis for SPN is favorable, with high rates of long-term survival reported in the literature. However, individual outcomes may vary based on tumor characteristics and treatment responses [47, 48].

7.7 Management of Metastatic SPN

Till date, there is no definite consensus or standardized approach for the treatment of metastatic SPN. For SPN with liver-limited metastasis, liver-directed therapies that include metastasectomy, radiofrequency ablation, chemotherapy, proton beam radiotherapy, partial liver resection, and liver transplantation can be considered [49–51].

Metastasectomy is recommended at the time of primary tumor resection or in cases of recurrence, if feasible. The roles of chemotherapy and radiation in the treatment of metastatic SPN remain unclear, but debulking surgery may be considered for metastases. There are reports in the literature, where the use of preoperative chemotherapy (either cisplatin- or 5-fluorouracil-based) was followed by surgical resection and intraoperative radiofrequency ablation of liver metastases resulting in successful outcomes [52, 53]. In cases of multiple liver metastases, partial liver resection, followed by postoperative chemotherapy with gemcitabine or paclitaxel has shown some success [54]. Extensive liver metastasis from SPN may also be managed with transarterial chemoembolization (TACE) with gemcitabine and lipiodol, followed by gelfoam embolization [55].

SPN is considered radiosensitive, so radiotherapy may be attempted for unresectable tumors. Peritoneal carcinomatosis (PC) can result from the intraoperative rupture of SPN, which may need cytoreductive surgery and hyperthermic intraperitoneal chemotherapy (HIPEC) using irinotecan and oxaliplatin resulting in successful outcomes, as shown by Honore et al. [56].

7.8 Prognostication

SPN, being an indolent tumor, has a good long-term prognosis, as shown by large-scale studies and meta-analyses, with the overall survival (OS) rate exceeding 97% at 10 years of follow-up. As SPN rarely invades surrounding vessels and has a very low incidence of metastasis to regional or distant lymph nodes, traditional staging systems like TNM are not helpful in the prognostication of these lesions [57].

Yang et al. identified that tumor size >9 cm and Ki-67 index >3% were independent predictors of lower recurrence-free survival (RFS) and developed the *Fudan Prognostic Index* (FPI) based on these factors. This grading system demonstrated a significant variation in RFS among the low-, intermediate-, and high-risk groups of SPN patients; however, no significant difference in overall survival (OS) was observed between the low- and intermediate-risk groups [58]. In a separate study, Chen et al. devised the *Peking Union Medical College Hospital (PUMCH)* model by incorporating lymphovascular invasion as an additional prognostic factor, further refining risk stratification for patients with SPN into low- and high-risk groups [59].

7.9 Postoperative Follow-Up

Currently, there are no established guidelines for the postoperative follow-up of SPN, leading to a lack of consensus in practice. Traditionally, postoperative regular check-ups are done every 3–6 months during the first 2 years, followed by semi-annually to annually, as deemed suitable. However, with the recent development of predictive models like FPI and the PUMCH index, follow-up protocols can now be tailored based on individual risk profiles. For low-risk patients, follow-up intervals can be extended to optimize healthcare utilization. Conversely, high-risk patients might need a more intensive and personalized plan to facilitate early detection of any recurrence. CT and MRI scans are considered the most effective modalities for monitoring recurrence. Since surgical intervention involves pancreatic resection, there is a need to monitor these patients for potential pancreatic endocrine and exocrine insufficiency, and follow-up should include assessment for steatorrhoea and monitoring of glycated hemoglobin.

7.10 Recent Advances in Research

Recent research has focused on elucidating the molecular mechanisms underlying SPN and improving diagnostic and therapeutic strategies. Advances in genomic sequencing and molecular profiling have provided insights into the genetic alterations associated with SPN, leading to a better understanding of their pathogenesis. Novel targeted therapies and immunotherapies are being explored in clinical trials to improve the outcomes for patients with advanced or recurrent SPN. Additionally, research into the development of more sensitive and specific diagnostic biomarkers is ongoing, with the goal of enhancing early detection and personalized treatment approaches [60, 61].

7.11 Conclusion

SPN is a rare, distinct pancreatic tumor with unique pathogenetic and histopathological features. Despite their rarity, due to more awareness and better imaging modalities, recently there has been a significant increase of SPN cases being reported in the literature. SPN should be considered as an important differential diagnosis for a mixed solid cystic pancreatic lesion, especially in young females. EUS-guided tissue acquisition with histopathology and IHC is the mainstay of diagnosis. With early detection and appropriate surgical intervention, patients can achieve excellent short- and long-term outcomes.

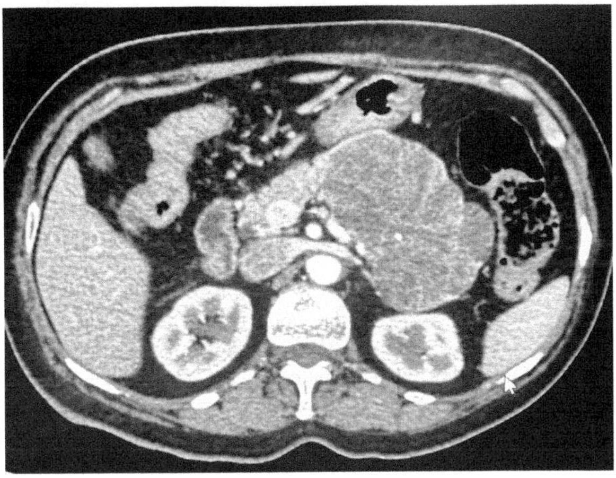

CT Scan
Well-encapsulated solid cystic heterogeneously enhancing lesion involving the body and tail of the pancreas shows peripheral enhancement with central cystic areas and thick enhancing internal septations

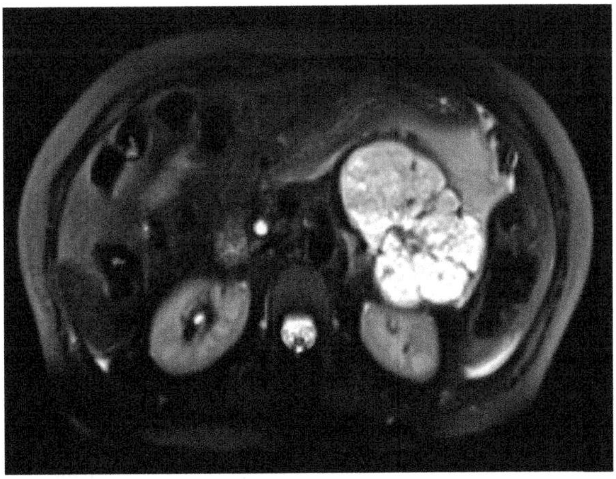

MRI Scan
Well-circumscribed lesion involving the body and tail of pancreas predominately solid in appearance with cystic spaces, showing heterogeneous to high signal on T2 W with central T2 hypointense strands

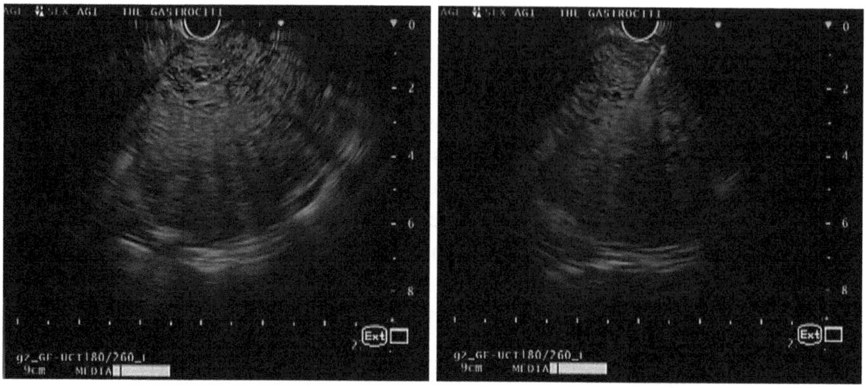

EUS Image
Well-defined heterogeneous, mixed to hypoechoic, solid cystic lesion involving the body and tail of the pancreas with hyperechoic internal strands. EUS-guided biopsy being performed using a 22 G Biopsy needle

References

1. Frantz VK. Tumors of the pancreas. Washington, DC: Armed Forced Institute of Pathology; 1959. Atlas of tumor pathology. Section VII-Fascicles 27 and 28; pp. 32–3.
2. Kloppel DG, Solcia DE, Sobin DLH, Longnecker DS, Capella DC. Histological typing of tumours of the exocrine pancreas. In Proceedings of the world health organization international histological classification of tumours; 1996: 14.
3. Bosman FT, Carneiro F, Hruban RH, Theise ND. WHO classification of tumours of the digestive system. In: WHO classification of tumours, vol. 3. 4th ed. IARC Publications; 2010.
4. Lu X, Chen H, Zhang T. Solid pseudopapillary neoplasm (SPN) of the pancreas: current understanding on its malignant potential and management. Discov Oncologia. 2024;15(1)
5. La Rosa S, Bongiovanni M. Pancreatic solid pseudopapillary neoplasm: key pathologic and genetic features. Arch Pathol Lab Med. 2020;144(7):829–37.
6. Valsangkar NP, Morales-Oyarvide V, Thayer SP, et al. 851 resected cystic tumors of the pancreas: a 33-year experience at the Massachusetts General Hospital. Surgery. 2012;152(3):S4–S12.
7. Antoniou EA, Damaskos C, Garmpis N, et al. Solid Pseudopapillary tumor of the pancreas: a single-center experience and review of the literature. In Vivo. 2017;31(4):501–10.
8. Zou Y, Huang Y, Hong B, Xiang X, Zhou B, Wei S. Comparison of the clinicopathological features of pancreatic solid pseudopapillary neoplasms between males and females: gender does matter. Histol Histopathol. 2020;35(3):257–68.
9. Serra S, Chetty R. Revision 2: an immunohistochemical approach and evaluation of solid pseudopapillary tumour of the pancreas. J Clin Pathol. 2008;61(11):1153–9.
10. Tanaka Y, Kato K, Notohara K, et al. Frequent beta-catenin mutation and cytoplasmic/nuclear accumulation in pancreatic solid-pseudopapillary neoplasm. Cancer Res. 2001;61:8401–4.
11. Abraham SC, Klimstra DS, Wilentz RE, et al. Solid-pseudopapillary tumors of the pancreas are genetically distinct from pancreatic ductal adenocarcinomas and almost always harbor beta-catenin mutations. Am J Pathol. 2002;160(4):1361–9.
12. Ohara Y, Oda T, Hashimoto S, et al. Pancreatic neuroendocrine tumor and solid-pseudopapillary neoplasm: key immunohistochemical profiles for differential diagnosis. World J Gastroenterol. 2016;22(38):8596–604.
13. Kosmahl M, Seada LS, Jänig U, Harms D, Klöppel G. Solid-pseudopapillary tumor of the pancreas: its origin revisited. Virchows Arch. 2000;436(5):473–80.

14. Yang F, Fu D, Jin C, et al. Clinical experiences of solid pseudopapillary tumors of the pancreas in China. J Gastroenterol Hepatol. 2008;23(12):1847–51.
15. Wang P, Wei J, Wu J, et al. Diagnosis and treatment of solid-pseudopapillary tumors of the pancreas: a single institution experience with 97 cases. Pancreatology. 2018;18(4):415–9.
16. Liu Q, Dai M, Guo J, et al. Long-term survival, quality of life, and molecular features of the patients with solid pseudopapillary neoplasm of the pancreas. Ann Surg. 2023;278(6):1009–17.
17. Cruz MAA, Moutinho-Ribeiro P, Costa-Moreira P, Macedo G. Solid pseudopapillary neoplasm of the pancreas: unfolding an intriguing condition. GE Port J Gastroenterol. 2021;29(3):151–62.
18. Estrella JS, Li L, Rashid A, et al. Solid pseudopapillary neoplasm of the pancreas: clinicopathologic and survival analyses of 64 cases from a single institution. Am J Surg Pathol. 2014;38(2):147–57.
19. Fan Z, Li Y, Yan K, et al. Application of contrast-enhanced ultrasound in the diagnosis of solid pancreatic lesions – a comparison of conventional ultrasound and contrast-enhanced CT. Eur J Radiol. 2013;82(9):1385–90.
20. Law JK, Ahmed A, Singh VK, et al. A systematic review of solid-pseudopapillary neoplasms. Pancreas. 2014;43(3):331–7.
21. Maimaijiang A, Wang H, Li W, Wang Y. Diagnosis and treatment of solid pseudopapillary neoplasm of the pancreas in children: a report of 18 cases. Front Pediatr. 2022;10:10.
22. Baek JH, Lee JM, Kim SH, et al. Small solid pseudopapillary tumors of the pancreas at multiphasic multidetector CT. Radiology. 2010;257(1):97–106.
23. Li DL, Li HS, Xu YK, Wang QS, Chen RY, Zhou F. Solid pseudopapillary tumor of the pancreas: clinical features and imaging findings. Clin Imaging. 2017;48:113–21.
24. De Robertis R, Marchegiani G, Catania M, et al. Solid pseudopapillary neoplasms of the pancreas: clinicopathologic and radiologic features according to size. Am J Roentgenol. 2019;213(5):1073–80.
25. Chi-Chang Y, Jeng-Hwei T, Chun-Nan Y, Tsann-Long H, Yi-Yin J. Clinicopathological study of solid and pseudopapillary tumor of pancreas: emphasis on magnetic resonance imaging findings. World J Gastroenterol. 2007;13(12):1811–5.
26. Schick V, Franzius C, Beyna T, et al. Diagnostic impact of 18F-FDG PET–CT evaluating solid pancreatic lesions versus endosonography, endoscopic retrograde cholangio-pancreatography with intraductal ultrasonography and abdominal ultrasound. Eur J Nucl Med Mol Imag. 2008;35(10):1775–85.
27. Liu W, Gong W, Zhang J, Ma J, Zhang C. 68GA-FAPI-04 PET/CT in the detection of non–FDG-Avid solid pseudopapillary neoplasm of the pancreas. Clin Nucl Med. 2022;48(1):100–2.
28. Banafea O, Mghanga FP, Zhao J, Zhao R, Zhu L. Endoscopic ultrasonography with fine-needle aspiration for histological diagnosis of solid pancreatic masses: a meta-analysis of diagnostic accuracy studies. BMC Gastroenterol. 2016;16(1):108.
29. Xu YC, Fu DL, Yang F. Unraveling the enigma: a comprehensive review of solid pseudopapillary tumor of the pancreas. World J Gastrointest Oncol. 2024;16(3):614–29.
30. Gonda TA, Cahen DL, Farrell JJ. Pancreatic cysts. N Engl J Med. 2024;391(9):832–43.
31. Pawlak KM, Tehami N, Maher B, et al. Role of endoscopic ultrasound in the characterization of solid pseudopapillary neoplasm of the pancreas. World J Gastrointest Endosc. 2023;15(4):273–84.
32. Khalyfa AA, Kapur U, Ayub K. The role of confocal endomicroscopy for diagnosis of solid pseudopapillary tumor of the pancreas. Endoscopy. 2022;54(S 02):E943–4.
33. Wu CCH, Lim SJM, Tan DMY. Endoscopic ultrasound-guided needle-based confocal laser endomicroscopy for pancreatic cystic lesions: current status and future prospects. Clin Endosc. 2024;57(4):434–45.
34. Wang BG, Mani H, Wang ZQ, Li W. Cytological diagnosis of pancreatic solid-pseudopapillary neoplasm: a single-institution community practice experience. Diagnostics. 2022;12(2):449.
35. Meriden Z, Shi C, Edil BH, et al. Hyaline globules in neuroendocrine and solid-pseudopapillary neoplasms of the pancreas. Am J Surg Pathol. 2011;35(7):981–8.
36. Burford H, Baloch Z, Liu X, Jhala D, Siegal GP, Jhala N. E-cadherin/beta-catenin and CD10: a limited immunohistochemical panel to distinguish pancreatic endocrine neoplasm from solid

pseudopapillary neoplasm of the pancreas on endoscopic ultrasound-guided fine-needle aspirates of the pancreas. Am J Clin Pathol. 2009;132(6):831–9.
37. Notohara K, Hamazaki S, Tsukayama C, et al. Solid-pseudopapillary tumor of the pancreas. Am J Surg Pathol. 2000;24(10):1361–71.
38. Hosokawa I, Shimizu H, Ohtsuka M, et al. Preoperative diagnosis and surgical management for solid pseudopapillary neoplasm of the pancreas. J Hepatobiliary Pancreat Sci. 2014;21(8):573–8.
39. Romics L, Oláh A, Belágyi T, Hajdú N, Gyűrűs P, Ruszinkó V. Solid pseudopapillary neoplasm of the pancreas – proposed algorithms for diagnosis and surgical treatment. Langenbeck's Arch Surg. 2010;395(6):747–55.
40. De Castro SMM, Singhal D, Aronson DC, et al. Management of Solid-pseudopapillary neoplasms of the pancreas: a comparison with standard pancreatic neoplasms. World J Surg. 2007;31(5):1130–5.
41. Lanke G, Ali FS, Lee JH. Clinical update on the management of pseudopapillary tumor of pancreas. World J Gastrointest Endosc. 2018;10(9):145–55.
42. Machado MCC, Machado MAC, Bacchella T, Jukemura J, Almeida JL, Cunha JEM. Solid pseudopapillary neoplasm of the pancreas: distinct patterns of onset, diagnosis, and prognosis for male versus female patients. Surgery. 2007;143(1):29–34.
43. Efron DT, Lillemoe KD, Cameron JL, Yeo CJ. Central pancreatectomy with pancreaticogastrostomy for benign pancreatic pathology. J Gastrointest Surg. 2004;8(5):532–8.
44. Grace PA, Pitt HA, Longmire WP. Pylorus preserving pancreatoduodenectomy: an overview. Br J Surg. 1990;77(9):968–74.
45. Coupier A, Khoury T, Gincul R, et al. Endoscopic ultrasound-guided radiofrequency ablation for solid pseudopapillary neoplasm of the pancreas. Endoscopy. 2023;55(S 01):E951–2.
46. Choi JH, Seo DW, Song TJ, et al. Endoscopic ultrasound-guided radiofrequency ablation for management of benign solid pancreatic tumors. Endoscopy. 2018;50(11):1099–104.
47. Coelho JCU, Da Costa M a R, Ramos EJB, Torres AR, Savio MC, Claus CMP. Surgical management of solid pseudopapillary tumor of the pancreas. J Soc Lap Surg. 2018;22(4):1–6.
48. Sreekanth A, Nagari B, Thumma V, et al. Treatment with long term follow-up of solid pseudopapillary tumor of pancreas – a single center experience from India. Ann Hepatobiliary Pancreat Surg. 2023;27(1):S404.
49. Kodama R, Koh Y, Midorikawa H, Yokota Y, Saegusa H, Ushimaru H. A case of recurrence of a solid pseudopapillary neoplasm of the pancreas effectively treated with proton beam radiotherapy. Clin J Gastroenterol. 2020;14(1):375–81.
50. Wang WB, Zhang TP, Sun MQ, Peng Z, Chen G, Zhao YP. Solid pseudopapillary tumor of the pancreas with liver metastasis: clinical features and management. Eur J Surg Oncol. 2014;40(11):1572–7.
51. Sumida W, Kaneko K, Tainaka T, Ono Y, Kiuchi T, Ando H. Liver transplantation for multiple liver metastases from solid pseudopapillary tumor of the pancreas. J Pediatr Surg. 2007;42(12):e27–31.
52. Maffuz A, De Thé Bustamante F, Silva JA, Torres-Vargas S. Preoperative gemcitabine for unresectable, solid pseudopapillary tumour of the pancreas. Lancet Oncol. 2005;6(3):185–6.
53. Hah JO, Park WK, Lee NH, Choi JH. Preoperative chemotherapy and intraoperative radiofrequency ablation for unresectable solid pseudopapillary tumor of the pancreas. J Pediatr Hematol Oncol. 2007;29(12):851–3.
54. Morikawa T, Onogawa T, Maeda S, et al. Solid pseudopapillary neoplasms of the pancreas: an 18-year experience at a single Japanese institution. Surg Today. 2012;43(1):26–32.
55. Prasad TV, Madhusudhan KS, Srivastava DN, Dash NR, Gupta AK. Transarterial chemoembolization for liver metastases from solid pseudopapillary epithelial neoplasm of pancreas: a case report. World J Radiol. 2015;7(3):61–5.
56. Honore C, Goere D, Dartigues P, Burtin P, Dumont F, Elias D. Peritoneal carcinomatosis from solid pseudopapillary neoplasm (Frantz's tumour) of the pancreas treated with HIPEC. Anticancer Res. 2012 Mar;32(3):1069–73.

57. You L, Yang F, Fu DL. Prediction of malignancy and adverse outcome of solid pseudopapillary tumor of the pancreas. World J Gastrointest Oncol. 2018;10(7):184–93.
58. Yang F, Wu W, Wang X, et al. Grading solid pseudopapillary tumors of the pancreas: the Fudan prognostic index. Ann Surg Oncol. 2020;28(1):550–9.
59. Chen J, Zong L, Wang P, et al. Solid pseudopapillary neoplasms of the pancreas: clinicopathologic analysis and a predictive model. Mod Pathol. 2023;36(6):1–12.
60. Wang X, Zhu D, Bao W, Li M, Wang S, Shen R. Case report: targeted therapy for metastatic solid pseudopapillary neoplasm of the pancreas with CTNNB1 and PTEN mutations. Front Oncologia. 2021:11.
61. Kornietskaya A, Evdokimova S, Kachmazov A, et al. Endocrine therapy for metastatic solid pseudopapillary neoplasm of the pancreas: a case report. Front Oncologia. 2022;12:12.

Management of Mucinous Cystic Neoplasms

8

Dinesh Walia, Samagra Agarwal, and Deepak Gunjan

Abstract

Pancreatic cystic lesions (PCLs) are commonly encountered as incidental radiological findings. The differentials include both neoplastic and neoplastic lesions. Management depends on identifying the type of cystic lesion based on a combination of clinical presentation, radiological characteristics, and cystic fluid and serum biomarkers. Mucinous cystic neoplasms represent neoplastic lesions with significant malignant potential. Clinically, they are usually asymptomatic and incidentally detected in middle-aged females. Morphologically, they are oligo-macrocystic with no communication with the main pancreatic duct. Adequate characterization is required to gauge the risk of malignancy and includes a combination of radiological findings on contrast-enhanced MRI or EUS with an option for EUS-guided sampling of the cystic fluid along with blood biomarkers. Patients with high-risk features warrant upfront surgical resection if they are fit for surgery. Those who are unfit for surgery or do not have high-risk stigmata or worrisome features may be kept on routine surveillance with CE-MRI or EUS at regular intervals, as suggested by various guidelines. Herein, we discuss the diagnosis and optimal management of mucinous cystic neoplasms along with the recommendations from various guidelines.

Keywords

Mucinous cystic neoplasms · Malignancy · Pancreatic carcinoma · Endoscopic ultrasound · Whipple's pancreatoduodenectomy

D. Walia · S. Agarwal · D. Gunjan (✉)
Department of Gastroenterology and HNU, All India Institute of Medical Sciences, New Delhi, India

R. K. Sharma et al. (eds.), *Differential Diagnosis and Management of Pancreatic Cystic Lesions*, https://doi.org/10.1007/978-981-92-0654-4_8

8.1 Introduction

Pancreatic cystic lesions (PCLs) encompass a variety of lesions including both benign and malignant. The incidental detection of PCLs has increased in the recent decades owing to increase in the life span of the population and the widespread use of various cross-sectional imaging modalities for other clinical indications [1]. They are broadly divided into mucinous cysts, which include intraductal papillary mucinous neoplasms (IPMN) and mucinous cystic neoplasms (MCN), and nonmucinous cysts, which include serous cystadenoma (SCN), solid pseudopapillary neoplasms (SPN), cystic neuroendocrine neoplasms, and other rare varieties.

MCNs are cystic-forming, mucin-producing neoplasms of pancreas and show "ovarian-type" stroma with mucin-producing epithelium on histology. Morphologically, MCNs are classically well-circumscribed cystic lesions that are either unilocular or multiloculated with macrocysts which may be greater than 2 cm in size [2]. Since MCNs are encapsulated lesions, they do not typically communicate with the MPD. They are usually asymptomatic and maybe quite large at initial presentation, with the mean diameter ranging from 6 to 11 cm [3]. This might be explained by the fact that the lesions are in the body or tail of the pancreas and may not elicit symptoms until they are quite large.

The mucinous PCLs have a propensity to develop malignancy. Adequate characterization of these lesions is critical for appropriate management. Major management decisions include either a conservative approach with regular surveillance or surgical or novel EUS-based ablative techniques for high-risk lesions. This decision is crucial since both methods have their own merits and demerits. The presence of high-risk stigmata and worrisome features warrants more definitive management like surgical resection, provided the patient is fit for surgery. Regular surveillance with cross-sectional imaging is recommended in low-risk lesions at different time intervals as given by various guidelines. Herein, we discuss the diagnosis, treatment, and surveillance of mucinous cystic neoplasms.

8.2 Epidemiology

MCNs occur in middle-aged females (99.4%) in the fourth to fifth decades [4]. Most of these lesions are in the body and tail (94.6%) of the pancreas [5]. The reported incidence of pancreatic cysts is highly variable among different studies and depends on the imaging modality used, the patient's age, and the population's ethnicity. The incidence increases from 1.2–2.6% on computed tomography (CT) to 2.4–49.1% on magnetic resonance imaging (MRI) [6–10]. The incedence of pancreatic cysts increased from 0% in 20s to 11% in the 70s in a Japanese hospital-based study [11]. The incidence also varied in different ethnic study populations, like 2.6% in Germany and 2.2% in Korea [12, 13]. A meta-analysis of 17 studies comprising more than 48,000 individuals showed that a pooled prevalence of incidentally detected pancreatic cysts was 8%, which was higher in studies that employed MRI (24.8% vs 2.7% with CT scan) as an imaging modality. Among these, mucinous lesions were most common with a prevalence of 4.3%, but only 0.7% had worrisome features or high-risk stigmata [14].

The data regarding the natural history and malignant transformation of cystic lesions is heterogeneous. Major limitations of these studies include lack of uniform definitions of malignancy, the use of variable modalities to identify malignancy like cytology, fluid markers, or molecular markers [15, 16]. The risk of MCN harboring invasive carcinoma ranged from 9.9% to 34% in various surgical series [17–20]. An incident risk of malignancy was estimated at 0.24% per year, and a prevalent malignant risk was 0.25% at the time of cyst detection in a study [21]. An overall risk of malignant transformation is low, with an estimated rate of 33 per 100,000, which increased with age, based on surveillance, epidemiology, and end results data [22]. A combination of clinical and imaging findings in addition to cyst fluid markers can help classify these cystic lesions appropriately and guide management. The previous studies showed a higher risk of malignancy, as these studies are mostly retrospective surgical studies; however, recent population-based studies had shown a lower risk of malignant transformation [23, 24].

8.3 Diagnosis

MCN is diagnosed by a combination of cross-sectional imaging, endoscopic ultrasound (EUS), and cyst fluid analysis.

8.3.1 Cross-Sectional Radiological Imaging

Cross-sectional imaging is used to distinguish mucinous lesions from other cysts, stratify the risk of malignancy, and detect serial interval changes that might require further investigation. The major features on imaging used to differentiate various cystic lesions include the location, size, morphology of the lesion, presence or absence of enhancing nodules or septa, relationship to the main pancreatic duct (MPD), MPD diameter, and morphology of the surrounding parenchymal and peripancreatic tissues.

Cystic lesions that are incidentally detected and are less than 10 mm in size remain a diagnostic ambiguity due to the poor sensitivity of cross-sectional imaging [25]. Contrast-enhanced MRI/magnetic resonance cholangiopancreatography (MRCP) is better than multidetector CT (MDCT) at characterizing the relationship of MPD with the cyst and identifying mural nodules and septations. MRI with diffusion-weighted imaging (DWI) can also help to distinguish benign from malignant lesions. The accuracy of MRI in correctly identifying and characterizing PCL is 50%–86%, and for CT, it is 39%–61.4% [26]. The sensitivity of MRI/MRCP to identify MPD communication and internal septa is 91% and 100%, respectively [27]. MRI is more sensitive than CT for detecting solid components or mural nodules [28]. Hence, CEMRI/MRCP is better for diagnosis and surveillance [29–31]. Peripheral cyst wall calcification, noted in 10%–25% of cases, is a classic feature of MCNs and is better appreciated on CECT examination [32].

8.3.2 Endoscopic Ultrasound

Despite significant advances in cross-sectional imaging techniques, the ability to accurately classify the cystic lesions on CT and MRI is, sometimes, limited. It is indicated specifically when the patient has worrisome features or difficult to characterize a lesion or require sampling.

EUS findings should note the number of cysts, including the size, and location of each cyst. Each cyst should be examined for septations, the thickness of each septum, the presence of a mural nodule, contrast enhancement of the nodule, or an associated mass. Pancreatic duct examination is indispensable and includes the size of the duct and its communication to the cyst. Rest of the pancreatic parenchyma must be examined as well, since some of PCLs, like IPMN, may be multifocal and can develop synchronous pancreatic ductal adenocarcinoma in areas away from the cyst (Fig. 8.1).

Multiple studies have demonstrated that EUS morphology alone cannot adequately distinguish different types of cysts, and benign from the malignant mucinous lesions reliably [23, 33–35]. Sometimes, it becomes difficult to distinguish a mural nodule from a mucin ball. Mucin ball shows a hypoechoic center with a well-demarcated hyperechoic rim. Also, a mucin ball is mobile and can move within the cysts by changing the patient's position or while targeting during FNA. On the contrary, a mural nodule is isoechoic or hyperechoic in the center and has an irregular non-hyperechoic rim [36]. Contrast-enhanced harmonic EUS (CEH-EUS) is not superior to EUS in identifying different types of PCLs. The role of CEH-EUS is to identify mural nodules and the enhancement of the nodules, septa, and cyst wall [37]. Contrast-enhanced harmonic EUS (CEH-EUS) differentiates mucin clots from

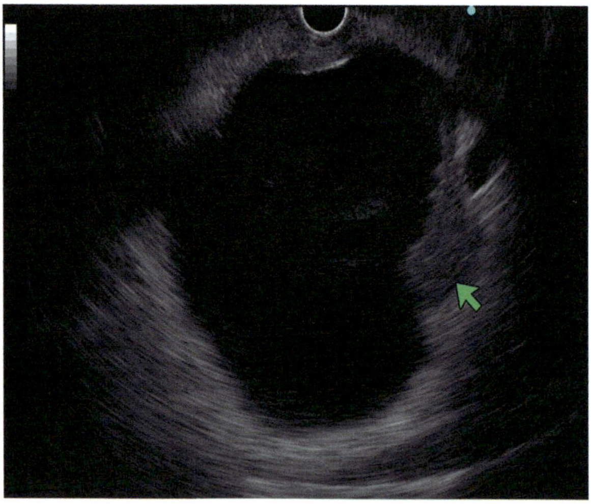

Fig. 8.1 Endoscopic ultrasound image of a mucinous cystic neoplasm, showing unilocular cyst with hypoechoic, irregular asymmetric wall thickening (green arrow). Asymmetric wall thickening is a worrisome feature that suggests potential malignant transformation

mural nodules, with sensitivity, specificity, positive predictive value, negative predictive value, and accuracy of 100%, 80%, 92%, 100%, and 94%, respectively, as shown in a meta-analysis [38]. The sensitivity of CEH-EUS and FNA from an enhancing mural nodule for any dysplasia or malignancy was 100%, and for HGD or malignancy, it was 76.9% [37]. Detecting a mural nodule increases the probability of detecting malignancy by 10 times [39].

If radiological and EUS findings are inconclusive, EUS-guided fine-needle aspiration (FNA) is indicated to obtain the cyst fluid for cytological, biochemical, and molecular analyses. EUS-FNA is done for definitive diagnosis when the suspicion for malignancy is high, like the presence of a solid component or enhancing mural nodule on cross-sectional imaging. Despite this, the ability of EUS to distinguish mucinous from nonmucinous cysts and to detect the presence of underlying malignancy is poor. The diagnostic accuracy was between 40% and 90% in various studies [21, 40]. The addition of EUS-FNA to imaging increases the diagnostic accuracy for detecting neoplastic MCN [41].

EUS-guided through-the-needle biopsy (EUS-TTNB) is used to obtain tissue from the cyst wall. The cyst is punctured with an FNA needle; then, a small-caliber forceps is passed through the needle to obtain tissue from the cyst wall [42]. EUS-TTNB was better than EUS-FNA in sample adequacy (OR—4.83) and diagnostic accuracy (OR—1.32) with a risk of mild bleeding and pancreatitis in 4% and 2% cases [43]. However, another meta-analysis reported an overall rate of adverse events as 8.6%, with 57.1% being self-limited bleeds, 14.3% abdominal pain, 24.5% mild acute pancreatitis, and 6.1% infections [44].

Needle-based confocal laser endomicroscopy (nCLE) is used to differentiate the PCN types. It enables real-time microscopic visualization of the lesion using an endoscopic probe through a 19-G FNA needle. MCN is characterized by single or multiple layers of nonpapillary epithelium [45, 46]. Although the interpretation of CLE is challenging, various studies report that its diagnostic accuracy is 71%–94% for differentiating between PCLs [47, 48]. However, its use is cumbersome, costly, and requires training to interpret the imaging.

8.3.3 Cyst Fluid Analysis

A. *Macroscopic:* "String sign" differentiates mucinous from nonmucinous PCL. Mucinous PCLs contain higha ly viscous cyst fluid [49]. A drop of cyst fluid aspirate is placed between the thumb and index finger and stretched; a string length > 3.5 mm indicates a mucinous PCN, with pooled sensitivity and specificity of 58% and 95%, respectively [50, 51]. A major limitation of the string sign is the subjective interpretation of the result and low sensitivity.
B. *Cytology:* In a systematic review of 13 studies with 5743 patients, the odds ratio (OR) to detect malignancy on cytology was 11, with the sensitivity and specificity of 57% and 84%, respectively [52]. The pooled sensitivity is 54%–63%, and specificity is 88%–93% for identifying IPMNs and MCNs, respectively [16]. EUS-guided brushing from the cyst wall has been studied to detect intracellular

mucin (ICM) to increase the sensitivity of cytology in diagnosing PCLs more than 2 cm. ICM was detected in 62% of brushings compared with 23% of FNA samples alone [53]. When EUS-guided brushings were compared to EUS-FNA cytology in PCLs more than 15 mm, the diagnostic accuracy of the brushings was only 44.8% compared to 41.1% in the FNA group in a recent RCT [54]. It is the most traditional method of cyst fluid analysis but suffers from a lack of sensitivity due to the low cellularity of fluid [55].

C. *Fluid* carcinoembryonic antigen (CEA): The mucinous neoplasms (IPMN and MCN) produce CEA from the endodermal-derived columnar epithelium. Compared to histology, the accuracy of CEA (79%) was significantly better than EUS morphology (51%) and cytology (59%) in differentiating mucinous from nonmucinous lesions [40]. The cyst fluid CEA level (>192 ng/mL) was the predictor of mucinous lesions with a diagnostic accuracy of 79% in a study [40]. CEA level of more than 800 ng/mL had a specificity of 98% but lower sensitivity (48%) [56]. An Indian study showed that cyst fluid CEA at a cutoff level of 45.0 ng/mL had a sensitivity, specificity, positive predictive value, and negative predictive value of 88.5%, 96.8%, 92.0%, and 95.3%, respectively, for differentiating mucinous from nonmucinous cystic lesions [57]. Studies have failed to show a correlation between the cyst fluid CEA level and dysplasia in patients with mucinous PCLs [58, 59]. Extremely low levels of CEA in the cyst fluid can rule out mucinous cysts. Cyst fluid CEA levels less than 5 ng/mL correlated with nonmucinous lesions with a sensitivity and specificity of 50% and 95%, respectively, in a study [56].

D. *Fluid amylase:* The exocrine pancreas produces amylase. It is usually elevated in lesions communicating with the ductal system like IPMN, pseudocysts, MCN, and ductal adenocarcinoma [60]. Although the cyst fluid amylase is elevated in IPMN, due to ductal communication, it has not been shown to distinguish IPMN from MCN [58, 59].

E. *Fluid inflammatory markers:* Malignancies, including PDAC, elicit antitumor immunity. Prostaglandin E2 (PGE2) is highly expressed in multiple cancers including PDAC. PGE2 levels in the cyst fluid of high-risk lesions were significantly higher than that in low-risk lesions in a study. A cystic fluid PGE2 cutoff of 1.1 pg/mL had sensitivity and specificity of 63% and 79%, respectively, to detect high-risk lesions but requires multicentric prospective validation [61].

F. *Molecular markers:* Cyst fluid is a rich source of DNA exfoliated from their lining epithelium. Mutated genes are released into the cyst fluid after cell death and have potential to serve as biomarkers. The most common mutations noted in PCLs include oncogenes, like kirsten rat sarcoma virus (KRAS) and guanine nucleotide-binding protein, alpha-stimulating (GNAS), and tumor suppressor genes like RNF43, CDKN2A, PTEN, TP53, and SMAD4 [62]. Mutations in *TP53, PIK3CA* (oncogene), deletions of *PTEN*, losses in *CDKN2A*, and *SMAD4* are noted in high-grade dysplasia and ductal adenocarcinoma [63]. Mutations in *KRAS* and/or *GNAS* are highly sensitive and specific for IPMN but not MCN [64]. Mutations in *KRAS* are most common in MCN, and their prevalence increases with the severity of dysplasia. *KRAS* mutations were seen in 13% with

LGD-MCN and 100% with HGD-MCN in a surgical series of 102 patients [64]. Mutations in *GNAS* are absent in MCN and could be used to distinguish IPMN from MCN [65]. *CDKN2A* and *TP53* are mutated in lesions with HGD or invasive carcinoma [66–69]. *SMAD4* expression is lost in most invasive carcinomas but remains normal in LGD or HGD-MCNs [70]. *RNF43* alterations are largely seen in noninvasive lesions [71].

Telomerase enzyme expression may be used as a surrogate of neoplastic progression. Cyst fluid telomerase activity is elevated in cystic neoplasm with high-grade dysplasia/malignant lesions. A telomerase cutoff value of 730 copies/L accurately identified high-risk lesions with a sensitivity and specificity of 74.2% and 93.2%, respectively, in a study that included 119 patients undergoing surgical resection or EUS-guided FNA, out of which 10 patients had MCN [63]. However, this requires external validation.

Next-generation sequencing (NGS) is a DNA mutational analysis technique. It requires a small quantity of cyst fluid and can detect multiple genes simultaneously. The amount of DNA shed into cyst fluid correlates with the degree of dysplasia. High DNA quantity in the cyst fluid had sensitivity and specificity of 78% and 53%, respectively, to detect high-risk IPMN when used alone with limited data on MCN [72]. Currently, available tests can identify the cyst type and stratify lesions according to grades of dysplasia. A 22-gene NGS panel had a sensitivity of 90% and specificity of 100% for diagnosing a mucinous cyst. This study had MCN in 12 patients out of 251 total surgical pancreatic cystic lesions. A combination of KRAS, GNAS, and the presence of TP53/SMAD4/CTNNB1/mTOR mutations had 88% sensitivity and 98% specificity for diagnosing high-grade dysplasia or early adenocarcinoma [73]. In the near future, this will help us to characterize and grade the lesion more accurately; however, availability, quality control, and cost are the issues.

G. *Metabolic markers:* Glucose levels in the mucinous PCLs are lower than that in nonmucinous cysts. Cyst fluid glucose concentration < 50 mg/dL had significantly better diagnostic accuracy than a CEA level >192 ng/mL for identifying mucinous cysts (94% vs 84%, respectively), as shown in a meta-analysis [74]. Onsite glucose measurement has been shown to have an excellent correlation with laboratory-based colorimetry. This is a point-of-care, easy-to-measure, and the most easily available test.

8.4 Blood-Based Tumor Markers

Carbohydrate antigen 19-9 (CA 19-9) is a tumor-associated glycoprotein used as a diagnostic and prognostic biomarker for ductal adenocarcinoma [75]. Elevated CA 19–9 levels are associated with HGD and invasive cancer [76]. Data on CA 19-9 in MCN is scarce since most of the studies have been conducted on IPMN [77]. Serum carcinoembryonic antigen (CEA) levels more than 5 ng/mL had poor sensitivity of 18%–40% and high specificity of 92%–95% to detect invasive lesions in a study [78]. It is less accurate than CA 19–9 and is therefore unsuitable for screening [79].

8.5 Risk Stratification

MCNs have been categorized as benign, premalignant, and malignant per the WHO classification based on histological features [80]. This is precisely possible only on surgically resected specimens. Histologically, the lesions may have low-grade dysplasia, high-grade dysplasia, or invasive carcinoma [81]. Predictors of malignancy are dynamic, hence the need for regular surveillance for those who do not undergo surgery. Several modalities are used to differentiate these, such as contrast-enhanced computed tomography (CECT), MRI with magnetic resonance cholangiopancreatography (MRCP), and contrast-enhanced ultrasonography EUS (CE-EUS) with cyst fluid aspiration. Correctly identifying malignancy-associated high-risk characteristics allows for increased diagnostic accuracy and reduces unnecessary surgical interventions and the need for surveillance. Several guidelines have demonstrated various high-risk features based on available evidence. These features are based on CECT, CEMRI with MRCP, CE-EUS, and EUS with cyst fluid aspirate.

Features associated with malignancy include invasion of adjacent structures, lymph nodal and distant metastases, lesion size ≥4 cm, thick irregular walls and septa >3 mm, enhancing soft-tissue components or mural nodules, peripheral calcifications, and pancreatic duct dilatation [82]. Male gender is at a higher risk for malignancy, as depicted in a hospital-based study of 329 cases of MCN with 15 years follow-up [24]. Metastases occur predominantly in the liver and may be cystic. In MCNs less than 4 cm in size and without worrisome features, malignant transformation occurred in 0.03% of cases in a study [82].

8.6 Clinical Management

Patients with benign or premalignant lesions, without worrisome features, are managed nonsurgically and kept on surveillance. Lesions with malignant or premalignant potential and high-grade dysplasia require surgical resection. Endoscopic ultrasound-guided ablative techniques have been recently introduced, including ethanol or paclitaxel/gemcitabine ablation. They are generally recommended for patients with premalignant lesions with high malignant potential but with a prohibitive risk for resection. EUS-cyst ablation is considered as definitive first-line therapy in surgically fit patients.

8.6.1 Surgery

Unlike IPMNs, MCNs do not have an increased risk of new lesions or malignancy in the remnant pancreas after surgery in the absence of invasive disease, as shown in a meta-analysis [82], while those with invasive disease at the time of surgery have a reported recurrence of up to 25% [24]. Therefore, resecting noninvasive MCN will cure the lesion, whereas the 5-year survival rate of invasive MCN is reported to be 30%–40% [18]. Surgical resection is indicated for patients with high-risk stigmata or worrisome features, with no contraindications to resection. High-risk features

Table 8.1 Indications for surgical resection of MCN as per various guidelines

Guideline	Indications of surgery
AGA 2015 [85]	Cyst >3 cm Dilated MPD Solid cystic component Cytology with high-grade dysplasia or invasive cancer
IAP 2017 [86]	All MCN
European Guidelines 2018 [83]	Cyst diameter ≥ 40 mm Enhancing mural nodule Symptoms (tumor-related jaundice, acute pancreatitis, new-onset diabetes mellitus)

Abbreviations: *AGA* American Gastroenterology Association, *IAP* International Association of Pancreatology, *MCN* mucinous cystic neoplasm, *MPD* main pancreatic duct

include jaundice, a contrast-enhancing mural nodule or solid component, or an MPD diameter of over 10 mm. Worrisome features include cyst size more than 3 cm, MPD size 5–9 mm, presence of an enhancing mural nodule <5 mm, history of acute pancreatitis, enhancing thickened cyst wall and septa (more than 3 mm), serum CA 19-9 >37 U/mL, cyst size growth of 5 mm over 2 years, lymphadenopathy, and MPD diameter change with distal pancreatic atrophy [83, 84]. Indications for surgical resection as given by various guidelines have been summarized in Table 8.1.

Different surgical procedures are available for the treatment of MCN. For MCN, located within the head or uncinate process of the pancreas, pancreatoduodenectomy is done, whereas distal pancreatectomy is done for lesions in the body or tail. Surgical resection is associated with perioperative morbidity of 20–40% and mortality of 1–3% for pancreatoduodenectomy and <1% for distal pancreatectomy [87–89]. Central pancreatectomy is a parenchyma-sparing technique that removes the neck and proximal body of the pancreas while preserving the head and tail. It is used to treat lesions in the neck and proximal body of the pancreas. It has an overall morbidity of 51% and pancreatic fistula in 35% of patients [90]. Central pancreatectomy is an alternative for young and fit patients capable of tolerating postoperative complications. It preserves the pancreatic exocrine and endocrine functions but at the cost of significant morbidity.

Resection of MCNs without an invasive malignancy is curative [91]. If the tumor is encapsulated within the cyst, 5-year survival may reach 100% even if an invasive component is present [92]. Patients with mucinous cystadenocarcinoma have a poor prognosis. About 16% of these have lymph nodes spread at the time of surgery, with a 5-year overall survival of only 35% [93]. Resected mucinous cystadenocarcinomas have a reported 3-year overall survival of 59% [94].

8.6.2 Endoscopic

EUS-guided pancreatic cystic ablation (EUS-PCA) is an alternative to surgery in high-surgical-risk patients. EUS-PCA is a minimally invasive intervention and is safe with fewer major adverse events. EUS-PCA is done by two major techniques:

EUS-guided fine-needle injection (EUS-FNI) using ethanol and/or any other ablative agent and EUS-guided radiofrequency ablation (EUS-RFA). The type of intervention depends on the characteristics of the lesion.

EUS-FNI may prevent malignant transformation of mucinous cysts. Indications include: (1) unilocular or oligolocular cystic (2–6 loculi) mucinous lesion, (2) largest single locule diameter of more than 2 cm, and (3) life expectancy of 3–5 years to benefit from treating a precancerous lesion. Contraindications include high-risk features indicative of invasive tumor, which include MPD >5 mm, mural nodules >3 mm, elevated CA 19-9, thickened cyst walls or septations >3 mm, common bile duct or pancreatic duct obstruction, pathologic lymphadenopathy, or multiloculated cysts with >4 noncommunicating loculi. Other contraindications include coagulopathy, high suspicion of malignancy, acute pancreatitis, or infected collections or necrosis [95].

After characterizing the lesion, the cyst is punctured by a 19-gauge needle with suction pressure under EUS guidance. Then, the maximum possible volume of cystic fluid is aspirated. The same amount of ablative agent should be prepared. Ablative agents include 99% ethanol or paclitaxel [96]. Ablative agent, equal to the volume of fluid aspirated, is injected into the cyst through the needle and re-aspirated immediately. This lavage with ablative fluid is repeated three to four times. After this, the injected ablative agent and total cystic fluid are aspirated, and the needle is removed. A meta-analysis of 15 studies showed complete cyst disappearance in 32% with ethanol, significantly better than 13% in RFA. The highest rate of complete cyst obliteration was noted with a combination of ethanol and paclitaxel (70%) [97]. Possible adverse events include fever, abdominal pain, acute pancreatitis, and infection [98]. The post-treatment response is categorized into complete resolution, partial resolution, or persistence, corresponding to less than 5%, 5%–25%, and more than 25% of the initial cyst size. Six-monthly follow-up CECT scans are done until cyst resolution and annually thereafter [95].

EUS-RFA is another option for minimally invasive ablation of PCLs. It delivers heat waves (between 350 and 500 kHz), with a high temperature between 60 and 100 °C that causes coagulation necrosis and apoptosis of the target neoplastic tissue [99]. Under EUS guidance, the RFA probe can be used percutaneously directly or through a 19G FNA needle to the target lesion. A systematic review of four studies on EUS-RFA was done for PCLs, with 38 patients who underwent 44 EUS-RFA sessions. Complete radiological cyst resolution was achieved in 36.8% cases at 10.2 months of follow-up. However, MCNs constituted only 5 out of 38 cases [100]. Adverse events reported with EUS-RFA for PCLs have 0% to 21% cases including abdominal pain, acute pancreatitis, and one case of perforation. Prophylactic endoscopic pancreatic duct stenting by ERCP (1 or 2 days before EUS-RFA) is recommended in case the PD is near the target lesion (<4 mm). EUS-RFA remains a management option for lesions not amenable to EUS-FNI like multilocular microcystic SCN, solid lesions like NETs close to CBD and PD [101]. The data of role of EUS-RFA in MCN is scarce currently.

Endoscopic interventions are upcoming modality with fewer experiences and done at only few centers. Multicentric RCTs are required to establish their widespread acceptance, and their availability at many centers remains challenging due to cost constraints.

8.7 Surveillance

Surveillance refers to an ongoing follow-up of patients at increased risk of disease. Surveillance is done for patients who do not have high-risk features warranting surgery. This helps to detect malignancy at an early and treatable stage, prevents the development of invasive cancer by finding high-risk features that might evolve into malignancy, and reassures the patient in case the disease is stable. Various disease-related and patient-related factors determine the surveillance strategies. Patient-related factors include age, comorbidities, fitness, and willingness for surgery.

8.7.1 Postoperative Surveillance

There was no risk of recurrence after the resection of MCN without invasive malignancy in a systematic review of 13 studies with 773 patients [82]. Therefore, patients with resected MCN with LGD, borderline dysplasia, or HGD do not warrant postoperative surveillance. The risk of recurrence in resected MCNs with invasive cancer has been shown up to 25% [92]. Thus, MCN-related malignancy should be followed up as ductal adenocarcinoma after pancreatectomy with CECT or CEMRI every 3–6 months for 2 years and then annually thereafter [102].

8.7.2 Surveillance for Nonresected MCN

Surveillance for presumed MCN may be considered in lesions less than 3 cm in size without any solid component, other worrisome features, or high-risk stigmata in surgically fit asymptomatic patients [83].

8.7.2.1 Surveillance Modalities

CEMRI is preferred due to its lack of ionizing radiation, better resolution for smaller cysts, is noninvasive, and delineates communication between a cyst and MPD [103]. Radiological surveillance aims to detect changes in cyst size, MPD morphology, and development of mass/septa/septal thickening/nodule. If a patient cannot undergo an MRI due to availability or patient preference, a pancreatic protocol multiphase contrast-enhanced CT scan is an alternative.

EUS may be used in surveillance, alternating with MRI or CT, in patients at a higher risk of developing malignancy who did not undergo surgery due to patients' preferences [104]. Such high-risk features include focal cyst wall thickening, non-enhancing mural nodule, solid component, MPD >5 mm, regional lymphadenopathy, cyst wall enhancement, elevated CA 19-9, and size >3 cm on cross-sectional imaging. Subsequently, FNA and cyst fluid analysis may be done in such cases. There is no current role of serial pancreatic cyst fluid analysis during the surveillance with EUS [92].

8.7.2.2 Surveillance Intervals

Various guidelines have given different surveillance intervals depending on the cyst size and other high-risk factors including mural nodules and MPD diameter. A summary of guidelines for surveillance has been shown in Table 8.2.

8.7.2.3 Surveillance Cessation

Initially, surveillance was done till the patient was fit to undergo surgery if any high-risk features developed. Recently, there has been an emphasis on stopping surveillance if there is no significant change in the characteristics of the cyst, but it comes at a cost and apprehension regarding the risk of progression and development of malignancy or high-risk features [107]. Guidelines for stopping surveillance in asymptomatic patients have been summarized in Table 8.3.

Table 8.2 Guidelines for surveillance modality and intervals for unresected MCNs

Cyst size	AGA 2015 [85]	ACR 2017 [105]	European 2018 [83]	ACG 2018 [106]
<1 cm	MRI at 1 year, then every 2 years	Cysts <1.5 cm: MRI/CT 1 year	EUS/MRI and CA19-9 for 1 year; then annually	MRI every 2 years, lengthen if stable
1–2 cm	MRI at 1 year, then every 2 years	Cysts 1.5–2.5 cm: MRI/CT 6 monthly ×4, then lengthen if stable	EUS/MRI and CA19-9 6 monthly for 1 year; then annually	MRI annually for 2 years., then every 2 years
2–3 cm	MRI at 1 year, then every 2 years	Cysts 2.5 cm: MRI/CT annually for 10 years	EUS/MRI and CA19-9 6 monthly for 1 year; then annually	EUS/MRI 6 monthly for 3 years then annually
>3 cm	MRI at 1 year, then every 2 years		EUS/MRI and CA19-9 6 monthly for 1 year; then annually	EUS/MRI 6 monthly for 3 years then annually

Abbreviations: *ACG* American College of Gastroenterology, *ACR* American College of Radiology, *AGA* American Gastroenterology Association, *CA 19-9* Cancer antigen 19-9, *CT* computed tomography, *EUS* endoscopic ultrasound, *MRI* magnetic resonance imaging

Table 8.3 Guidelines for surveillance cessation in asymptomatic MCNs

Guideline	When to stop surveillance
AGA 2015 [85]	No significant change in cyst characteristics of the cyst after 5 years or the patient is no longer a surgical candidate
ACR 2017 [105]	Cyst <1.5 cm after a minimum 10 years
ACG 2018 [106]	If the patient is no longer a surgical candidate For patients between 75–85 years, an individualized approach is to be adopted depending on performance status and surgical candidacy
European 2018 [83]	Continue surveillance until the patient is no longer fit for surgery

Abbreviations: *ACG* American College of Gastroenterology, *ACR* American College of Radiology, *AGA* American Gastroenterology Association

8.8 Conclusion

MCNs are mucin-producing cystic neoplasms of pancreas almost exclusively seen in middle-aged females with no communication with the ductal system. They have a macro-oligocystic morphology with a characteristic ovarian-type stroma on histology. They are usually asymptomatic and detected incidentally with a higher incidence in the body and tail. Diagnosis is made on a combination of radiological imaging and EUS with or without cyst fluid analysis. Various radiological high-risk features and worrisome features are associated with malignancy. Surgery is the mainstay of management for lesions more than 4 cm or smaller lesions with high-risk features like solid components or mural nodules, with a negligible risk of recurrence for noninvasive lesions. Nonresected lesions require long-term surveillance with radiological imaging or EUS, which may be stopped in a subset of cases as given by various guidelines.

Conflict of Interest No conflict of interest

References

1. Canto MI, Hruban RH, Fishman EK, Kamel IR, Schulick R, Zhang Z, et al. Frequent detection of pancreatic lesions in asymptomatic high-risk individuals. Gastroenterology. 2012;142(4):796–804; quiz e14–15
2. Buetow PC, Rao P, Thompson LD. From the archives of the AFIP. Mucinous cystic neoplasms of the pancreas: radiologic-pathologic correlation. Radiogr Rev Publ Radiol Soc N Am Inc. 1998;18(2):433–49.
3. Khan A, Khosa F, Eisenberg RL. Cystic lesions of the pancreas. AJR Am J Roentgenol. 2011;196(6):W668–77.
4. Taya M, Hecht EM, Huang C, Lo GC. Pancreatic cystic lesions: imaging techniques and diagnostic features. Gastrointest Endosc Clin N Am. 2023;33(3):497–518.
5. van Huijgevoort NCM, Del Chiaro M, Wolfgang CL, van Hooft JE, Besselink MG. Diagnosis and management of pancreatic cystic neoplasms: current evidence and guidelines. Nat Rev Gastroenterol Hepatol. 2019;16(11):676–89.

6. de Oliveira PB, Puchnick A, Szejnfeld J, Goldman SM. Prevalence of incidental pancreatic cysts on 3 tesla magnetic resonance. PLoS One. 2015;10(3):e0121317.
7. Megibow AJ, Baker ME, Gore RM, Taylor A. The incidental pancreatic cyst. Radiol Clin North Am. 2011;49(2):349–59.
8. Chu LC, Singhi AD, Haroun RR, Hruban RH, Fishman EK. The many faces of pancreatic serous cystadenoma: radiologic and pathologic correlation. Diagn Interv Imaging. 2017;98(3):191–202.
9. Lee KS, Sekhar A, Rofsky NM, Pedrosa I. Prevalence of incidental pancreatic cysts in the adult population on MR imaging. Off J Am Coll Gastroenterol ACG. 2010;105(9):2079.
10. Girometti R, Intini S, Brondani G, Como G, Londero F, Bresadola F, et al. Incidental pancreatic cysts on 3D turbo spin echo magnetic resonance cholangiopancreatography: prevalence and relation with clinical and imaging features. Abdom Imaging. 2011;36(2):196–205.
11. Tanaka S, Tsujimae M, Masuda A, Inoue J, Inomata N, Uemura H, et al. Metabolic syndrome accelerates the age-related increase of Intraductal papillary mucinous neoplasm of the pancreas. Pancreas. 2024;53(1):e9–15.
12. Chang YR, Park JK, Jang JY, Kwon W, Yoon JH, Kim SW. Incidental pancreatic cystic neoplasms in an asymptomatic healthy population of 21,745 individuals: large-scale, single-center cohort study. Medicine (Baltimore). 2016;95(51):e5535.
13. Kromrey ML, Bülow R, Hübner J, Paperlein C, Lerch MM, Ittermann T, et al. Prospective study on the incidence, prevalence and 5-year pancreatic-related mortality of pancreatic cysts in a population-based study. Gut. 2018;67(1):138–45.
14. Zerboni G, Signoretti M, Crippa S, Falconi M, Arcidiacono PG, Capurso G. Systematic review and meta-analysis: prevalence of incidentally detected pancreatic cystic lesions in asymptomatic individuals. Pancreatology. 2019;19(1):2–9.
15. Thornton GD, McPhail MJW, Nayagam S, Hewitt MJ, Vlavianos P, Monahan KJ. Endoscopic ultrasound guided fine needle aspiration for the diagnosis of pancreatic cystic neoplasms: a meta-analysis. Pancreatology. 2013;13(1):48–57.
16. Thosani N, Thosani S, Qiao W, Fleming JB, Bhutani MS, Guha S. Role of EUS-FNA-based cytology in the diagnosis of mucinous pancreatic cystic lesions: a systematic review and meta-analysis. Dig Dis Sci. 2010;55(10):2756–66.
17. Jang KT, Park SM, Basturk O, Bagci P, Bandyopadhyay S, Stelow EB, et al. Clinicopathologic characteristics of 29 invasive carcinomas arising in 178 pancreatic mucinous cystic neoplasms with ovarian-type stroma: implications for management and prognosis. Am J Surg Pathol. 2015;39(2):179–87.
18. Zamboni G, Scarpa A, Bogina G, Iacono C, Bassi C, Talamini G, et al. Mucinous cystic tumors of the pancreas: clinicopathological features, prognosis, and relationship to other mucinous cystic tumors. Am J Surg Pathol. 1999;23(4):410–22.
19. Sarr MG, Carpenter HA, Prabhakar LP, Orchard TF, Hughes S, van Heerden JA, et al. Clinical and pathologic correlation of 84 mucinous cystic neoplasms of the pancreas: can one reliably differentiate benign from malignant (or premalignant) neoplasms? Ann Surg. 2000;231(2):205–12.
20. Park JW, Jang JY, Kang MJ, Kwon W, Chang YR, Kim SW. Mucinous cystic neoplasm of the pancreas: is surgical resection recommended for all surgically fit patients? Pancreatology. 2014;14(2):131–6.
21. Scheiman JM, Hwang JH, Moayyedi P. American gastroenterological association technical review on the diagnosis and management of asymptomatic neoplastic pancreatic cysts. Gastroenterology. 2015;148(4):824–848.e22.
22. Gardner TB, Glass LM, Smith KD, Ripple GH, Barth RJ, Klibansky DA, et al. Pancreatic cyst prevalence and the risk of mucin-producing adenocarcinoma in US adults. Am J Gastroenterol. 2013;108(10):1546–50.
23. Cellier C, Cuillerier E, Palazzo L, Rickaert F, Flejou JF, Napoleon B, et al. Intraductal papillary and mucinous tumors of the pancreas: accuracy of preoperative computed tomography, endoscopic retrograde pancreatography and endoscopic ultrasonography, and long-term outcome in a large surgical series. Gastrointest Endosc. 1998;47(1):42–9.

24. Ethun CG, Postlewait LM, McInnis MR, Merchant N, Parikh A, Idrees K, et al. The diagnosis of pancreatic mucinous cystic neoplasm and associated adenocarcinoma in males: an eight-institution study of 349 patients over 15 years. J Surg Oncol [Internet]. 2017 Jun [cited 2024 Sep 3];115(7). Available from: https://pubmed.ncbi.nlm.nih.gov/28211072/
25. Udare A, Agarwal M, Alabousi M, McInnes M, Rubino JG, Marcaccio M, et al. Diagnostic accuracy of MRI for differentiation of benign and malignant pancreatic cystic lesions compared to CT and endoscopic ultrasound: systematic review and meta-analysis. J Magn Reson Imaging JMRI. 2021;54(4):1126–37.
26. Mohamed E, Jackson R, Halloran CM, Ghaneh P. Role of radiological imaging in the diagnosis and characterization of pancreatic cystic lesions: a systematic review. Pancreas. 2018;47(9):1055–64.
27. Alwahbi O, Ghumman Z, van der Pol CB, Patlas MN, Gopee-Ramanan P. Pancreatic cystic lesions: review of the current state of diagnosis and surveillance. Can Assoc Radiol J. 2023;74(3):557–69.
28. Sahani DV, Kambadakone A, Macari M, Takahashi N, Chari S, Fernandez-del CC. Diagnosis and management of cystic pancreatic lesions. AJR Am J Roentgenol. 2013;200(2):343–54.
29. Hecht EM, Khatri G, Morgan D, Kang S, Bhosale PR, Francis IR, et al. Intraductal papillary mucinous neoplasm (IPMN) of the pancreas: recommendations for standardized imaging and reporting from the Society of Abdominal Radiology IPMN disease focused panel. Abdom Radiol NY. 2021;46(4):1586–606.
30. Tirkes T, Menias CO, Sandrasegaran K. MR imaging techniques for pancreas. Radiol Clin North Am. 2012;50(3):379–93.
31. Jang KM, Kim SH, Min JH, Lee SJ, Kang TW, Lim S, et al. Value of diffusion-weighted MRI for differentiating malignant from benign intraductal papillary mucinous neoplasms of the pancreas. AJR Am J Roentgenol. 2014;203(5):992–1000.
32. Lee LS. Updates in diagnosis and management of pancreatic cysts. World J Gastroenterol. 2021;27(34):5700–14.
33. Song MH, Lee SK, Kim MH, Lee HJ, Kim KP, Kim HJ, et al. EUS in the evaluation of pancreatic cystic lesions. Gastrointest Endosc. 2003;57(7):891–6.
34. Sugiyama M, Atomi Y, Saito M. Intraductal papillary tumors of the pancreas: evaluation with endoscopic ultrasonography. Gastrointest Endosc. 1998;48(2):164–71.
35. Kubo H, Chijiiwa Y, Akahoshi K, Hamada S, Harada N, Sumii T, et al. Intraductal papillary-mucinous tumors of the pancreas: differential diagnosis between benign and malignant tumors by endoscopic ultrasonography. Am J Gastroenterol. 2001;96(5):1429–34.
36. Al-Taee AM, Taylor JR. Endoscopic imaging of pancreatic cysts. Gastrointest Endosc Clin N Am. 2023;33(3):583–98.
37. Olar MP, Bolboacă SD, Pojoga C, Moşteanu O, Gheorghiu M, Seicean R, et al. Clinical utility of the contrast-enhanced endoscopic ultrasound guided fine needle aspiration in the diagnosis of pancreatic cyst. Diagn Basel Switz. 2022;12(9):2209.
38. Yamashita Y, Ueda K, Itonaga M, Yoshida T, Maeda H, Maekita T, et al. Usefulness of contrast-enhanced endoscopic sonography for discriminating mural nodules from mucous clots in intraductal papillary mucinous neoplasms: a single-center prospective study. J Ultrasound Med Off. 2013;32(1):61–8.
39. Chon HK, Song TJ, Yoo KH, Hwang JS, Kim MH, Choi EK, et al. Enhancing mural nodules in the Main pancreatic duct of main and mixed types of intraductal papillary mucinous neoplasms: does size matter in malignancy risk? Gut Liver. 2023;17(6):942–8.
40. Brugge WR, Lewandrowski K, Lee-Lewandrowski E, Centeno BA, Szydlo T, Regan S, et al. Diagnosis of pancreatic cystic neoplasms: a report of the cooperative pancreatic cyst study. Gastroenterology. 2004;126(5):1330–6.
41. Khashab MA, Kim K, Lennon AM, Shin EJ, Tignor AS, Amateau SK, et al. Should we do EUS/FNA on patients with pancreatic cysts? The incremental diagnostic yield of EUS over CT/MRI for prediction of cystic neoplasms. Pancreas. 2013;42(4):717–21.

42. Manfrin E, Perini C, Di Stefano S, Bernardoni L, Parisi A, Frulloni L, et al. Pseudo solid-appearing pancreatic serous microcystic adenomas: histologic diagnosis with the EUS core biopsy fork-tip needle. Endosc Ultrasound. 2019;8(5):334–41.
43. Facciorusso A, Del Prete V, Antonino M, Buccino VR, Wani S. Diagnostic yield of EUS-guided through-the-needle biopsy in pancreatic cysts: a meta-analysis. Gastrointest Endosc. 2020;92(1):1–8.e3.
44. Tacelli M, Celsa C, Magro B, Barchiesi M, Barresi L, Capurso G, et al. Diagnostic performance of endoscopic ultrasound through-the-needle microforceps biopsy of pancreatic cystic lesions: systematic review with meta-analysis. Dig Endosc. 2020;32(7):1018–30.
45. Konda VJA, Meining A, Jamil LH, Giovannini M, Hwang JH, Wallace MB, et al. A pilot study of in vivo identification of pancreatic cystic neoplasms with needle-based confocal laser endomicroscopy under endosonographic guidance. Endoscopy. 2013;45(12):1006–13.
46. Modi RM, Kamboj AK, Swanson B, Conwell DL, Krishna SG. Novel technique for diagnosis of mucinous cystic neoplasms: in vivo and ex vivo confocal laser endomicroscopy. VideoGIE. 2017;2(3):55–6.
47. Napoleon B, Lemaistre AI, Pujol B, Caillol F, Lucidarme D, Bourdariat R, et al. In vivo characterization of pancreatic cystic lesions by needle-based confocal laser endomicroscopy (nCLE): proposition of a comprehensive nCLE classification confirmed by an external retrospective evaluation. Surg Endosc. 2016;30(6):2603–12.
48. Krishna SG, Swanson B, Hart PA, El-Dika S, Walker JP, McCarthy ST, et al. Validation of diagnostic characteristics of needle based confocal laser endomicroscopy in differentiation of pancreatic cystic lesions. Endosc Int Open. 2016;4(11):E1124–35.
49. Leung KK, Ross WA, Evans D, Fleming J, Lin E, Tamm EP, et al. Pancreatic cystic neoplasm: the role of cyst morphology, cyst fluid analysis, and expectant management. Ann Surg Oncol. 2009;16(10):2818–24.
50. Bick BL, Enders FT, Levy MJ, Zhang L, Henry MR, Abu Dayyeh BK, et al. The string sign for diagnosis of mucinous pancreatic cysts. Endoscopy. 2015;47(7):626–31.
51. Khamaysi I, Abu Ammar A, Vasilyev G, Arinstein A, Chowers Y, Zussman E. Differentiation of pancreatic cyst types by analysis of rheological behavior of pancreatic cyst fluid. Sci Rep. 2017;7:45589.
52. Tanaka M, Heckler M, Liu B, Heger U, Hackert T, Michalski CW. Cytologic analysis of pancreatic juice increases specificity of detection of malignant IPMN-A systematic review. Clin Gastroenterol Hepatol. 2019;17(11):2199–211.e21.
53. Al-Haddad M, Gill KR, Raimondo M, Woodward TA, Krishna M, Crook JE, et al. Safety and efficacy of cytology brushings versus standard fine-needle aspiration in evaluating cystic pancreatic lesions: a controlled study. Endoscopy. 2010;42(2):127–32.
54. Lariño-Noia J, de la Iglesia D, Iglesias-García J, Macías M, López Martín A, Legaz ML, et al. Endoscopic ultrasound cytologic brushing vs endoscopic ultrasound - fine needle aspiration for cytological diagnosis of cystic pancreatic lesions. A multicenter, randomized open-label trial. Rev Esp Enferm Dig. 2018;110(8):478–84.
55. Centeno BA, Warshaw AL, Mayo-Smith W, Southern JF, Lewandrowski K. Cytologic diagnosis of pancreatic cystic lesions. A prospective study of 28 percutaneous aspirates. Acta Cytol. 1997;41(4):972–80.
56. van der Waaij LA, van Dullemen HM, Porte RJ. Cyst fluid analysis in the differential diagnosis of pancreatic cystic lesions: a pooled analysis. Gastrointest Endosc. 2005;62(3):383–9.
57. Sharma RK, Bush N, Rana SS, Srinivasan R, Nada R, Gupta R, et al. Lower cyst fluid carcinoembryonic antigen cutoff is helpful in the differential diagnosis of mucinous versus non-mucinous pancreatic cysts. Indian J Gastroenterol. 2022;41(4):397–404.
58. Cizginer S, Turner BG, Bilge AR, Karaca C, Pitman MB, Brugge WR. Cyst fluid carcinoembryonic antigen is an accurate diagnostic marker of pancreatic mucinous cysts. Pancreas. 2011;40(7):1024–8.
59. Ngamruengphong S, Bartel MJ, Raimondo M. Cyst carcinoembryonic antigen in differentiating pancreatic cysts: a meta-analysis. Dig Liver Dis. 2013;45(11):920–6.

60. Park WGU, Mascarenhas R, Palaez-Luna M, Smyrk TC, O'Kane D, Clain JE, et al. Diagnostic performance of cyst fluid carcinoembryonic antigen and amylase in histologically confirmed pancreatic cysts. Pancreas. 2011;40(1):42–5.
61. Yip-Schneider MT, Barnard DS, Billings SD, Cheng L, Heilman DK, Lin A, et al. Cyclooxygenase-2 expression in human pancreatic adenocarcinomas. Carcinogenesis. 2000;21(2):139–46.
62. Singhi AD, Wood LD. Early detection of pancreatic cancer using DNA-based molecular approaches. Nat Rev Gastroenterol Hepatol. 2021;18(7):457–68.
63. Hata T, Dal Molin M, Suenaga M, Yu J, Pittman M, Weiss M, et al. Cyst fluid telomerase activity predicts the histologic grade of cystic neoplasms of the pancreas. Clin Cancer Res. 2016;22(20):5141–51.
64. Singhi AD, Nikiforova MN, Fasanella KE, McGrath KM, Pai RK, Ohori NP, et al. Preoperative GNAS and KRAS testing in the diagnosis of pancreatic mucinous cysts. Clin Cancer Res. 2014;20(16):4381–9.
65. Wu J, Matthaei H, Maitra A, Dal Molin M, Wood LD, Eshleman JR, et al. Recurrent GNAS mutations define an unexpected pathway for pancreatic cyst development. Sci Transl Med. 2011;3(92):92ra66.
66. Conner JR, Mariño-Enríquez A, Mino-Kenudson M, Garcia E, Pitman MB, Sholl LM, et al. Genomic characterization of low- and high-grade pancreatic mucinous cystic neoplasms reveals recurrent KRAS alterations in "high-risk" lesions. Pancreas. 2017;46(5):665–71.
67. Fischer CG, Wood LD. From somatic mutation to early detection: insights from molecular characterization of pancreatic cancer precursor lesions. J Pathol. 2018;246(4):395–404.
68. Gnoni A, Licchetta A, Scarpa A, Azzariti A, Brunetti AE, Simone G, et al. Carcinogenesis of pancreatic adenocarcinoma: precursor lesions. Int J Mol Sci. 2013;14(10):19731–62.
69. Gerdes B, Wild A, Wittenberg J, Barth P, Ramaswamy A, Kersting M, et al. Tumor-suppressing pathways in cystic pancreatic tumors. Pancreas. 2003;26(1):42–8.
70. Iacobuzio-Donahue CA, Wilentz RE, Argani P, Yeo CJ, Cameron JL, Kern SE, et al. Dpc4 protein in mucinous cystic neoplasms of the pancreas: frequent loss of expression in invasive carcinomas suggests a role in genetic progression. Am J Surg Pathol. 2000;24(11):1544–8.
71. Wu J, Jiao Y, Dal Molin M, Maitra A, de Wilde RF, Wood LD, et al. Whole-exome sequencing of neoplastic cysts of the pancreas reveals recurrent mutations in components of ubiquitin-dependent pathways. Proc Natl Acad Sci USA. 2011;108(52):21188–93.
72. Khalid A, Zahid M, Finkelstein SD, LeBlanc JK, Kaushik N, Ahmad N, et al. Pancreatic cyst fluid DNA analysis in evaluating pancreatic cysts: a report of the PANDA study. Gastrointest Endosc. 2009;69(6):1095–102.
73. Paniccia A, Polanco PM, Boone BA, Wald AI, McGrath K, Brand RE, et al. Prospective, multi-institutional, real-time next-generation sequencing of pancreatic cyst fluid reveals diverse genomic alterations that improve the clinical management of pancreatic cysts. Gastroenterology. 2023;164(1):117–133.e7.
74. McCarty TR, Garg R, Rustagi T. Pancreatic cyst fluid glucose in differentiating mucinous from nonmucinous pancreatic cysts: a systematic review and meta-analysis. Gastrointest Endosc. 2021;94(4):698–712.e6.
75. Groot VP, Gemenetzis G, Blair AB, Rivero-Soto RJ, Yu J, Javed AA, et al. Defining and predicting early recurrence in 957 patients with resected pancreatic ductal adenocarcinoma. Ann Surg. 2019;269(6):1154–62.
76. Del Chiaro M, Verbeke C, Salvia R, Klöppel G, Werner J, McKay C, et al. European experts consensus statement on cystic tumours of the pancreas. Dig Liver Dis. 2013;45(9):703–11.
77. Fritz S, Hackert T, Hinz U, Hartwig W, Büchler MW, Werner J. Role of serum carbohydrate antigen 19-9 and carcinoembryonic antigen in distinguishing between benign and invasive intraductal papillary mucinous neoplasm of the pancreas. Br J Surg. 2011;98(1):104–10.
78. Wang W, Zhang L, Chen L, Wei J, Sun Q, Xie Q, et al. Serum carcinoembryonic antigen and carbohydrate antigen 19-9 for prediction of malignancy and invasiveness in intraductal papillary mucinous neoplasms of the pancreas: a meta-analysis. Biomed Rep. 2015;3(1):43–50.

79. Moris D, Damaskos C, Spartalis E, Papalampros A, Vernadakis S, Dimitroulis D, et al. Updates and critical evaluation on novel biomarkers for the malignant progression of Intraductal papillary mucinous neoplasms of the pancreas. Anticancer Res. 2017;37(5):2185–94.
80. Nagtegaal ID, Odze RD, Klimstra D, Paradis V, Rugge M, Schirmacher P, et al. The 2019 WHO classification of tumours of the digestive system. Histopathology. 2020;76(2):182–8.
81. Tjaden C, Sandini M, Mihaljevic AL, Kaiser J, Khristenko E, Mayer P, et al. Risk of the watch-and-wait concept in surgical treatment of intraductal papillary mucinous neoplasm. JAMA Surg. 2021;156(9):818–25.
82. Nilsson LN, Keane MG, Shamali A, Millastre Bocos J, Marijinissen van Zanten M, Antila A, et al. Nature and management of pancreatic mucinous cystic neoplasm (MCN): a systematic review of the literature. Pancreatology. 2016;16(6):1028–36.
83. European study group on cystic Tumours of the pancreas. European evidence-based guidelines on pancreatic cystic neoplasms. Gut. 2018;67(5):789–804.
84. Ohtsuka T, Fernandez-Del Castillo C, Furukawa T, Hijioka S, Jang JY, Lennon AM, et al. International evidence-based Kyoto guidelines for the management of intraductal papillary mucinous neoplasm of the pancreas. Pancreatology. 2024;24(2):255–70.
85. Vege SS, Ziring B, Jain R, Moayyedi P, Clinical Guidelines Committee, American Gastroenterology Association. American gastroenterological association institute guideline on the diagnosis and management of asymptomatic neoplastic pancreatic cysts. Gastroenterology. 2015;148(4):819–22; quize12–13.
86. Tanaka M, Fernández-Del Castillo C, Kamisawa T, Jang JY, Levy P, Ohtsuka T, et al. Revisions of international consensus Fukuoka guidelines for the management of IPMN of the pancreas. Pancreatology. 2017;17(5):738–53.
87. Allen PJ, D'Angelica M, Gonen M, Jaques DP, Coit DG, Jarnagin WR, et al. A selective approach to the resection of cystic lesions of the pancreas: results from 539 consecutive patients. Ann Surg. 2006;244(4):572–82.
88. Clancy TE. Surgery for pancreatic cancer. Hematol Oncol Clin North Am. 2015;29(4):701–16.
89. McPhee JT, Hill JS, Whalen GF, Zayaruzny M, Litwin DE, Sullivan ME, et al. Perioperative mortality for pancreatectomy: a national perspective. Ann Surg [Internet]. 2007 [cited 2024 Sep 4];246(2). Available from: https://pubmed.ncbi.nlm.nih.gov/17667503/
90. Xiao W, Zhu J, Peng L, Hong L, Sun G, Li Y. The role of central pancreatectomy in pancreatic surgery: a systematic review and meta-analysis. HPB [Internet]. 2018 [cited 2024 Sep 4];20(10). Available from: https://pubmed.ncbi.nlm.nih.gov/29886106/
91. Liang H, Xie W, Lin X, Wang T, Xie J, Wang C, et al. Pathologic T1 and T2 encapsulated invasive carcinomas arising from mucinous cystic neoplasms of the pancreas have favorable prognosis and might be treated conservatively. J Pathol Clin Res. 2021;7(5):507–16.
92. Postlewait LM, Ethun CG, McInnis MR, Merchant N, Parikh A, Idrees K, et al. Association of preoperative risk factors with malignancy in pancreatic mucinous cystic neoplasms: a multicenter study. JAMA Surg. 2017;152(1):19–25.
93. Ahmad M, Maegawa FB, De La Rosa E, Davis B, Tyroch A, Konstantinidis IT. Mucinous cystic neoplasms of the pancreas in the modern era. Experience with 707 patients. Am J Surg. 2020;220(6):1433–7.
94. Keane MG, Shamali A, Nilsson LN, Antila A, Millastre Bocos J, Marijinissen Van Zanten M, et al. Risk of malignancy in resected pancreatic mucinous cystic neoplasms. Br J Surg. 2018;105(4):439–46.
95. Teoh AYB, Seo DW, Brugge W, Dewitt J, Kongkam P, Linghu E, et al. Position statement on EUS-guided ablation of pancreatic cystic neoplasms from an international expert panel. Endosc Int Open. 2019;7(9):E1064–77.
96. Oh HC, Seo DW, Song TJ, Moon SH, Park DH, Soo Lee S, et al. Endoscopic ultrasonography-guided ethanol lavage with paclitaxel injection treats patients with pancreatic cysts. Gastroenterology. 2011;140(1):172–9.
97. Papaefthymiou A, Johnson GJ, Maida M, Gkolfakis P, Ramai D, Facciorusso A, et al. Performance and safety of EUS ablation techniques for pancreatic cystic lesions: a systematic review and meta-analysis. Cancer. 2023;15(9):2627.

98. Choi JH, Seo DW, Song TJ, Park DH, Lee SS, Lee SK, et al. Long-term outcomes after endoscopic ultrasound-guided ablation of pancreatic cysts. Endoscopy. 2017;49(9):866–73.
99. Paiella S, Salvia R, Ramera M, Girelli R, Frigerio I, Giardino A, et al. Local ablative strategies for ductal pancreatic cancer (radiofrequency ablation, irreversible electroporation): a review. Gastroenterol Res Pract. 2016;2016(1):4508376.
100. Khoury T, Sbeit W, Napoléon B. Endoscopic ultrasound guided radiofrequency ablation for pancreatic tumors: a critical review focusing on safety, efficacy and controversies. World J Gastroenterol. 2023;29(1):157–70.
101. Moyer MT, Canakis A. Endoscopic ultrasound-guided ablation of pancreatic mucinous cysts. Gastrointest Endosc Clin N Am. 2024;34(3):537–52.
102. Castellanos JA, Merchant NB. Intensity of follow-up after pancreatic cancer resection. Ann Surg Oncol. 2014;21(3):747–51.
103. Luk L, Hecht EM, Kang S, Bhosale PR, Francis IR, Gandhi N, et al. Society of Abdominal Radiology disease focused panel survey on clinical utilization of incidental pancreatic cyst management recommendations and template reporting. J Am Coll Radiol. 2021;18(9):1324–31.
104. Madhani K, Yousaf M, Aamar A, Ooka K, Muniraj T, Aslanian H, et al. Impact of endoscopic ultrasound on diagnosis and management of presumed mucinous neoplasms when done for pancreatic cyst morphology change on non-invasive surveillance imaging. Endosc Int Open. 2019;7(4):E389–95.
105. Megibow AJ, Baker ME, Morgan DE, Kamel IR, Sahani DV, Newman E, et al. Management of incidental pancreatic cysts: a white paper of the ACR incidental findings committee. J Am Coll Radiol. 2017;14(7):911–23.
106. Elta GH, Enestvedt BK, Sauer BG, Lennon AM. ACG clinical guideline: diagnosis and Management of Pancreatic Cysts. Am J Gastroenterol. 2018;113(4):464–79.
107. Chhoda A, Singh S, Sheth AH, Grimshaw AA, Gunderson CG, Sharma P, et al. Benefit of extended surveillance of low-risk pancreatic cysts after 5-year stability: a systematic review and meta-analysis. Clin Gastroenterol Hepatol. 2023;21(6):1430–46.

Comprehensive Management of Serous Cystic Neoplasm of the Pancreas

9

Kartikeya Mathur, Chhagan Lal Birda, Ankit Agarwal, and Ashish Agarwal

Abstract

The widespread use of high-resolution cross-sectional imaging and the progressive aging of the population have led to a marked increase in the detection of pancreatic cystic lesions (PCLs), the majority of which are detected incidentally. These lesions encompass a heterogeneous spectrum ranging from benign, premalignant, and malignant, posing significant diagnostic and management challenges. Serous cystic neoplasms (SCNs) represent the most common benign PCLs predominantly detected in older women, frequent involvement of the pancreatic body and tail, and an indolent clinical course with a very low risk of malignant transformation. Most SCNs remain asymptomatic and can be safely managed conservatively once an accurate diagnosis is established. However, differentiating SCNs from mucinous and malignant cystic neoplasms remains a critical challenge, as management strategies differ substantially. Diagnostic uncertainty often necessitates a nuanced approach that balances the risks of unnecessary surgical intervention against the potential consequences of missed malignancy. This chapter provides a comprehensive and up-to-date review of serous cystic neoplasms, focusing on their epidemiology, pathogenesis, clinical presentation, and natural history. It critically discusses current diagnostic strategies, including advanced imaging modalities and adjunctive tools, outlines surgical and nonsurgical management options, and highlights emerging developments in diagnostics and therapeutics.

K. Mathur · C. L. Birda · A. Agarwal · A. Agarwal (✉)
Department of Gastroenterology, All India Institute of Medical Sciences, Jodhpur, Rajasthan, India
e-mail: drkartikeyamathur@geetanjaliuniversity.com; ankitagarwal@aiims.edu; agarwal_a@aiimsjodhpur.edu.in

R. K. Sharma et al. (eds.), *Differential Diagnosis and Management of Pancreatic Cystic Lesions*, https://doi.org/10.1007/978-981-92-0654-4_9

Keywords

Serous cystadenoma · Non malignant cyst · Non mucinous cyst · Diagnosis · Benign pancreatic cyst

Abbreviations

ACG	American College of Gastroenterology
ACR	American College of Radiology
AI	Artificial Intelligence
AUC	area under curve
CEA	carcinoembryonic antigen
CLE	confocal laser endomicroscopy
CNN	convolutional neural network
CT	computed tomography
CP	chronic pancreatitis
EUS	endoscopic ultrasound
FNA	fine-needle aspiration
GNAS	GNAS complex Locus (originally named after the G-protein alpha-stimulatory subunit)
IPMN	intraductal papillary mucinous neoplasm
KRAS	Kirsten rat sarcoma viral oncogene homolog
MCN	mucinous cystic neoplasm
MFB	micro forceps biopsy
MPD	main pancreatic duct
MRI	magnetic resonance imaging
PCL	pancreatic cystic lesions
RNF43	ring finger protein 43
SCN	serous cystic neoplasms
TTNB	through-the-needle micro biopsy
VEGF	vascular endothelial growth factor

9.1 Introduction

There has been an increase in the incidence and prevalence of pancreatic cystic lesions (PCLs) due to the increasing availability of high-quality cross-sectional imaging and the aging population. Most of these cysts are detected incidentally during scans done for unrelated reasons [1]. These cysts are characterized as benign, precancerous, and cancerous. Serous cystic neoplasms (SCNs) are the most common benign PCL, and approximately 60% of them would continue to be asymptomatic over a long period [2]. They primarily affect older women and are predominantly seen in the body or tail of the pancreas, although 40% of cases can be present in the head of the pancreas. They are often sporadic, though the prevalence is higher in patients with Von Hippel–Lindau disease [2]. SCNs have a low risk of malignant potential and a slow growth rate. The main challenge lies in differentiating a benign cyst from a precancerous and a cancerous cyst since the management differs drastically.

Thus, once confident about the diagnosis, most asymptomatic cases do not require any intervention. In cases where the diagnosis is uncertain, management can be challenging and calls for a careful balance between action and observation. With the help of pertinent references and illustrations, this chapter offers a thorough review of SCN care, including diagnosis, imaging methods, surgical procedures, and the most recent developments in therapy and research.

9.2 Diagnosis

9.2.1 Presentation

SCNs are mostly identified in women in the fifth to seventh decade, although they can be diagnosed at any age. Most patients with SCNs are asymptomatic, and the lesion is often identified incidentally. In a large multicenter study that recruited more than 2600 patients, up to 60% of the cases with SCN were asymptomatic, 27% had nonspecific abdominal pain, 5% had diabetes, and only 9% had pancreaticobiliary symptoms [2]. Examination in patients with SCN is mostly unremarkable except in patients with larger cysts where a vague abdominal lump may be palpable. In all patients with PCLs, a detailed medical history should be taken to uncover any history of acute or chronic pancreatitis and any underlying familial pancreatic cancer syndromes. If available, previous imaging should also be reviewed as it may be useful to narrow down the differentials and provide invaluable insights into the growth rate and the inherent malignant potential associated with the PCL. Patients with a significant family history of pancreatic cancer should consider undergoing complete genetic counselling and testing [3].

9.2.2 Imaging Techniques

Diagnosis of SCN relies heavily on imaging modalities, including computed tomography (CT), magnetic resonance imaging (MRI), and endoscopic ultrasound (EUS). Although the overall diagnostic accuracy of cross-sectional imaging modalities is generally low for PCLs, it is highest in the case of SCN [4]. In most cases, SCN can be diagnosed with certainty using these imaging modalities, and no further intervention is required. The cysts can have one of the following four morphological patterns on imaging: microcystic, macrocystic, mixed, and solid. Multiple cysts less than 2 cm apart, spaced by fibrous, very thin septa that may converge into a *central stellate scar* that may calcify, make up the more prevalent microcystic pattern. The lesion takes on a "honeycomb" form when the cysts are numerous and smaller than a centimeter [5]. The macrocystic pattern, characterized by a small number of cysts measuring less than 2 cm and lacking a central scar, can frequently be confused with other PCLs. A few bigger cysts (> 2 cm) are found peripherally in the less common mixed form. The solid variant, also called as solid serous adenoma, has no cystic component on imaging. In a multinational review of 2622 patients with SCA [2], the authors observed that the most frequent pattern was microcystic (45%), followed by macrocystic (32%), mixed type (18%), and honeycomb pattern (5%). Each imaging modality provides distinct advantages and limitations in identifying the unique characteristics of SCN.

9.2.2.1 Computed Tomography

Because of its accessibility and high spatial resolution, dedicated pancreatic protocol contrast-enhanced CT is frequently utilized as the first imaging modality to evaluate PCLs. SCNs appear as distinct polycystic lesions with lobulated contours on CT scans with a central fibrous scar. The lesions resemble honeycombs or spongy patches because they comprise multiple tiny cysts (less than 2 cm). The central fibrous scar shows early enhancement with contrast injection and persistent enhancement on delayed imaging, a feature unique to SCN. When calcified, the central scar can take on the characteristics of a *sunburst or starburst pattern*, which is also unique to SCN (Fig. 9.1).

For the diagnosis of SCN, the combination of lobulated margins and microcystic appearance has a sensitivity of 68%, a specificity of 100%, and a positive predictive value of 100%. On the other hand, the values for the central scar are 32.4%, 100%, and 100%, respectively [6], suggesting that the central scar, microcystic appearance, and lobulated borders are pathognomonic for SCN. Nevertheless, these features have a limited sensitivity (30–70%); therefore, their absence does not rule out SCN as a diagnosis. According to some authors, the "circumvascular sign"—that is, the presence of some aberrant arteries encircling the lesion on the arterial

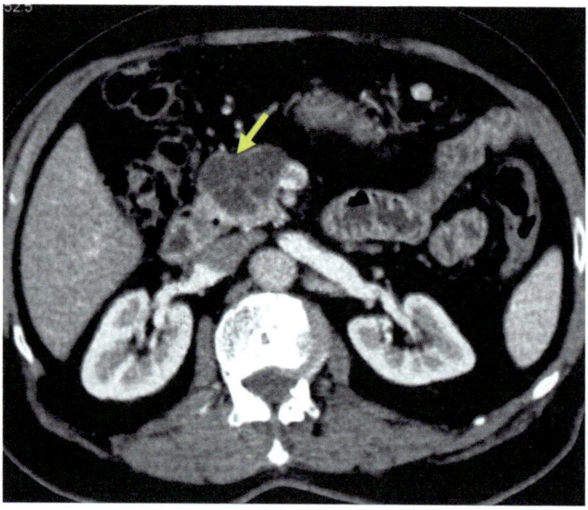

Fig. 9.1 Axial contrast-enhanced CT shows a polycystic mass within the head of the pancreas, with lobulated margins giving the "bunch of grapes"/ "honeycomb" appearance (arrow). No enhancement was noted within the lesion. Features suggest pancreatic serous cystadenoma

phase—and the presence of a central calcification are both pathognomonic for SCN on MDCT (100% specificity) [7].

MRI is more sensitive than CT in identifying noncalcified central scars. It can be challenging to diagnose uncommon and atypical presentations of SCN with CT alone, such as macrocystic variants or those with a primarily solid appearance. These cases should be further evaluated with MRI or EUS [4].

9.2.2.2 MRI Findings

In comparison to CT, MRI is more sensitive in detecting PCLs and provides a more accurate internal structure characterization of SCNs. According to 19 studies in a systematic review, CT had a sensitivity and specificity of 36.3–71.4% and 64–100% in identifying a benign disease and an accuracy of 39–45% in making a specific diagnosis, but MRI had a 89.7% and 91.4–100% sensitivity and specificity, respectively, in evaluating the main pancreatic duct connectivity [8]. SCNs typically show up on MRI as well-circumscribed, polycystic, or lobulated masses. They can be hyperintense on T2-weighted scans and show varying intensities on T1-weighted imaging, depending on the protein content of the cyst fluid. On T2-weighted imaging, the core scar is often hypointense, but it exhibits contrast enhancement and thin septation enhancement. These characteristic features help differentiate SCNs from MCNs or IPMNs (Fig. 9.2).

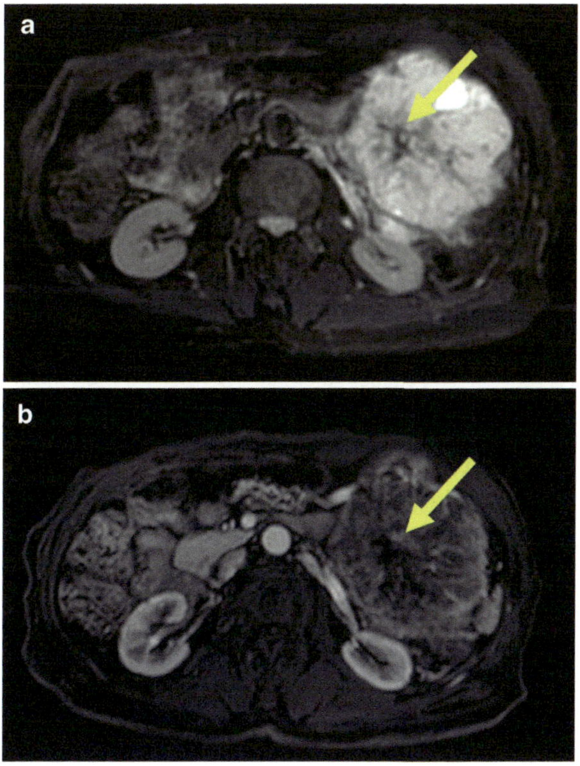

Fig. 9.2 Axial T2W MR (**a**) and post-contrast T1-weighted MR (**b**); images show a microcystic mass within the tail region of the pancreas with fine external lobulations and multiple thin enhancing internal septations. Fibrous central scar with calcification showing no post-contrast enhancement (arrow) is a classic feature of serous cystadenoma

Often, the macrocystic pattern is mistaken for other PCLs, especially intraductal papillary mucinous neoplasms (IPMN) and mucinous cystic neoplasms (MCN). Differential diagnosis is important since SCN is often benign, while MCN and IPMN can act like malignant tumors. A set of 41 PCLs showed significant differences in lesion morphology between SCN, MCN, and IPMN: MCN has a smooth contour with or without septation, while macrocystic SCN has a multicystic or lobulated contour with or without septation, while IPMN has either a pleomorphic or a clubbed finger-like cystic shape [9]. Furthermore, since IPMN interacts with the main pancreatic duct and makes this communication evident at MRCP, it can be differentiated from SCN. However, a definite diagnosis is not always possible, and thus further evaluation, including sampling, is sometimes needed.

Also, a pseudosolid form is an uncommon variant of SCN. Under the microscope, the serous solid adenoma resembles the serous microcystic cystadenoma in architecture and cytology. This is because the solid adenoma lacks secretory activity, which results in a more compact structure than the cystic, and the cystic spaces are small, consisting of cuboid cells derived from the ductular epithelium. A substantial contrast enhancement in the stromal components of these lesions can lead to an inaccurate diagnosis of a neuroendocrine tumor on MDCT; however, MRI's high sensitivity to static fluids makes it easy to identify this variation [10, 11].

Each imaging modality has its own merits and demerits. While CT can depict calcifications and hypervascularity, it provides insufficient soft tissue contrast and spatial resolution, which does not allow for the identification of the microcystic appearance and SCAs less than 2 cm in size [8]. MRI, conversely, is superior to CT when identifying septations, the presence of a solid component, pancreatic ductal communication, and magnification of the macrocystic nature [8]. However, it is limited by its availability and is prone to motion artefícts. Due to their complementary nature, the best strategy is usually a combination of both CT and MRI. Most cases can be definitively diagnosed using a combination of CT and MRI examination; further evaluation is generally needed in a few patients to further characterize the nature of the cystic lesion.

9.2.2.3 Endoscopic Ultrasound (EUS) Findings

EUS has now become a more widely utilized modality in distinguishing benign, precancerous, and malignant PCLs with a diagnostic accuracy of around 50–75% [12]. The major limitation of EUS is that it is operator-dependent and is affected by variable interobserver agreement. The better resolution and the additional option to perform cyst fluid sampling for biochemical and cytological examination make EUS the gold standard for examining PCLs. The characteristics of SCN in EUS findings include the following:

(i) *Microcystic (honeycomb) appearance*: The microcystic pattern, which is typified by a large number of tiny, anechoic cysts (less than 2 cm) grouped in a honeycomb-like structure, is the most typical EUS finding in SCN (Fig. 9.3).

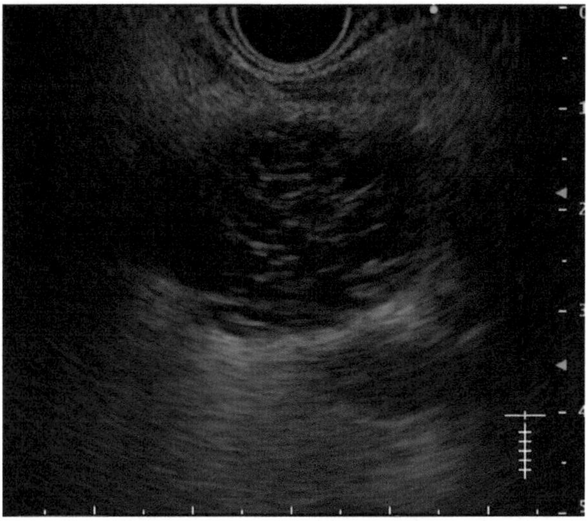

Fig. 9.3 Endoscopic ultrasound in a patient with a small pancreatic cyst shows anechoic cysts grouped in a honeycomb-like structure in the body of the pancreas, which is highly typical of SCN

This pattern distinguishes SCN from mucinous cystic lesions and strongly indicates SCN.

(ii) *Central stellate scar*: Hypervascular central scars can be a crucial diagnostic indicator for differentiating SCN from other cystic lesions on EUS. Calcifications may be present in a central stellate scar, which is observed as a hyperechoic region on EUS.

(iii) *Thin, regular septations*: Thin, well-defined septations within the cyst can be seen with EUS. These septations are homogeneous and regular, contrasting the more irregular and thicker septations found in mucinous tumors. Further, the septations are often hypervascular on Doppler examination in patients with SCN (Fig. 9.4).

(iv) *Absence of solid nodules*: SCNs typically do not have solid components or mural nodules, unlike potentially malignant cystic lesions like MCNs or IPMNs. The lack of these characteristics on EUS strongly points to a benign origin.

Indications for EUS-Guided Sampling Although EUS is operator-dependent with variable interobserver agreement, a large study has shown that the interobserver agreement is highest between endosonographers for diagnosing SCN with certainty [13]. Also, due to the presence of multiple tiny cysts and high vascularity of the epithelium and septa, sampling in cases with microcystic SCN is generally avoided. However, a fine-needle aspiration/biopsy may be helpful in cases with oligocystic variants, cysts with thicker walls, or cases where a carcinomatous transformation of the cyst is suspected. Although the findings are not specific to SCA, they can help differentiate benign and precancerous (mucinous) cysts and thus guide further management.

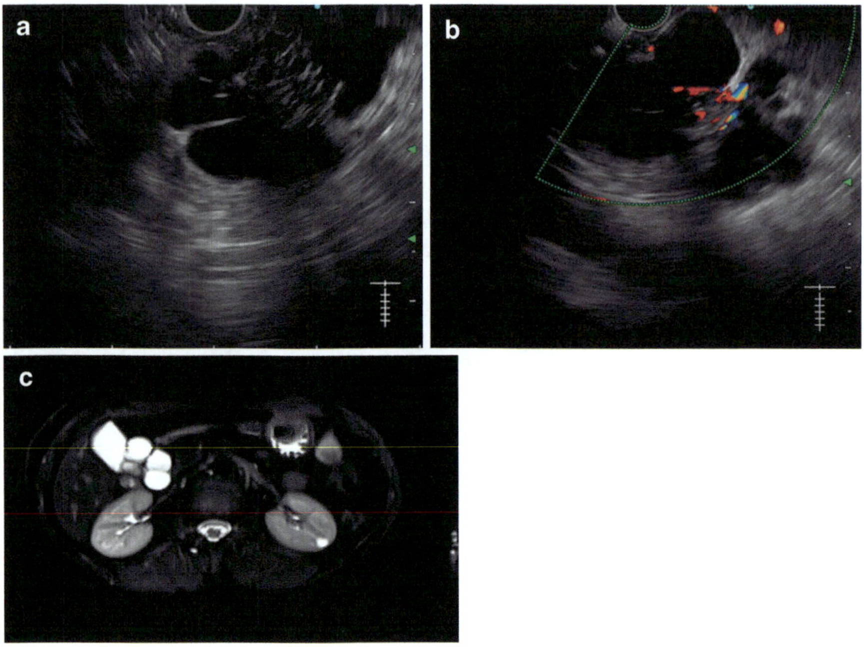

Fig. 9.4 Endoscopic ultrasound shows (**a**) multiple large cysts with thin septae in the periphery with a honeycomb appearance in the center with (**b**) Doppler showing high vascularity in the septae. Both features are suggestive of mixed variant of SCN. (**c**) CEMR image of the same patient showing a multilocular cyst with septations in the head of pancreas

9.2.2.4 Cyst Fluid Characteristics

Gross Examination

On gross appearance, SCN cyst fluid is generally described as *low-viscosity or watery due to the absence of mucin*. This contrasts with the *high-viscosity (thick, mucinous)* fluid in mucinous cysts (IPMNs and MCNs). The samples may be hemorrhagic due to the presence of highly vascular epithelium and septa.

Biochemical Analysis

Amylase As amylase is a digestive enzyme secreted by the pancreas, levels are higher in PCLs, with ductal communication (pseudocyst, IPMN). The amylase levels in SCN fluid are typically *low or normal*. However, there are no specific cutoffs for SCN.

Carcinoembryonic Antigen (CEA) CEA levels in the SCN cyst fluid are typically *very low or undetectable*, usually below 5 ng/mL. This finding is highly suggestive of SCN. Interestingly, one study showed that in a cohort of patients with cyst fluid CEA levels <30 ng/mL and amylase levels <350 U/L, 85% of cases were diagnosed as SCN [14].

Glucose Levels Cyst fluid glucose level is rapidly gaining attention in the differential diagnosis of PCLs as it is rapid, readily available, and inexpensive. Mucinous cysts often have low or undetectable glucose levels in the cyst fluid. This feature helps differentiate MCNs from SCNs, which generally have a higher glucose level. While not always specific, low glucose levels may assist in distinguishing mucinous PCLs from SCNs and pseudocysts. A recent systematic review and meta-analysis showed that intracystic glucose ≤50 mg/dL has a pooled sensitivity and specificity of 90.5% and 88%, respectively, for differentiating mucinous and nonmucinous PCLs [15]. A study by Park et al. has also shown that the mean cyst fluid glucose levels for SCA are higher compared to pseudocysts (98 mg/dL and 23 mg/dL, respectively) [16]. Although promising, very few studies have shown the utility of cyst fluid glucose levels for differentiating different benign PCLs.

Cyst Fluid Cytology

SCN fluid aspirates are generally acellular or paucicellular with a clear or hemorrhagic background and an absence of necrosis, atypia, and mitoses. Occasionally, glycogen-rich cuboidal epithelial cells may be identified, which, though specific for SCN, may not always be found. Some studies have also shown that the presence of hemosiderin-laden macrophages in the cyst fluid, although uncommon, can provide a clue to the diagnosis of SCN [14, 17].

9.2.2.5 Others—New and Investigational Modalities

Molecular Analysis

While biochemical tests cannot identify specific cyst types, molecular markers can be used to diagnose specific types of cysts definitively. SCNs are generally negative for KRAS and GNAS mutations, which are commonly seen in mucinous neoplasms (IPMNs and MCNs). VHL gene inactivation or loss of heterozygosity is highly sensitive and specific for the diagnosis of SCN, and the presence of VHL mutation with an absence of KRAS, GNAS, and RNF43 mutation can preoperatively diagnose SCN with high sensitivity (71–100%) and specificity (91–100%) [18, 19]. However, VHL mutation may not be seen in many patients with SCN, and there is no other available marker specific for SCN. The diagnosis thus can be made only by the absence of markers specific for other cyst variants (KRAS and GNAS—mucinous cysts, CTNNB1—solid pseudopapillary neoplasm).

Proteomic and Metabolomic Studies

Recent studies have explored the cyst fluid's proteomic and metabolomic profiles in SCNs. Specific proteins like vascular endothelial growth factor (VEGF) may be elevated in SCNs compared to mucinous neoplasms. Carcinoembryonic antigen 19–9 (CA 19–9) is low or undetectable in the SCN cyst fluid, further helping to differentiate it from mucinous neoplasms [20]. Further, some studies have shown differences in the lipid composition of the SCN cyst fluid compared to other cyst types, though this is not widely used in routine practice [21].

EUS-Through-the-Needle Micro Biopsy Forceps

Recently, there has been a growing interest in tissue acquisition in cystic lesions of the pancreas, and diagnosis has evolved from cyst fluid sampling to histological criteria using needle-based confocal endomicroscopy, through-the-needle cystoscopy, and through-the-needle intracystic biopsy [22]. Cyst wall sampling using through-the-needle micro biopsy (TTNB) forceps has gained the most interest among these techniques. The Moray micro forceps biopsy (MFB) device (US Endoscopy, Ohio, US) is a disposable tissue acquisition device that can be passed through a 19G needle, allowing for tissue sampling of the cyst wall. In a systematic review of 463 patients, EUS-guided MFB was able to establish the correct final diagnosis in 312 out of 455 (diagnostic accuracy 68.6%; 95% CI, 61%–76%) PCLs and concluded that MFB is better than EUS-FNA in differentiating non-neoplastic from neoplastic PCLs and diagnosing the specific type of cyst [23].

High-Risk Features

SCNs generally have nonspecific symptoms that are similar to those of other cystic neoplasms. Macrocystic SCNs are a rare presentation that resemble MCNs but might be unilocular or have a few big locules [24]. Features such as the development of weight loss/jaundice, rapid growth of cyst, features of gastric outlet obstruction or biliary obstruction, or pancreatobiliary pain on imaging features such as unilocular cysts or cysts with the involvement of surrounding structures suggesting local invasion are high-risk features and require consideration of surgical intervention.

Differential Diagnosis

The differential diagnosis of SCN includes other cystic pancreatic lesions such as:

- *Mucinous cystic neoplasms (MCNs)*: Differentiated by the presence of ovarian-type stroma and a higher propensity for malignancy. MCNs are typically unilocular with thick walls and often present in the body and tail of the pancreas.
- *Intraductal papillary mucinous neoplasms (IPMNs)*: Distinguished by communication with the pancreatic duct and the presence of mucin-producing epithelium. Main duct IPMNs exhibit dilated pancreatic ducts, while branch-duct IPMNs show cysts that branch off from the main duct.
- *Pseudocysts*: Usually associated with a history of pancreatitis and lack internal septations or cystic locules typical of neoplastic cysts. Unlike the clear fluid seen in SCNs, they may contain debris or hemorrhage.

9.3 Management

9.3.1 Natural Course of SCN

The natural history of patients with SCN was investigated in a retrospective international study involving 2622 patients [2]. They comprised all SCN cases identified by radiology or histology from 1994 to 2014. The median age at diagnosis in this study was 58 years, and 74% of the patients were female. 39% of patients had no surgery, 9% had resection after a year of follow-up (median: 3 years, size at diagnosis: 25 mm), and 52% had surgery during the first year following diagnosis (median cyst size was 40 mm). Uncertain diagnosis (60%), symptoms (23%), size rise (12%), excessive size (6%), and compression of surrounding organs (5%) were surgical indications. Size grew 37% in patients who were monitored for more than a year (n = 1271) (growth rate: 4 mm/year), was stable in 57%, and decreased in 6%. Only three cases of serous cystadenocarcinomas were recorded (0.1%).

A three-decade experience at a single center with 1290 resections of pancreatic cysts by Roldán, Jorge et al. [25] had 62% female patients with a mean age of 60 years. Fifty-seven percent of tumors were incidentally discovered, of which 13% were SCN. The study suggests that resections done for MCN and SCN have decreased significantly over the three decades. Resections done for benign non-neoplastic lesions have also decreased (13%–5.5%, P = 0.004), signifying better imaging modalities to diagnose SCN correctly, and the majority are being followed up with imaging.

SCN was diagnosed in 273 out of 1177 (23.1%) patients undergoing surveillance and in 27 patients requiring resection for incidental PCLs, according to a retrospective review of a prospectively kept database of all patients referred for PCL between January 2005 and March 2016 [26]. Overall, 300 out of 1271 patients (23.6%) who presented with an accidental PCL had a suspected or confirmed diagnosis of SCA. After an average follow-up of 36 months, no adverse events were noted in patients receiving surveillance with a suspected diagnosis of SCN. This data demonstrates that a diagnostic error typically does not lead to incorrect management when there are no concerning features or high-risk stigmata.

These studies thus suggest that (1) A majority of patients with SCN are asymptomatic. (2) SCN has a low growth rate, and new onset symptoms in a previously asymptomatic patient are rare. (3) SCN has very low malignant progression. (4) SCN is associated with almost nil disease-specific mortality.

Currently, there is a lack of coherence among the guidelines regarding the optimal duration, interval, and mode of follow-up imaging of SCN. For people with "asymptomatic" SCN, the American College of Gastroenterology (ACG) advises against follow-up. But symptoms lack a definite definition [27]. Only when blockage symptoms (bile duct, stomach, duodenum, portal vein) are present is surgical resection recommended by the European guidelines, which also call for a 1-year follow-up [28]. Similar to ACG, the American College of Radiology (ACR) does not specify symptoms but advises against additional surveillance for SCAs unless they are symptomatic [29]. Regular imaging is associated with increased healthcare costs, so a conscious decision should be made regarding follow-up imaging if a diagnosis of SCN is certain. Furthermore surgery for PCL's comes with their own set of complications including pancreatic leak and exocrine and endocrine insufficiency.

Management protocol for SCN varies depending on the policies of the center and includes the following (Fig. 9.5).

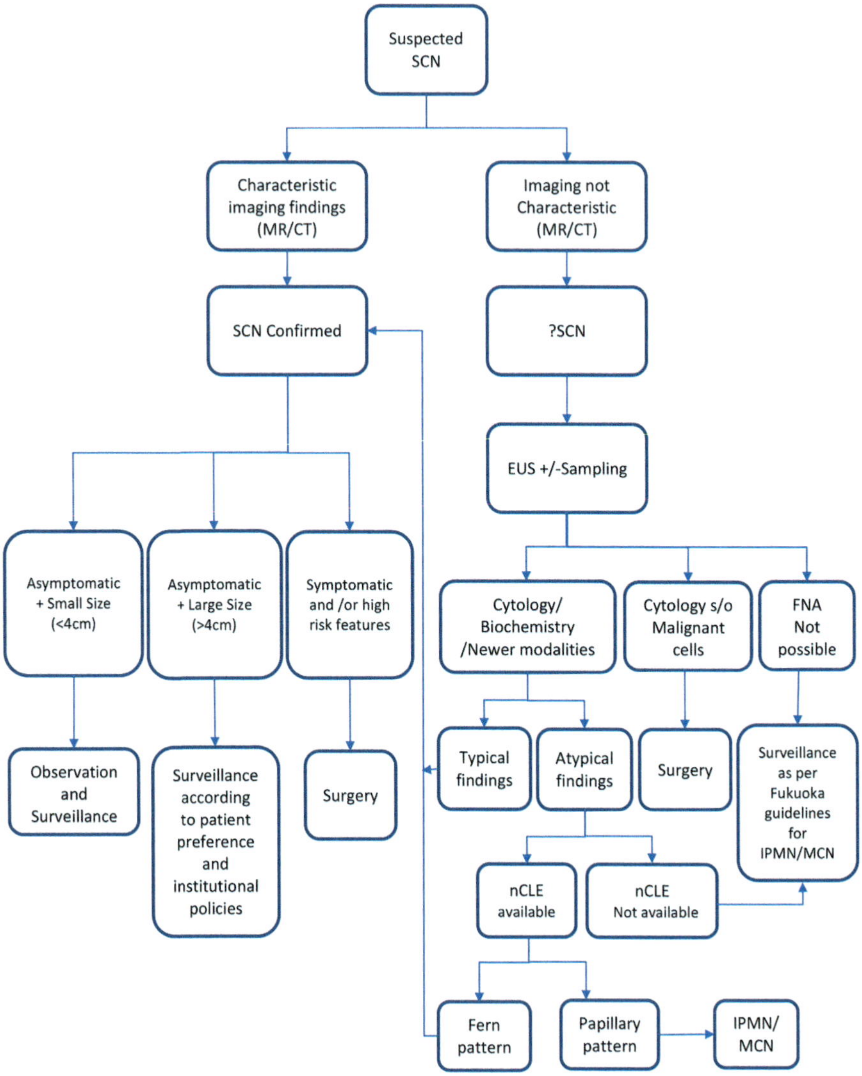

CT (Computed Tomography); EUS (Endoscopic Ultrasound); IPMN (Intraductal Papillary Mucinous neoplasm); MCN (Mucinous cystic neoplasm); MR (Magnetic Resonance Imaging); nCLE (Confocal laser endomicroscopy); SCN (Serous cystic neoplasm).

Fig. 9.5 Approach to pancreatic cystic lesion suspected of SCN

9.3.2 Observation

Observation is generally recommended for asymptomatic SCNs smaller than 4 cm without worrisome features such as rapid growth or the presence of solid components [30]. This cautious approach is recommended primarily based on SCNs' modest development rate and low risk of cancer. Evidence that most SCNs remain stable over time supports the choice to watch rather than perform surgery. These patients should only be reviewed in the case of appearance of symptoms, and then further imaging should be done for evaluation.

9.3.3 Surgical Management

Surgical intervention is indicated for:

- Symptomatic SCNs causing pain or obstructive jaundice or symptoms likely arising from SCN directly.
- Rapidly growing cysts on follow-up imaging.
- Diagnostic uncertainty.
- Features suggestive of malignant transformation [31].

Surgery is often indicated for SCN that presents a serious risk or produces a great deal of symptoms, making its removal necessary to enhance the patient's quality of life or rule out cancer.

9.3.4 Types of Surgery

Enucleation: Suitable for small, easily accessible lesions involving careful dissection from surrounding pancreatic tissue. This procedure preserves most of the pancreatic tissue, reducing the risk of postoperative pancreatic insufficiency.
Distal pancreatectomy: Removal of the distal portion of the pancreas, often with the spleen, for tumors located in the body or tail of the pancreas. This approach is indicated for larger lesions or those with a higher risk of malignancy.
Whipple procedure (pancreaticoduodenectomy): Extensive surgery for tumors in the head of the pancreas, involving removal of the head of the pancreas, duodenum, bile duct, and sometimes part of the stomach. This procedure is more complex and is associated with higher morbidity and mortality rates, but it is necessary for large or symptomatic lesions in the pancreatic head.
Laparoscopic approach: Minimally invasive option for suitable candidates, offering advantages such as reduced postoperative pain, shorter hospital stay, and quicker recovery [32]. Advances in laparoscopic techniques and robotic surgery have made these approaches increasingly feasible for SCNs, with outcomes comparable to open surgery.

It is pretty much clear that any asymptomatic SCN of size <4 cm can be safely observed, and SCNs with high-risk features or symptoms should be subjected to surgery. However, there is a lack of consensus regarding patients with asymptomatic large SCN with size >6 cm. The cyst size does not always correlate with the growth rate of the cyst [33]. If the diagnosis is certain with imaging, surveillance of SCN is not needed most of the time as these cysts, irrespective of their size, have a slow growth rate and rarely turn malignant [2]. For large asymptomatic cysts, annual CT or MRI imaging is suggested to track any changes in the lesion's size or development of alarm features. The follow-up intervals may be extended if the lesion stays stable over several years. If the lesion shows a rapid growth rate, shows high-risk features on imaging, or the patient becomes symptomatic, surgery may be indicated on follow-up [34]. The decision to intervene or not should also be taken considering patient-specific characteristics, taking into account age (younger patients might opt for surgical intervention considering long follow-up and radiation exposure over the long term and better surgical outcomes), comorbidities, and most importantly, patient's preference and expertise available at that center.

Thus, most patients without any symptoms and with small cysts and classical imaging findings of SCN can be managed conservatively and may not even require follow-up imaging. Surgery is indicated in a small proportion of patients where the diagnosis is unclear, the presence of high-risk or worrisome features, or significant and related symptoms.

9.4 Future Research Areas/Avenues/Directions

9.4.1 Newer Molecular Biomarkers

Ongoing research aims to identify specific biomarkers that can definitively differentiate SCNs from other cystic lesions and predict the risk of malignancy [35]. The identification of trustworthy biomarkers can transform pancreatic cystic lesion detection and treatment, eliminating the need for invasive operations and enhancing patient outcomes. In a study done by Chikashi Watase et al. [36], the gene expression profiles of SCN was compared with that of normal pancreatic tissue and pancreatic ductal adenocarcinoma. The expression of the molecules that were upregulated in SCN was then compared with that in other types of PCLS. They found that Aquaporin 1 (AQP1) and STRC were highly upregulated in SCN and were not seen commonly in other PCLs or were expressed in very low quantities, suggesting that these markers could potentially be used as SCN markers. Similarly, multiple other studies are underway to identify a molecular marker that can identify various PCL subtypes to guide definite management and avoid unnecessary confusion and anxiety [37–39].

9.4.2 Advanced Imaging Techniques

A new technique for assessing and subtyping PCLs is confocal laser endomicroscopy (CLE). A 19-gauge FNA needle is used to introduce a tiny probe, which takes microscopic pictures of the cyst's epithelial lining. The effectiveness of nCLE in treating indeterminate cystic lesions of the pancreas, particularly those with concerning characteristics, has now been documented in a number of investigations. To offer accepted classifications, nCLE findings in cyst subtypes have been well associated with pathological findings [40]. An SCN is identified by the presence of a superficial vascular network or fern-like pattern; an IPMN is identified by papillary projections; an MCN is identified by a dark band; a pseudocyst is identified by bright particles; and malignancy is identified by dark patches [41]. It offers a noninvasive and real-time assessment of tissue morphology, providing a "virtual biopsy" that can help differentiate benign from malignant lesions. CLE can also guide fine-needle aspirations, assess surgical margins, and monitor disease progression. While CLE has limitations, such as being operator-dependent and having a limited penetration depth, it remains a promising technology for improving the diagnosis and management of SCNs. According to a study, nCLE's diagnostic accuracy was comparable to that of standard cytology (77% vs. 66%; $P = 0.12$). With only one case of severe pancreatitis and one instance of transitory pruritis and an infected pseudocyst, the study's adverse effects were minimal at 3.5%. According to the studies, 4.3% of PCLs experienced post-procedural acute pancreatitis on average [40].

Recent studies have also demonstrated the potential of radiomics and FDG-PET in improving the characterization, differentiation, and prediction of malignant transformation in SCNs of the pancreas. Radiomics, a quantitative analysis technique, extracts features from medical images that can help differentiate SCNs from other PCLs and identify high-risk subgroups [42]. FDG-PET, a functional imaging technique, measures the metabolic activity of SCNs, which can aid in distinguishing benign from malignant lesions [43]. Combined radiomics and FDG-PET analysis can predict the risk of malignant transformation, evaluate treatment response, and develop prognostic models for SCNs. However, further research is needed to standardize radiomic feature extraction and analysis methods and to validate these techniques in larger datasets [44].

In a study, Leang Sim Nguon [45] examined the use of artificial intelligence (AI) to distinguish between SCN and MCN. To do so, he used a convolutional neural network (CNN) model with ResNet50. Retrospective data collection was done on 49 SCN and 59 MCN patients from two hospitals. The suggested network model had an accuracy of up to 82.75% and an area under the curve (AUC) score of 0.88 (95% CI: 0.817–0.930) (Fig. 9.5).

9.5 Conclusion

Although typical SCNs are easy to diagnose using the available imaging modalities, they often have atypical presentation and thus pose a diagnostic dilemma. Technological advancements in cross-sectional imaging, endoscopic examination, and molecular marker emergence have made a definitive diagnosis of SCN feasible in most cases. A balanced strategy combining surveillance and surgical intervention depending on lesion characteristics and patient considerations is needed to manage SCNs. Improved results are anticipated as minimally invasive procedures and imaging methods continue to develop with the emergence of new molecular markers. Optimizing management methods is the goal of ongoing research into biomarkers and long-term outcomes. In order to provide patients with SCNs with individualized therapy and the best potential results, multidisciplinary collaboration is crucial.

Disclosures We declare no competing interests.

References

1. Kromrey ML, Bülow R, Hübner J, Paperlein C, Lerch MM, Ittermann T, et al. Prospective study on the incidence, prevalence and 5-year pancreatic-related mortality of pancreatic cysts in a population-based study. Gut. 2018;67(1):138–45.
2. Jais B, Rebours V, Malleo G, Salvia R, Fontana M, Maggino L, et al. Serous cystic neoplasm of the pancreas: a multinational study of 2622 patients under the auspices of the International Association of Pancreatology and European Pancreatic Club (European Study Group on Cystic Tumors of the Pancreas). Gut. 2016;65(2):305–12.
3. Yang J, Xu R, Wang C, Qiu J, Ren B, You L. Early screening and diagnosis strategies of pancreatic cancer: a comprehensive review. Cancer Commun. 2021;41(12):1257–74.
4. Hu F, Hu Y, Wang D, Ma X, Yue Y, Tang W, et al. Cystic neoplasms of the pancreas: differential diagnosis and radiology correlation. Front Oncol. 2022;12:860740.
5. Choi JY, Kim MJ, Lee JY, Lim JS, Chung JJ, Kim KW, et al. Typical and atypical manifestations of serous Cystadenoma of the pancreas: imaging findings with pathologic correlation. Am J Roentgenol. 2009;193(1):136–42.
6. Shah AA, Sainani NI, Ramesh AK, Shah ZK, Deshpande V, Hahn PF, et al. Predictive value of multi-detector computed tomography for accurate diagnosis of serous cystadenoma: radiologic-pathologic correlation. WJG. 2009;15(22):2739.
7. Wang G-X, Wang Z-P, Chen H-L, Zhang D, Wen L. Discrimination of serous cystadenoma from mucinous cystic neoplasm and branch duct intraductal papillary mucinous neoplasm in the pancreas with CT. Abdom Radiol. 2020;45(9):2772–8.
8. Jones MJ, Buchanan AS, Neal CP, Dennison AR, Metcalfe MS, Garcea G. Imaging of indeterminate pancreatic cystic lesions: a systematic review. Pancreatology. 2013;13(4):436–42.
9. Kim SY, Lee JM, Kim SH, Shin KS, Kim YJ, An SK, et al. Macrocystic neoplasms of the pancreas: CT differentiation of serous Oligocystic adenoma from mucinous Cystadenoma and Intraductal papillary mucinous tumor. Am J Roentgenol. 2006;187(5):1192–8.
10. Chu LC, Singhi AD, Haroun RR, Hruban RH, Fishman EK. The many faces of pancreatic serous cystadenoma: radiologic and pathologic correlation. Diagn Interv Imaging. 2017;98(3):191–202.
11. Park HS, Kim SY, Hong SM, Park SH, Lee SS, Byun JH, et al. Hypervascular solid-appearing serous cystic neoplasms of the pancreas: differential diagnosis with neuroendocrine tumours. Eur Radiol. 2016;26(5):1348–58.

12. Sedlack R, Affi A, Vazquez-Sequeiros E, Norton ID, Clain JE, Wiersema MJ. Utility of EUS in the evaluation of cystic pancreatic lesions. Gastrointest Endosc. 2002;56(4):543–7.
13. Ahmad NA, Kochman ML, Brensinger C, Brugge WR, Faigel DO, Gress FG, et al. Interobserver agreement among endosonographers for the diagnosis of neoplastic versus non-neoplastic pancreatic cystic lesions. Gastrointest Endosc. 2003;58(1):59–64.
14. Lilo MT, VandenBussche CJ, Allison DB, Lennon AM, Younes BK, Hruban RH, et al. Serous Cystadenoma of the pancreas: potentials and pitfalls of a preoperative Cytopathologic diagnosis. Acta Cytol. 2017;61(1):27–33.
15. Guzmán-Calderón E, Md BMM, Casellas JA, Aparicio JR. Intracystic glucose levels appear useful for diagnosis of pancreatic cystic lesions: a systematic review and meta-analysis. Dig Dis Sci. 2022;67(6):2562–70.
16. Park WG, Wu M, Bowen R, Zheng M, Fitch WL, Pai RK, et al. Metabolomic-derived novel cyst fluid biomarkers for pancreatic cysts: glucose and kynurenine. Gastrointest Endosc. 2013;78(2):295–302.e2.
17. Belsley NA, Pitman MB, Lauwers GY, Brugge WR, Deshpande V. Serous cystadenoma of the pancreas: limitations and pitfalls of endoscopic ultrasound-guided fine-needle aspiration biopsy. Cancer. 2008;114(2):102–10.
18. Springer S, Wang Y, Dal Molin M, Masica DL, Jiao Y, Kinde I, et al. A combination of molecular markers and clinical features improve the classification of pancreatic cysts. Gastroenterology. 2015;149(6):1501–10.
19. Paniccia A, Polanco PM, Boone BA, Wald AI, McGrath K, Brand RE, et al. Prospective, multi-institutional, real-time next-generation sequencing of pancreatic cyst fluid reveals diverse genomic alterations that improve the clinical Management of Pancreatic Cysts. Gastroenterology. 2023;164(1):117–133.e7.
20. Lee T, Teng TZJ, Shelat VG. Carbohydrate antigen 19-9 — tumor marker: Past, present, and future. WJGS. 2020;12(12):468–90.
21. Thornton GD, McPhail MJW, Nayagam S, Hewitt MJ, Vlavianos P, Monahan KJ. Endoscopic ultrasound guided fine needle aspiration for the diagnosis of pancreatic cystic neoplasms: a meta-analysis. Pancreatology. 2013;13(1):48–57.
22. Palma GDD. Confocal laser endomicroscopy in the "in vivo" histologicaldiagnosis of the gastrointestinal tract. WJG. 2009;15(46):5770.
23. Balaban V, Cazacu I, Pinte L, Jinga M, Bhutani M, Saftoiu A. EUS-through-the-needle microbiopsy forceps in pancreatic cystic lesions: a systematic review. Endosc Ultrasound. 2021;10(1):19.
24. Hijioka S, Hara K, Mizuno N, Imaoka H, Bhatia V, Yamao K. Morphological differentiation and follow-up of pancreatic cystic neoplasms using endoscopic ultrasound. Endosc Ultrasound. 2015;4(4):312–8.
25. Roldán J, Harrison JM, Qadan M, Bolm L, Baba T, Brugge WR, et al. Evolving trends in pancreatic cystic Tumors: a 3-decade single-Center experience with 1290 resections. Ann Surg. 2023;277(3):491–7.
26. Lombardo C, Iacopi S, Menonna F, Napoli N, Kauffmann E, Bernardini J, et al. Incidence and reasons of pancreatic resection in patients with asymptomatic serous cystadenoma. Pancreatology. 2018;18(5):577–84.
27. Khalid A, Brugge W. ACG practice guidelines for the diagnosis and management of neoplastic pancreatic cysts. Am J Gastroenterol. 2007;102(10):2339–49.
28. Del Chiaro M, Verbeke C, Salvia R, Klöppel G, Werner J, McKay C, et al. European experts consensus statement on cystic tumours of the pancreas. Dig Liver Dis. 2013;45(9):703–11.
29. Megibow AJ, Baker ME, Morgan DE, Kamel IR, Sahani DV, Newman E, et al. Management of incidental pancreatic cysts: a white paper of the ACR incidental findings committee. J Am Coll Radiol. 2017;14(7):911–23.
30. Pfister M, Probst P, Müller PC, Antony P, Klotz R, Kalkum E, et al. Minimally invasive versus open pancreatic surgery: meta-analysis of randomized clinical trials. BJS Open. 2023;7(2):zrad007.

31. Kadiyala V, Lee LS. Endosonography in the diagnosis and management of pancreatic cysts. World J Gastrointest Endosc. 2015;7(3):213–23.
32. Lin R, Lin X, Pan M, Lu F, Yang Y, Wang C, et al. Perioperative outcomes of robotic pancreaticoduodenectomy: a single surgeon's experience with 55 consecutive cases. Gland Surg. 2021;10(1):122–9.
33. El-Hayek KM, Brown N, O'Rourke C, Falk G, Morris-Stiff G, Walsh RM. Rate of growth of pancreatic serous cystadenoma as an indication for resection. Surgery. 2013;154(4):794–802.
34. Zhang J, Wu WM, You L, Zhao YP. Robotic versus open pancreatectomy: a systematic review and meta-analysis. Ann Surg Oncol. 2013;20(6):1774–80.
35. Permuth-Wey J, Egan KM. Family history is a significant risk factor for pancreatic cancer: results from a systematic review and meta-analysis. Fam Cancer. 2009;8(2):109–17.
36. Watase C, Fuse M, Ino Y, Naito C, Hiraoka N. Novel insights into immunohistochemical analysis for diagnosing serous neoplasm of the pancreas: aquaporin 1, stereocilin, and transmembrane protein 255B. Histopathology. 2021;79(5):872–9.
37. McCarty TR, Paleti S, Rustagi T. Molecular analysis of EUS-acquired pancreatic cyst fluid for KRAS and GNAS mutations for diagnosis of intraductal papillary mucinous neoplasia and mucinous cystic lesions: a systematic review and meta-analysis. Gastrointest Endosc. 2021;93(5):1019–1033.e5.
38. Ren R, Krishna SG, Chen W, Frankel WL, Shen R, Zhao W, et al. Activation of the RAS pathway through uncommon BRAF mutations in mucinous pancreatic cysts without KRAS mutation. Mod Pathol. 2021;34(2):438–44.
39. Singhi AD, McGrath K, Brand RE, Khalid A, Zeh HJ, Chennat JS, et al. Preoperative next-generation sequencing of pancreatic cyst fluid is highly accurate in cyst classification and detection of advanced neoplasia. Gut. 2018;67(12):2131–41.
40. Keane MG, Wehnert N, Perez-Machado M, Fusai GK, Thorburn D, Oppong KW, et al. A prospective trial of CONfocal endomicroscopy in CYSTic lesions of the pancreas: CONCYST-01. Endosc Int Open. 2019;07(09):E1117–22.
41. Kovacevic B, Antonelli G, Klausen P, Hassan C, Larghi A, Vilmann P, et al. EUS-guided biopsy versus confocal laser endomicroscopy in patients with pancreatic cystic lesions: a systematic review and meta-analysis. Endosc Ultrasound. 2021;10(4):270–9.
42. Tomaszewski MR, Gillies RJ. The biological meaning of Radiomic features. Radiology. 2021;298(3):505–16.
43. Huang S, Chong H, Sun X, Wu Z, Jia Q, Zhang Y, et al. The value of 18F-FDG PET/CT in diagnosing pancreatic lesions: comparison with CA19-9, enhanced CT or enhanced MR. Front Med (Lausanne). 2021;8:668697.
44. Cobo M, Menéndez Fernández-Miranda P, Bastarrika G, Lloret IL. Enhancing radiomics and deep learning systems through the standardization of medical imaging workflows. Sci Data. 2023;10(1):732.
45. Nguon LS, Seo K, Lim JH, Song TJ, Cho SH, Park JS, et al. Deep learning-based differentiation between mucinous cystic neoplasm and serous cystic neoplasm in the pancreas using endoscopic ultrasonography. Diagnostics (Basel). 2021;11(6):1052.

Management Strategies of Intrapancreatic Mucinous Neoplasms (IPMNs)

10

Vijant Singh Chandail, Vinu Jamwal, and Shreenidhi Chandail

Abstract

An effective management of IPMNs requires a balance between the risk of malignant transformation and regular follow-up. It is influenced by lesion characteristics, patient health, and risk stratification. The key factors are High-Risk Stigmata: Main pancreatic duct diameter >10 mm, presence of an enhancing solid nodule, or obstructive jaundice associated with the cyst.

Worrisome Features: Main pancreatic duct dilation (5–9 mm), mural nodules (<5 mm), cyst size >3 cm, or thickened cyst walls. Surveillance Protocols include as Low-risk IPMNs (no worrisome features): Monitor with annual magnetic resonance imaging (MRI) or endoscopic ultrasound (EUS). Moderate-risk IPMNs (worrisome features): Close monitoring every 3–6 months with MRI/EUS and biochemical markers like CA19-9. High-risk IPMNs: Immediate surgical evaluation and management. Surgical excision continues to be the mainstay of treatment for high-risk IPMNs. The location, size, and general health of the patient all influence the surgical treatment that is selected. Pancreaticoduodenectomy (Whipple Procedure) is ideal for lesions in the pancreatic head. Distal pancreatectomy is preferred for lesions in the body or tail, and total pancreatectomy is reserved for multifocal disease or extensive involvement but associated with significant morbidity, including diabetes and exocrine insufficiency.

V. S. Chandail (✉)
PG Department of Medicine, Govt Medical College Jammu, Jammu, J&K, India

V. Jamwal
PG Department of Medicine, ASCOMS & Hospital Jammu, Jammu, J&K, India

S. Chandail
Acharya Shri Chander College of Medical Sciences, Jammu, J&K, India

R. K. Sharma et al. (eds.), *Differential Diagnosis and Management of Pancreatic Cystic Lesions*, https://doi.org/10.1007/978-981-92-0654-4_10

Keywords

Intrapancreatic mucinous neoplasms (IPMNs) · Stigmata · Surveillance · Surgery

10.1 Introduction

Intraductal papillary mucinous neoplasms (IPMNs) are an important group of pancreatic cystic lesions that can turn into cancer. Their detection has grown significantly with the wider use of high-resolution imaging, often found by chance. The main challenge in managing IPMNs is finding the right time for intervention to prevent pancreatic cancer while avoiding unnecessary surgery and preserving pancreatic function [1]. Risk assessment takes into account imaging features, duct involvement, and patient specifics; it serves as the basis for management and follows international recommendations [2]. However, the difficulty in accurately predicting the potential for cancer often results in overtreatment or delayed diagnoses. Recent improvements in imaging, endoscopic evaluation, and molecular markers have helped with lesion assessment and personalized risk evaluation [3]. This chapter discusses current methods for monitoring and treating IPMNs, focusing on management based on guidelines and new strategies to enhance clinical outcomes.

10.2 Risk Assessment and Surveillance

Risk stratification forms the cornerstone of IPMN management, helping to identify patients who require immediate intervention versus those suitable for surveillance [2].

Key Risk Factors

- *High-risk stigmata:* Main pancreatic duct diameter >10 mm, presence of an enhancing solid nodule, or obstructive jaundice associated with the cyst
- *Worrisome features:* Main pancreatic duct dilation (5–9 mm), mural nodules (<5 mm), cyst size >3 cm, or thickened cyst walls

Surveillance Protocols

- Low-risk IPMNs (no worrisome features): Monitor with annual magnetic resonance imaging (MRI) or endoscopic ultrasound (EUS).
- Moderate-risk IPMNs (worrisome features): Close monitoring every 3–6 months with MRI/EUS and biochemical markers like CA19-9.

Table 10.1 Risk stratification criteria for IPMNs

Risk category	Key features	Management strategy
Low risk	Small cysts (<3 cm), no worrisome features	Annual imaging surveillance
Moderate risk	Cysts >3 cm, mild duct dilation (5–9 mm)	Imaging every 3–6 months, evaluate CA19-9
High risk	Solid nodules, duct dilation >10 mm, jaundice	Consider surgery

- High-risk IPMNs: Immediate surgical evaluation and management (Table 10.1).

Conservative treatment is often used for low-risk lesions, which are characterized by their modest size, lack of symptoms, and lack of high-risk characteristics including solid components or dilation of the main pancreatic duct. These individuals are routinely monitored for any changes that could be signs of progression, utilizing imaging modalities such as computed tomography (CT) or magnetic resonance imaging (MRI). This method ensures prompt diagnosis of malignant transformation while reducing needless surgical risks [3].

10.3 Surgical Management

Surgical excision continues to be the mainstay of treatment for high-risk IPMNs. The location, size, and general health of the patient all influence the surgical treatment that is selected [4, 5] (Table 10.2).

Types of Surgical Interventions

1. *Pancreaticoduodenectomy (Whipple Procedure):* Ideal for lesions in the pancreatic head
2. *Distal Pancreatectomy:* Preferred for lesions in the body or tail
3. *Total Pancreatectomy:* Reserved for multifocal disease or extensive involvement but associated with significant morbidity, including diabetes and exocrine insufficiency

Table 10.2 Indications for surgery in IPMNs

Parameter	Indications	Clinical relevance
Symptoms	Obstructive jaundice, recurrent pancreatitis, weight loss, abdominal pain	Strong predictors of malignant transformation or symptomatic progression
Imaging findings	Mural nodules >5 mm, thickened cyst walls, main pancreatic duct dilation (5–9 mm)	Indicators of "worrisome features," warranting closer evaluation and possible surgical intervention
High-risk stigmata	Main duct diameter >10 mm, enhancing mural nodules, obstructive jaundice with a cystic lesion	Strongly suggestive of malignancy, requiring immediate surgical resection
Cytological analysis	Presence of high-grade dysplasia or carcinoma in cyst fluid	Confirms malignancy or high-risk pathology, necessitating surgical management
Patient factors	Age, comorbidities, patient preferences	Important for balancing risks of surgery against expected outcomes

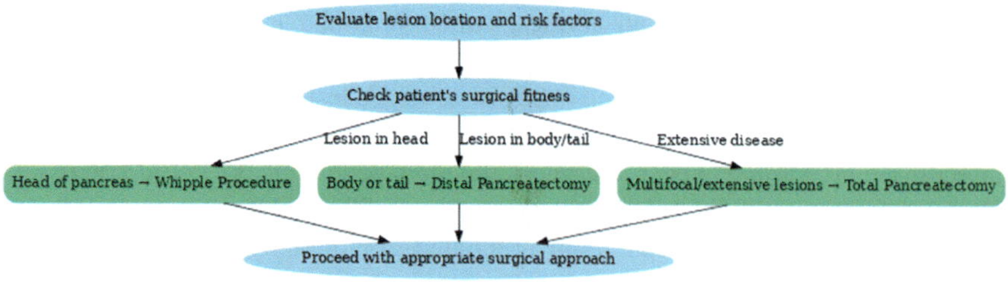

Intraoperative Techniques

- Frozen section analysis ensures negative surgical margins.
- Minimally invasive options (laparoscopic or robotic surgery) are increasingly preferred for select patients to reduce the recovery time [6].

10.4 Emerging Endoscopic Therapies

For patients unfit for surgery, endoscopic techniques offer promising alternatives.

Techniques

1. *EUS-guided fine needle aspiration (FNA):* For diagnosis and cyst fluid analysis [7]
2. *Endoscopic cyst ablation:* Utilizes ethanol injection or radiofrequency ablation to reduce the cyst volume and malignant potential [8]

Indications for Endoscopic Therapy

- Symptomatic low-risk lesions
- Inoperable candidates with minimal risk of malignancy (Table 10.3)

These techniques are still experimental, nevertheless, and should only be used in carefully chosen situations when surgery is not recommended and the danger of cancer is minimal [9].

Table 10.3 Comparison of surgical and endoscopic approaches

Parameter	Surgical resection	Endoscopic therapy
Indications	High-risk, invasive IPMNs	Low-risk, symptomatic IPMNs
Procedure invasiveness	High	Minimal
Recovery time	Prolonged	Short
Risk of malignant progression	Negligible (if complete)	Moderate

Table 10.4 Prognostic outcomes based on lesion type

Lesion type	5-year survival rate	Prognostic considerations
Low-grade IPMNs	>90%	Complete resection ensures good outcomes
High-grade IPMNs	50–70%	Risk of recurrence if margins positive
Invasive IPMNs	30–60%	Early detection critical

10.5 Postoperative Management and Surveillance

Despite advancements, surgical risks such as pancreatic fistula, delayed gastric emptying, and infections remain concerns. Postoperative management focuses on mitigating these complications and ensuring long-term functional preservation.

Monitoring Schedule

- Imaging (MRI/EUS) every 6–12 months
- CA19-9 levels as an adjunct for recurrence detection

Complications

- *Exocrine insufficiency:* Managed with pancreatic enzyme replacement therapy
- *Endocrine dysfunction:* Lifelong insulin therapy in total pancreatectomy cases

10.6 Prognostic Factors and Outcomes

The prognosis depends on the lesion's histopathological grade and presence of invasive carcinoma. Noninvasive IPMNs have excellent outcomes post-resection, with 5-year survival rates exceeding 90%. In contrast, invasive lesions show poorer survival rates (30–60%) [3, 9] (Table 10.4).

10.7 Molecular and Biomarker-Based Advances

Molecular Profiling

- Detection of KRAS and TP53 mutations to predict malignant transformation.
- GNAS mutations indicate cystic lesions with lower malignancy risk.

Emerging Biomarkers

- Circulating tumor DNA (ctDNA) and microRNAs offer noninvasive methods for risk prediction and monitoring.

Future Directions

- Integrating AI into imaging for enhanced detection and risk stratification
- Development of nanotechnology-based localized therapies

10.8 Current Guidelines Regarding Treatment Modalities

1. *European Evidence-Based Guidelines (2022)*
   - Highlight multidisciplinary team involvement for decision-making.
   - Recommend integrating molecular diagnostics (e.g., KRAS, GNAS mutations) into risk assessment protocols
2. *Fukuoka Guidelines (2017 Update)* [11]
   - Emphasize risk stratification based on high-risk stigmata (e.g., mural nodules, MPD >10 mm) and worrisome features.
   - Recommend surgical resection for high-risk IPMNs and close monitoring for low- to moderate-risk cases with imaging and biomarkers.
3. *American Gastroenterological Association (AGA) Guidelines (2015)* [12]
   - Suggest limiting surveillance to cysts >3 cm or those with worrisome features.
   - Endorse surgical intervention for patients with high-risk features but recommend against routine resection of all cysts.
4. *International Consensus Guidelines (Tanaka et al. 2012)* [10]
   - Focus on early detection of malignancy through imaging, cytology, and surveillance intervals based on risk categories.
   - Provide specific surgical recommendations for main-duct and branch-duct IPMNs.
5. *Japanese Pancreatic Society (JPS) Guidelines*
   - Advocate for individualized management plans, integrating genetic profiling and long-term follow-up protocols.
6. *National Comprehensive Cancer Network (NCCN) Guidelines*
   - Emphasize the role of EUS-FNA for cyst fluid analysis in determining malignancy potential.
   - Support tailored management plans incorporating patient comorbidities and preferences.

These guidelines collectively underscore the importance of risk stratification, multidisciplinary care, and emerging diagnostic tools to optimize IPMN management.

10.9 Future Directions in Research and Innovation

1. *Integration of molecular biomarkers:*

   Ongoing research focuses on identifying molecular markers such as KRAS, GNAS, and TP53 mutations for improved risk stratification and early detection of malignancy. Biomarkers like circulating tumor DNA (ctDNA) and microRNAs are gaining attention for their potential to offer noninvasive diagnostic and monitoring options.
2. *Advancements in artificial intelligence (AI):*

   AI and machine learning are being developed to enhance diagnostic accuracy by integrating clinical, imaging, and genomic data. These tools aim to personalize risk assessment, identify malignancy patterns, and optimize surveillance strategies, potentially reducing unnecessary interventions.

3. *Emerging nonsurgical therapies:*

   Minimally invasive approaches, such as endoscopic cyst ablation with ethanol or radiofrequency, are being explored for patients unsuitable for surgery. Nanotechnology and drug delivery innovations also show promise for targeted therapy, preserving pancreatic function and improving patient outcomes.

10.10 Challenges in Long-Term Surveillance and Follow-Up

1. *Uncertainty in progression risk:*

   The unpredictable progression of IPMNs complicates surveillance strategies. While some lesions remain stable for years, others rapidly transform into malignancies, necessitating robust risk assessment models integrating biomarkers and imaging.
2. *Patient compliance and standardization:*

   Ensuring adherence to follow-up protocols is challenging, especially for asymptomatic patients. Variability in recommendations across guidelines further complicates standardization, often leading to over- or under-surveillance. Patient education and personalized care plans are critical in addressing this issue.
3. *Resource limitations and accessibility:*

   Limited access to advanced imaging and molecular diagnostics in resource-poor settings creates disparities in care. Telemedicine and mobile health technologies offer potential solutions to enhance accessibility, but global efforts are needed to standardize and distribute affordable diagnostic tools.

Bibliography

1. Moris D, Liapis I, Gupta P, Ziogas IA, Karachaliou GS, Dimitrokallis N, Nguyen B, Radkani P. An overview for clinicians on Intraductal papillary mucinous neoplasms (IPMNs) of the pancreas. Cancer. 2024;16(22):3825.
2. Del Chiaro M, Ateeb Z, Hansson MR, Rangelova E, Segersvärd R, Kartalis N, Ansorge C, Löhr MJ, Arnelo U, Verbeke C. Survival analysis and risk for progression of intraductal papillary mucinous neoplasia of the pancreas (IPMN) under surveillance: a single-institution experience. Ann Surg Oncol. 2017;24:1120–6.
3. Higashi M, Yokoyama S, Yamamoto T, Goto Y, Kitazono I, Hiraki T, Taguchi H, Hashimoto S, Fukukura Y, Koriyama C, Mataki Y. Mucin expression in endoscopic ultrasound-guided fine-needle aspiration specimens is a useful prognostic factor in pancreatic ductal adenocarcinoma. Pancreas. 2015;44(5):728–34.
4. Kimura W, Kuroda A, Makuuchi M. Problems in the diagnosis and treatment of a so-called mucin-producing tumor of the pancreas. Pancreas. 1998;16(3):363–9.
5. Malleo G, Marchegiani G, Borin A, Capelli P, Accordini F, Butturini G, Pederzoli P, Bassi C, Salvia R. Observational study of the incidence of pancreatic and extrapancreatic malignancies during surveillance of patients with branch-duct intraductal papillary mucinous neoplasm. Ann Surg. 2015;261(5):984–90.

6. Tonutti M, Elson DS, Yang GZ, Darzi AW, Sodergren MH. The role of technology in minimally invasive surgery: state of the art, recent developments and future directions. Postgrad Med J. 2017;93(1097):159–67.
7. Suzuki R, Thosani N, Annangi S, Guha S, Bhutani MS. Diagnostic yield of EUS-FNA-based cytology distinguishing malignant and benign IPMNs: a systematic review and meta-analysis. Pancreatology. 2014;14(5):380–4.
8. Matsumoto K, Kato H. Endoscopic ablation therapy for the pancreatic neoplasms. Dig Endosc. 2023;35(4):430–42.
9. Ahmad M, Maegawa FB, De La Rosa E, Davis B, Tyroch A, Konstantinidis IT. Mucinous cystic neoplasms of the pancreas in the modern era. Experience with 707 patients. Am J Surg. 2020;220(6):1433–7.
10. Tanaka M, Fernández-del Castillo C, Adsay V, Chari S, Falconi M, Jang JY, Kimura W, Levy P, Pitman MB, Schmidt CM, Shimizu M. International consensus guidelines 2012 for the management of IPMN and MCN of the pancreas. Pancreatology. 2012;12(3):183–97.
11. Tanaka M, Fernández-del Castillo C, Kamisawa T, Jang JY, Levy P, Ohtsuka T, Salvia R, Shimizu Y, Tada M, Wolfgang CL. Revisions of international consensus Fukuoka guidelines for the management of IPMN of the pancreas. Pancreatology. 2017;17(5):738–53.
12. Lennon AM, Ahuja N, Wolfgang CL. AGA guidelines for the management of pancreatic cysts. Gastroenterology. 2015;149(3):825.

Surgical Management of Pancreatic Cystic Neoplasms (PCNs)

11

Venu Bhargava, Surinder Singh Rana, and Rajesh Gupta

Abstract

Pancreatic cystic neoplasms (PCNs) are being identified more often today, largely because of the widespread use of high-quality imaging. These cysts range from harmless serous lesions to mucinous and solid tumors that carry a real risk of cancer. Because of this wide spectrum, recognizing the exact subtype is crucial for choosing the right management approach.

This chapter offers a clear and practical overview of how each major type of PCN is surgically managed—IPMNs, MCNs, SCNs, and SPNs. It brings together the latest international guidelines, current evidence, and real-world decision-making strategies. Readers will learn why MCNs nearly always require removal, why IPMNs demand a careful balance between surveillance and timely surgery, why most SCNs can be safely observed, and why complete resection cures the vast majority of SPNs. The chapter also highlights how minimally invasive, robotic, and parenchyma-preserving operations are transforming surgical practice. Key challenges—such as interpreting frozen sections and planning postoperative follow-up—are explained in a practical manner. Emerging innovations like radiomics, molecular profiling, artificial intelligence, and liquid biopsy are introduced as tools that will soon reshape how surgeons assess risk and individualize treatment.

V. Bhargava
Department of Surgical Gastroenterology, ESIC Medical College and Hospital, Hyderabad, India

S. S. Rana
Department of Gastroenterology, Postgraduate Institute of Medical Education and Research, Chandigarh, India

R. Gupta (✉)
Department of GI Surgery, HPB and Liver Transplantation, Postgraduate Institute of Medical Education and Research, Chandigarh, India

R. K. Sharma et al. (eds.), *Differential Diagnosis and Management of Pancreatic Cystic Lesions*, https://doi.org/10.1007/978-981-92-0654-4_11

As diagnostic tools advance, surgical strategies are becoming more tailored, less invasive, and more focused on preserving pancreatic function without compromising cancer control.

Keywords

Pancreatic cystic neoplasms · Intraductal papillary mucinous neoplasm (IPMN) Mucinous cystic neoplasm (MCN) · Serous cystic neoplasm (SCN) · Solid pseudopapillary neoplasm (SPN) · Pancreatic surgery · Minimally invasive pancreatic surgery · Robotic distal pancreatectomy · Parenchyma-sparing surgery Pancreatic risk stratification · Radiomics · Artificial intelligence in pancreatic disease · Molecular profiling · Pancreatic cancer prevention · Surgical decision-making

Pancreatic cystic neoplasms (PCNs) encompass a diverse group of lesions ranging from benign cystadenomas to potentially malignant and malignant tumors, such as mucinous cystic neoplasms (MCNs), intraductal papillary mucinous neoplasms (IPMNs), and solid pseudopapillary neoplasms (SPNs). The prevalence of these lesions has risen markedly in recent decades, attributed largely to the widespread use of cross-sectional imaging such as CT and MRI [1, 2]. Up to 50% of PCNs are discovered incidentally, often in asymptomatic individuals. Despite this, the malignant potential of certain PCNs necessitates a meticulous and individualized surgical approach based on histologic subtype, anatomic location, lesion size, presence of high-risk features, patient fitness, and goals of care [3–6].

11.1 Surgical Management of IPMNs

In the current medical landscape, the widespread use of high-resolution imaging has uncovered a “pandemic” of incidentally discovered pancreatic cystic neoplasms (PCNs), among which intraductal papillary mucinous neoplasms (IPMNs) are most common [4]. IPMNs are unique as they straddle the line between benign cysts and precursor lesions to pancreatic ductal adenocarcinoma (PDAC) [5, 6]. Their natural history, diverse morphology, and varying malignant potential render a singular management strategy elusive. Originally managed aggressively due to the presumed high risk of malignancy, treatment of IPMNs has shifted toward a more conservative, evidence-based approach, especially for low-risk lesions [7, 8]. However, the balance between overtreatment and missed opportunities for cancer prevention continues to pose significant clinical dilemmas.

IPMNs are mucin-producing epithelial neoplasms originating from the pancreatic ductal system, with the potential to progress via the adenoma–carcinoma sequence [9]. Prevalence increases with age [10], with no strong gender predilection. Morphologically, IPMNs are subclassified into main-duct (MD), branch-duct (BD), and mixed-type (MT). Surgical series highlight a higher malignant potential for MD-IPMN (up to 92%) and MT-IPMN compared to BD-IPMN (6–46%)

[11–13]. Histologically, IPMNs are graded into low-grade (LGD) or high-grade dysplasia (HGD), with subtypes including gastric, intestinal, pancreatobiliary, and oncocytic [14–16], and associated invasive components like tubular or colloid carcinoma. The molecular heterogeneity of IPMNs supports a more nuanced understanding of progression risk and justifies stratified surgical strategies.

Symptoms are often nonspecific, with the majority of IPMNs incidentally detected [17]. However, obstructive jaundice and pancreatitis may suggest higher-grade dysplasia or invasion. Radiologically, MRI with MRCP and contrast-enhanced EUS (CE-EUS) provide vital insights into ductal communication, mural nodules, and cyst complexity [18, 19]. Despite technological advancements, diagnostic specificity remains modest [20, 21]. EUS-FNA offers cytology and cyst fluid analysis—CEA >192 ng/mL, low glucose [22–28], and elevated amylase levels can support mucinous origin [27], though cytologic sensitivity is hindered by locular heterogeneity [2].

Three major guidelines inform IPMN management: the International Association of Pancreatology (IAP, 2016 and 2024 update) [2, 29], European Evidence-Based Guidelines (2018) [13], and American Gastroenterological Association (AGA, 2015, updated 2024) [4, 30]. Across the guidelines, key absolute indications for surgery (or "high-risk stigmata") include MPD ≥10 mm, enhancing mural nodules ≥5 mm, obstructive jaundice, and positive cytology [31–34]. Relative indications ("worrisome features") include cyst size ≥3–4 cm, elevated serum markers, and cyst growth >5 mm/year. The updated 2024 AGA guidelines remain conservative but slightly broaden the criteria for EUS evaluation while refining surgical criteria, now recognizing specific combinations of cyst size, ductal dilation, and nodule presence for early referral. The AGA now recommends multidisciplinary review for equivocal cysts and emphasizes shared decision-making [AGA 2024].

The 2024 AGA guidelines also contribute new surveillance algorithms, offering risk-based stratification for cysts based on imaging, cytology, and patient factors, promoting individualized follow-up duration and intensity. Compared to the 2012 Fukuoka guidelines, newer evidence shows the AGA guideline offers high specificity but reduced sensitivity in selecting cysts for EUS or surgery, while Fukuoka performs better in detecting malignancy at the cost of increased intervention rates [30]. These differences reinforce the need to integrate radiologic, clinical, and patient-specific factors, avoiding a one-size-fits-all approach. The 2023 surveillance study led by the Verona group further suggests that stable BD-IPMNs <30 mm in patients >75 years and <15 mm in patients >65 years over 5 years of follow-up can safely discontinue surveillance without increased cancer risk [41]. The IAP 2024 surveillance criteria also support surveillance cessation in elderly, stable BD-IPMN cases without high-risk features, strengthening this patient-tailored approach [29].

Surveillance for BD-IPMN has evolved substantially in the past decade. Current consensus recommends MRI or EUS-based follow-up every 6–24 months depending on the lesion size and stability. For BD-IPMNs <10 mm, surveillance intervals can extend to 24 months, whereas cysts >20 mm or with evolving features require closer observation. Patient age and comorbidities heavily influence surveillance duration [30–35]. Discontinuation of surveillance is advised for elderly patients (>75–80 years) with stable small cysts and no high-risk features for over 5 years, as endorsed by the 2024 IAP update and Verona consensus. The role of CA 19-9 in surveillance remains adjunctive, primarily guiding further imaging in rising values without imaging correlation [35–40].

In a recent longitudinal cohort study by Hamada et al. [37], the risk of developing pancreatic cancer is primarily influenced by cyst size and growth rate within the first 5 years of surveillance. An IPMN growth rate ≥ 2.5 mm/year or size ≥40 mm during this period significantly increases cancer risk and may warrant surgical evaluation. However, beyond 5 years, these features lose predictive value. Instead, the main pancreatic duct (MPD) diameter at 5 years becomes the most reliable long-term predictor—MPD ≥5 mm correlates with a sharply increased cancer risk. Surveillance should thus be personalized: initially guided by cyst dynamics, then by MPD diameter in extended follow-up.

The Verona group advanced the concept of dynamic risk assessment by evaluating "crossover" cases that shifted from surveillance to surgery [40–43]. They concluded that evolving features (e.g., new mural nodules or MPD dilation) portended higher malignancy, while stable BD-IPMNs carried low risk, particularly in patients >65 years without worrisome features for ≥5 years [41–43]. Conversely, the Heidelberg group, in a landmark surgical series ($n = 1439$), categorized surgery timing as too early (LGD), timely (HGD), and too late (IC) [41]. Only 34% of "timely" and 88% of "too late" surgeries showed radiographic criteria, underscoring poor correlation between imaging and pathology. These findings reinforce the need for careful timing and individualized decision-making. This large international study [44] compared pancreatic cancers arising from IPMN and PanIN precursors. It found that IPMN-derived pancreatic cancer has significantly better survival than PanIN-derived cancer (median OS: 43.1 vs. 23.0 months). Colloid-type IPMN cancers have the best prognosis, while tubular types are more aggressive but still outperform PanIN-derived cancers if detected early. After adjusting for tumor stage and biology, tubular and colloid subtypes showed similar survival, highlighting the value of early detection and resection. The study supports developing separate, tailored guidelines for IPMN-derived PDAC, rather than extrapolating from PanIN-based protocols.

11.1.1 Surgical Strategy

Surgery for IPMN must be oncologically sound, technically meticulous, and tailored to the patient's anatomy and risk profile. The physiologic condition of the patient plays a pivotal role in surgical decision-making. Frailty scores, nutritional status, cardiorespiratory reserve, glycemic control, and sarcopenia all significantly impact operative outcomes. In elderly or comorbid patients, extensive resections like total pancreatectomy require careful deliberation, balancing cancer control with postoperative quality of life. Enhanced prehabilitation strategies, including nutritional optimization, smoking cessation, and physiotherapy, have shown to improve postoperative recovery in such high-risk groups [41–45].

Intraoperatively, frozen section analysis of the pancreatic transection margin is a critical determinant of oncologic adequacy. A positive frozen section showing high-grade dysplasia necessitates further resection to achieve negative margins, particularly if adjacent parenchyma or ducts show involvement. However, low-grade dysplasia at the resection margin typically does not require extension. Complexities arise in cases with denuded epithelium in dilated ducts, as such findings may obscure residual high-grade disease and have been associated with postoperative recurrence. In these ambiguous scenarios, the decision to proceed with further resection must weigh lesion biology, the presence of multifocality, margin proximity, and patient comorbidity status [40, 43, 44].

Postoperatively, complications remain a major consideration. Pancreatic fistula is the most frequent complication, particularly after pancreatoduodenectomy, and is strongly influenced by gland texture and duct diameter. Delayed gastric emptying, hemorrhage, bile leak, and intraabdominal abscess formation are additional concerns. These complications can impact not only the immediate recovery but also long-term pancreatic function and quality of life. Risk stratification using the Fistula Risk Score (FRS) and the application of Enhanced Recovery After Surgery (ERAS) pathways have reduced complication rates in specialized centers [45].

The post-resection surveillance plan includes periodic imaging (MRI or CT), CA 19-9 monitoring, and symptom assessment. For patients histologically diagnosed as high-risk or invasive lesions in the surgical specimen, surveillance is intensified. In cases where residual pancreatic parenchyma shows low-risk features post-resection, a watch-and-wait approach with semi-annual imaging may be reasonable. However, the risk of recurrence or metachronous lesion formation in the remnant pancreas mandates long-term vigilance [46].

Watchful waiting in patients unfit for surgery or with low-risk BD-IPMN has become an acceptable standard, provided there is robust surveillance. This approach is increasingly supported by data showing that many BD-IPMNs remain stable for over a decade, particularly in elderly patients. Importantly, this strategy requires strict adherence to follow-up protocols and a low threshold for intervention upon emergence of high-risk features.

Recent developments have highlighted the potential of artificial intelligence (AI) and radiomics in enhancing IPMN risk stratification and surgical decision-making. Balduzzi et al. [47] introduced an AI-based predictive model using radiomic features extracted from preoperative imaging. Their model demonstrated an AUC of 0.81 for predicting malignancy, outperforming traditional guideline-based assessments in external validation. Such tools leverage machine learning algorithms trained on large imaging datasets to detect subtle features beyond human perception [47].

Other models, such as those by Chakraborty et al. and Permuth et al. [48, 49], utilized deep learning and integrated molecular profiling with imaging data to improve predictive accuracy. Chakraborty's multi-institutional model achieved AUCs >0.85 in identifying high-grade dysplasia, while Permuth demonstrated utility in combining KRAS/GNAS mutations with radiologic phenotypes to predict malignancy risk. A 2023 meta-analysis confirmed the superior specificity and positive predictive value of AI-enhanced diagnostics compared to existing guidelines.

These AI models not only aid in predicting dysplasia grade but also help distinguish indeterminate lesions, improving diagnostic confidence in borderline cases. Importantly, their real-world applicability is currently limited by the lack of standardized image acquisition protocols and multicenter prospective validation. However, as evidence accumulates, AI integration into routine clinical pathways appears increasingly viable.

Several studies comparing guideline-based decision-making versus AI-driven tools show that while guidelines emphasize sensitivity for malignancy, AI models offer improved specificity and individualized predictions. The convergence of guideline criteria with AI-enhanced imaging is expected to redefine future surveillance and resection strategies for IPMNs [32, 49–53].

The growing recognition of molecular profiling, imaging-based deep learning, and patient-specific clinical modeling suggests that the next frontier in IPMN management will be precision oncology. Future guideline iterations will likely incorporate these tools, allowing for better identification of candidates for surgery versus surveillance and minimizing both overtreatment and undertreatment [54–56].

Surgical management thus demands a holistic understanding of IPMN biology, imaging correlates, patient physiology, operative risk, and technological advancements. Increasing incorporation of minimally invasive techniques, robotics, radiomics, and artificial intelligence continues to refine outcomes, reduce morbidity, and preserve quality of life in this complex and heterogeneous disease.

11.2 Surgical Management of Mucinous Cystic Neoplasms (MCNs)

Surgical resection of mucinous cystic neoplasms (MCNs) is broadly endorsed by all major international guidelines due to their premalignant nature and histologic hallmark of ovarian-type stroma, which cannot be definitively identified without excision. The International Association of Pancreatology (IAP) and Kyoto guidelines are unequivocal in recommending surgical resection for all fit patients diagnosed with MCNs, regardless of size, symptoms, or cyst characteristics. This recommendation stems from the understanding that MCNs carry a substantial risk of harboring high-grade dysplasia or invasive carcinoma, particularly when left untreated. Similarly, the Verona consensus strongly supports universal resection in surgically fit individuals, with particular emphasis on younger, premenopausal women and lesions that exhibit radiologic features such as mural nodules, septations, or wall thickening. These groups discourage surveillance once the diagnosis of MCN is established, even in the absence of symptoms or worrisome features. The European evidence-based guidelines align closely with these recommendations, promoting resection in nearly all cases, though they allow for observation in select patients who are elderly, frail, or carry small (<40 mm), asymptomatic lesions without high-risk features. In contrast, American guidelines—particularly those from the

American Gastroenterological Association (AGA)—take a more conservative stance, recommending surgery only when specific criteria are met, such as cysts larger than 3 cm with enhancing solid components, positive cytology, or clinical symptoms like pain or pancreatitis. The American College of Gastroenterology (ACG), however, leans toward a more proactive surgical approach than AGA, supporting resection in most patients with suspected MCNs. The Heidelberg consensus also advocates for resection in all radiologically or clinically suspected MCNs, particularly when mural nodules, cyst wall enhancement, or elevated serum tumor markers are present. Across these guidelines, key surgical indications consistently include cyst size greater than 40 mm, presence of mural nodules, cyst wall thickening, symptoms, and elevated CA19–9 levels. While some divergence exists in the threshold for intervention—particularly between European–Asian and American guidelines—the overarching consensus remains that surgery is the standard of care for MCNs in fit patients, with observation reserved only for very specific, low-risk clinical scenarios. Recent research into the management of mucinous cystic neoplasms (MCNs) has sought to refine the criteria for surgical intervention beyond traditional guideline-based triggers like size, symptoms, or imaging features. One of the key areas of evolution involves *molecular and cyst fluid biomarker analysis*, which aims to enhance diagnostic precision and risk stratification. Studies have shown that *mutations in KRAS and GNAS* are often present in mucinous lesions, but high-risk lesions—especially those with invasive potential—are more likely to harbor additional alterations such as *TP53, SMAD4, and RNF43.* While these genetic markers are not yet standard in clinical decision-making, they offer promising avenues for preoperative differentiation between low-risk and high-risk MCNs [57–61].

Additionally, *radiomics and machine learning approaches* have gained traction in predicting malignancy in pancreatic cysts, including MCNs. By analyzing high-dimensional features from CT and MRI imaging—such as texture, shape, and enhancement patterns—AI-based models have shown improved accuracy in identifying high-grade dysplasia or invasive carcinoma. Some of these models demonstrate area under the curve (AUC) values exceeding 0.85, outperforming traditional radiologic assessment. However, most models are still in the validation phase and have not been incorporated into clinical guidelines due to variability across institutions and imaging protocols [57–59].

Recent studies also emphasize the *limited role of surveillance* once a diagnosis of MCN is established. A 2023 multicenter cohort study reaffirmed that even small, asymptomatic MCNs may harbor invasive components, which are often underestimated on imaging. Importantly, this study found that *up to 20% of resected MCNs < 3 cm* had high-grade dysplasia or invasive carcinoma, reinforcing the rationale for early surgical intervention, especially in younger patients. Conversely, certain subgroups—particularly elderly patients with stable, cystic lesions <3 cm lacking mural nodules—have shown low progression risk in observational cohorts, suggesting potential for individualized surveillance in select scenarios [62, 63].

Moreover, emerging interest surrounds *liquid biopsy techniques*, including analysis of circulating tumor DNA (ctDNA) and exosomal RNA in cyst fluid or peripheral blood. Preliminary findings indicate that the presence of ctDNA with high-risk mutations correlates strongly with malignant transformation, offering a noninvasive adjunct to current risk stratification methods. Though not yet clinically adopted, these biomarkers may eventually help avoid unnecessary surgery in indolent MCNs and prioritize intervention in those with subclinical malignant evolution [64].

In summary, while surgery remains the mainstay of management for MCNs in most patients, newer research is gradually reshaping the landscape. Integration of molecular diagnostics, AI-driven imaging analytics, and liquid biopsy techniques holds promise for more personalized, biology-based surgical decision-making. However, these tools still require larger prospective validation and guideline endorsement before they can reliably supplant the current morphology-based paradigm.

Surgical approaches for mucinous cystic neoplasms (MCNs) vary slightly across different international and regional guidelines, reflecting differences in oncologic philosophy, institutional expertise, and healthcare infrastructure. However, the unifying principle across all guidelines is that resection is warranted in surgically fit patients, with emphasis on minimizing recurrence while preserving pancreatic function. The choice of surgical procedure depends on tumor location, size, morphology, and invasiveness and is shaped by each guideline's threshold for intervention and philosophy on parenchymal preservation.

Globally, the most commonly performed surgery for MCNs is *distal pancreatectomy*, as the majority of MCNs are located in the body and tail of the pancreas. The *Kyoto guidelines (2024)* and *Japanese Pancreatic Society recommendations* strongly endorse *spleen-preserving distal pancreatectomy* where feasible, especially for benign or low-grade lesions, to reduce immunologic compromise and long-term morbidity. In Japan and much of East Asia, there is a clear preference for *parenchyma- and organ-preserving surgeries*, including *laparoscopic and robotic distal pancreatectomy*, which are now routinely used in high-volume centers. The Japanese approach also emphasizes accurate preoperative imaging and intraoperative navigation, with high utilization of intraoperative frozen sections and selective central pancreatectomy in younger patients when lesions are close to the neck [65–70].

The *American guidelines (AGA, ACG)* tend to emphasize oncologic safety but also promote *minimally invasive approaches*. In the United States, *laparoscopic distal pancreatectomy* has become the standard of care in most tertiary centers for resectable MCNs, and *robotic surgery* is increasingly common, particularly in academic institutions. Central pancreatectomy is rarely used due to concerns about postoperative pancreatic fistula, although it remains an option for carefully selected patients with mid-body lesions. The *AGA* is more conservative in recommending surgery; thus, the operations performed tend to be for lesions already exhibiting high-risk features, where a more formal oncologic resection is indicated.

In *European centers*, particularly those aligned with the *European Study Group on Cystic Tumours of the Pancreas*, there is a balanced approach favoring resection with the preservation of function. Laparoscopic surgery is standard, and *spleen-preserving techniques* are favored where oncologically acceptable. *Parenchyma-sparing techniques*, including enucleation or central pancreatectomy, are considered in low-grade, small MCNs in younger patients. The *Verona guidelines* endorse these techniques and emphasize individualized decision-making based on tumor biology, location, and patient age. *Intraoperative frozen section analysis* is standard practice across Europe to guide margin decisions and confirm the nature of the lesion.

Overall, while distal pancreatectomy remains the cornerstone surgery for MCNs globally, variations exist in the extent of resection, spleen preservation, use of minimally invasive techniques, and application of parenchyma-sparing surgery. The *Kyoto and Asian guidelines* emphasize function-preserving and minimally invasive surgery, the *American and ACG approach* leans toward definitive resection with oncologic safety, and *European and Verona strategies* strike a balance between oncologic radicality and organ preservation. These differing philosophies illustrate the global evolution toward more tailored, patient-centered surgical management of MCNs, with increasing use of technology and emphasis on preserving quality of life post-resection [67–70].

Margin assessment during resection of mucinous cystic neoplasms (MCNs) is a critical component of surgical management, especially when there is suspicion of invasive carcinoma. The goal of resection is to achieve negative surgical margins (R0), as positive margins (R1) are associated with a higher risk of local recurrence and poorer long-term outcomes. Intraoperatively, frozen section analysis of the pancreatic transection margin is frequently employed when there are high-risk features such as mural nodules, thickened cyst walls, or radiologic signs suggestive of malignancy. If frozen section reveals only noninvasive MCN, further resection is usually unnecessary. However, if invasive carcinoma is detected at the margin, the surgeon may consider extending the resection [71].

The diagnostic accuracy of frozen sections is generally high, but interpretation challenges may arise, particularly in distinguishing high-grade dysplasia from early invasive components. Among international guidelines, the IAP and Verona consensus encourage routine frozen section analysis for margin assessment, while the European guidelines recommend its use in selected cases with worrisome features. The AGA and ACG take a more conservative view, advocating selective use based on operative findings or preoperative suspicion. The Kyoto guidelines support intraoperative histology where available, especially if it alters the extent of surgery. Postoperatively, final pathological evaluation confirms margin status. An R0 resection in noninvasive MCNs usually does not require further treatment, and the prognosis is excellent. In contrast, R1 resections in the setting of invasive carcinoma may necessitate adjuvant chemotherapy, and further surgery may be considered in selected cases. Overall, margin assessment remains essential for ensuring oncologically adequate resections and guiding further management, particularly in cases where malignancy cannot be definitively excluded intraoperatively [72, 73].

Surveillance following surgical resection of mucinous cystic neoplasms (MCNs) varies across major international guidelines, with differences reflecting attitudes toward recurrence risk, resource availability, and philosophical approaches to post-oncologic monitoring. The key determinant of postoperative follow-up is whether the resected MCN was *noninvasive* or had features of *invasive carcinoma*, with most guidelines aligning on limited or no surveillance for benign disease and structured surveillance for malignancy.

According to the *Kyoto guidelines (2024)* and *Japanese consensus statements, no postoperative surveillance is required* for completely resected, noninvasive MCNs with negative margins (R0 resection). These guidelines emphasize that once an MCN has been resected and histologically confirmed as noninvasive, the risk of recurrence is exceedingly low, and further imaging or tumor marker monitoring offers little clinical value. However, in cases where the lesion demonstrates *invasive carcinoma*, Japanese guidelines recommend a *structured follow-up schedule* similar to that used for pancreatic ductal adenocarcinoma, including *CT or MRI imaging every 3–6 months for the first 2 years*, and annually thereafter for up to 5 years, along with *tumor marker surveillance* (e.g., CA19-9).

The *AGA and ACG* also state that *no surveillance is necessary* following resection of a *noninvasive MCN*, particularly if the surgical pathology confirms low-grade or borderline features without any lymphovascular or perineural invasion. For *invasive MCNs*, American protocols recommend *regular imaging (CT or MRI)* every 6 months for at least 2–3 years, with *annual scans* up to 5 years in patients with high-risk histologic features. Tumor markers such as *CA19-9 and CEA* are commonly included in follow-up, although they are not used in isolation to dictate further treatment.

European guidelines from the *European Study Group on Cystic Tumours of the Pancreas* similarly advocate *no surveillance* for patients who undergo complete resection of noninvasive MCNs. However, they recommend *oncology-guided follow-up* for patients with high-grade dysplasia or invasive cancer. The typical European surveillance strategy includes *biannual imaging for the first 2 years*, followed by *annual imaging up to 5 years*, particularly when R1 resection, lymph node involvement, or perineural invasion is present. European centers often employ *cross-sectional imaging with MRI or CT* and tumor marker monitoring as part of a multidisciplinary postoperative strategy. The *Verona consensus group* and the *Heidelberg group* strongly support this risk-stratified approach. However, the *Heidelberg group* in patients with borderline resection margins or high-grade dysplasia sometimes extends follow-up to *10 years*, particularly in younger individuals [13, 73, 74].

In summary, all major guidelines converge on the principle that *noninvasive MCNs resected with negative margins do not require routine surveillance*, reflecting their excellent prognosis. Conversely, *invasive MCNs or those with high-risk features* mandate structured oncologic follow-up, typically involving *CT or MRI every 6–12 months*, *tumor marker monitoring*, and *multidisciplinary evaluation*. The approach is most stringent in *European and Heidelberg centers*, risk-adapted in *Verona and American guidelines*, and conservative but precise in *Asian practices*, in which case follow-up is solely employed on malignant potential rather than routine imaging.

11.3 Surgical Management of Serous Cystic Neoplasms (SCNs)

SCNs are benign epithelial neoplasms representing 15–35% of PCNs. They comprise multiple small cysts (<2 cm), often forming a microcystic mass with a central stellate scar. SCNs are predominantly diagnosed in older women (60–70 years) and are usually asymptomatic. Indications for surgery in serous cystic neoplasms (SCNs) of the pancreas vary significantly across international guidelines, reflecting their overwhelmingly benign nature and the near-zero risk of malignant transformation. The International Association of Pancreatology (IAP) and Kyoto guidelines are conservative in this regard, clearly stating that surgery is not indicated for asymptomatic SCNs, regardless of size, as long as malignancy is not suspected. They emphasize that most SCNs are indolent and incidentally detected, and even large lesions can often be safely observed. Similarly, the Verona consensus supports nonoperative management in the majority of patients, recommending surgery only in cases where the diagnosis is uncertain, symptoms are present, or the lesion is causing compressive effects on adjacent structures. The European evidence-based guidelines mirror this view, advising against resection in asymptomatic individuals and recommending intervention only for symptomatic patients, rapidly growing lesions, or those with atypical features suggesting an alternative diagnosis such as mucinous cystic neoplasm or cystic neuroendocrine tumor.

The AGA and ACG (American guidelines) align with this conservative approach, stressing that SCNs do not warrant surgery unless they cause significant symptoms like pain, biliary obstruction, or gastric outlet obstruction, or when the diagnosis remains indeterminate after thorough imaging and cyst fluid analysis. The Heidelberg group, although based in a high-volume surgical center, similarly reserves surgery for symptomatic lesions, emphasizing that resection should not be offered solely based on cyst size and cautioning against unnecessary surgery in elderly or comorbid patients. Across the board, there is consensus that the presence of diagnostic uncertainty, such as overlapping imaging features with mucinous neoplasms, remains one of the most common indications for resection, often to exclude malignancy rather than treat it.

In some Asian centers, particularly those influenced by Japanese and Korean protocols, a watchful waiting approach is favored, with resection considered only if the lesion becomes symptomatic or exceeds 10 cm, given the rare but documented complications such as hemorrhage or compression. Collectively, all major guidelines endorse a nonoperative strategy for definitively diagnosed, asymptomatic SCNs and reserve surgical resection for select cases with uncertain diagnosis, significant symptoms, or risk of complications due to large size or local mass effect compressing adjacent structures such as the stomach, duodenum, or bile duct. This unified but conservative management paradigm reflects the biological indolence of SCNs and the growing emphasis on avoiding overtreatment. Surgical approaches for serous cystic neoplasms (SCNs) of the pancreas are dictated less by oncologic necessity and more by symptom burden, diagnostic uncertainty, or mass effect on adjacent organs. When surgery is indicated, Japanese centers prioritize *minimally invasive techniques*, often performing *laparoscopic distal pancreatectomy* or *spleen-preserving pancreatectomy* if the lesion is in the body or tail. In rare cases where the lesion is in the head, *pancreaticoduodenectomy* is performed, although this is approached with caution given the benign nature of SCNs.

In *European practice*, particularly within centers adhering to *European evidence-based guidelines* and the *Verona consensus [74]*, the approach is highly individualized. Surgery is avoided unless there is significant mass effect or suspicion of an alternate diagnosis. When required, *spleen-preserving distal pancreatectomy* is favored for left-sided lesions, and *laparoscopic techniques* are strongly encouraged to minimize morbidity. The Verona group also emphasizes the use of *central pancreatectomy* in highly selected patients when the lesion is localized to the neck or proximal body, especially in younger individuals where pancreatic parenchyma preservation is prioritized.

In summary, while the *type of surgery performed for SCNs globally is influenced by lesion location*, the *overarching principle is surgical minimalism*—intervening only when necessary and favoring *minimally invasive, organ-preserving techniques. Distal pancreatectomy (often laparoscopic or robotic and spleen-preserving)* remains the most frequently performed procedure. *Central pancreatectomy* is selectively employed in Europe and Asia for lesions in the neck or proximal body, while *pancreaticoduodenectomy* is a rare last resort for large, symptomatic head lesions or when malignancy cannot be excluded.

Routine surveillance following surgical resection of serous cystic neoplasms is unnecessary when benign histology and complete excision are confirmed. Exceptions to this practice are rare and usually pertain to *uncertain diagnoses, incomplete resections, or atypical pathology*, in which case short-term individualized follow-up may be employed. This uniform approach underscores the benign nature of SCNs and the collective aim to minimize overtreatment and post-surgical burden in patients with nonmalignant pancreatic cystic disease.

11.4 Surgical Management of Solid Pseudopapillary Neoplasms (SPNs)

Solid pseudopapillary neoplasms (SPENs) are rare tumors, accounting for 1–2% of exocrine pancreatic neoplasms, and occur predominantly in young women between 20 and 30 years of age. Despite their potential for local invasion or metastasis, they typically exhibit indolent behavior. Surgical resection provides a cure in the vast majority of cases. However, when SPENs exhibit local vascular involvement, surgery becomes more complex, requiring a balance between achieving R0 resection and minimizing perioperative morbidity. Although SPENs rarely invade surrounding tissues aggressively, large or centrally located tumors may abut or encase major vessels, such as the portal vein, splenic vein, or superior mesenteric vein, presenting significant intraoperative challenges. Studies such as Wang et al. [74] have shown that even in the presence of vascular involvement, complete resection can yield long-term survival rates exceeding 95%, with minimal recurrence when negative margins are achieved.

Distal pancreatectomy remains the most commonly performed surgical procedure for SPENs located in the body or tail of the pancreas, even when the tumors abut the splenic vessels. In a retrospective analysis of 195 patients, Wang et al. [74] reported that vascular involvement—particularly of the splenic vein—was present in approximately 12% of cases. When en bloc resection, including vessel removal, was performed, survival outcomes were not adversely affected. Lu et al. [75] similarly found that tumors larger than 5 cm and those with a Ki-67 index above 3% were more likely to exhibit venous invasion and require more extensive resection. Despite this, favorable oncologic outcomes were consistently achieved when surgeries were performed in high-volume centers.

SPENs involving the pancreatic head and in proximity to the portal or superior mesenteric vein often necessitate pancreaticoduodenectomy, sometimes combined with venous resection and reconstruction. A multicenter study by Yang et al. [76] reported that vascular resection was required in 8% of SPEN surgeries, with no significant increase in postoperative mortality or long-term recurrence. SPENs usually displace rather than encase vessels, facilitating safer dissection. This has been corroborated by the Heidelberg group [77], who noted the absence of the dense desmoplastic reaction commonly seen in pancreatic adenocarcinoma, allowing for safer vascular dissection or segmental resection.

Central pancreatectomy may be technically feasible for SPENs in the neck or proximal body, even with limited venous involvement. However, Zhou et al. [78] cautioned that such procedures carry an increased risk of postoperative pancreatic fistula, with reported rates exceeding 30%, due to the presence of two pancreatic transection sites and proximity to major vascular structures.

Enucleation is not recommended when SPENs are near major vessels or if vascular invasion is suspected. It may be considered for small (<3 cm), well-encapsulated lesions located away from critical structures, but several studies, including Zhou et al. [79] and Wang et al. [80], have demonstrated higher rates of incomplete resection and postoperative pancreatic fistula in such cases. As a result, most institutions advise against enucleation in tumors with vascular proximity.

Another intraoperative concern is tumor rupture, particularly in hemorrhagic or cystic SPENs. Machado et al. [81], in a large multi-institutional review, reported that intraoperative rupture during dissection near vascular structures may increase the risk of peritoneal dissemination. However, long-term recurrence remains rare if meticulous handling and complete resection are achieved.

Lymphadenectomy is generally not required, even in cases of vessel involvement, as lymph node metastasis is uncommon (<5%). Martin et al. [82] confirmed that routine lymph node dissection offers no survival benefit, even in aggressive SPEN variants.

Following complete resection of noninvasive SPENs with negative margins, intensive long-term surveillance is not typically required due to the extremely low risk of recurrence. Most guidelines support limited postoperative imaging to monitor for early recurrence, with extended follow-up reserved for patients with high-risk histological features.

According to Japanese guidelines and the Kyoto consensus [1, 2, 83], no surveillance is needed after R0 resection of a low-grade SPEN, particularly in young women. However, in cases of capsular breach, Ki-67 index greater than 10%, or positive margins, imaging at 6-month intervals for 2 years is suggested, with discontinuation thereafter if no recurrence is detected.

The American approach (AGA/ACG) is less standardized, with most academic centers recommending CT or MRI at 6–12 months postoperatively, followed by annual imaging for up to 3 years in patients with high-risk features such as large tumor size (>8 cm), lymphovascular invasion, or incomplete resection. For patients with completely resected low-risk tumors, further imaging beyond the first postoperative year is usually not required.

European consensus, including from the Verona group [84, 85], supports a risk-stratified surveillance model. A single postoperative MRI or CT at 6 months is generally recommended. If the tumor is confirmed to be low risk and imaging is normal, no further surveillance is indicated. In contrast, if vascular invasion, margin positivity, or a Ki-67 index above 10% is noted, annual imaging for 5 years is advised. Tumor markers such as CA19–9 and CEA are not used in surveillance due to their lack of relevance in SPENs.

The Heidelberg group [85] recommends structured surveillance in high-risk or atypical cases, including those with nodal involvement, invasion into adjacent organs, or positive surgical margins. Their protocol includes MRI or CT imaging every 6 months for 2 years, followed by annual imaging for 3 years.

In other Asian countries, such as South Korea, China, and Singapore, a modified version of the Japanese protocol is commonly followed. Imaging at 6 months and 1 year postoperatively is standard, with follow-up discontinued in low-risk cases. However, longer surveillance may be employed for larger tumors (>10 cm), those with intraoperative rupture, or surgeries involving vascular resection.

In rare instances of metastatic SPEN, particularly to the liver, prolonged surveillance is warranted. In such cases, imaging every 6 months for 5 years is generally recommended, sometimes supplemented with PET or functional imaging based on institutional preference.

11.5 Role of Enucleation of Pancreatic Cystic Lesions

Enucleation is a pancreas-sparing surgical technique that involves removal of a cystic lesion without formal pancreatic resection. It is most suitable for small, benign, exophytic lesions that are located away from the main pancreatic duct (MPD) and have low malignant potential. Across the world, its use is selective and individualized, varying by cyst type, institutional experience, and proximity to ductal and vascular structures.

In *serous cystic neoplasms (SCNs)*, enucleation is occasionally performed for small, symptomatic lesions, especially when they are exophytic and located in the body or tail. Since SCNs are nearly always benign, enucleation offers the benefit of preserving pancreatic parenchyma and minimizing morbidity. However, because SCNs often have a rich vascular stroma, bleeding risk is higher, and in deeper or central lesions, distal pancreatectomy is often favored. Studies like El-Hayek et al. [86] and others suggest that enucleation of SCNs is safe in expert hands but has higher rates of pancreatic fistula (20–30%) due to inadequate sealing of transected tissue near the ductal system.

In *mucinous cystic neoplasms (MCNs)*, enucleation is not recommended by major guidelines (AGA, IAP, Kyoto, Verona, Heidelberg), due to the premalignant or malignant potential of MCNs and their characteristic ovarian-type stroma. Complete oncologic resection—typically distal pancreatectomy—is the standard of care. Studies have shown that enucleation may lead to incomplete resection and failure to properly evaluate the lesion's invasive component. Therefore, formal anatomic resection remains the preferred approach for all MCNs, even when small and superficially located [87, 88].

In *intraductal papillary mucinous neoplasms (IPMNs)*, especially branch-duct (BD) types, enucleation has a limited role. It may be considered in highly selected patients with solitary, small (<2–3 cm), non-enhancing BD-IPMN that is clearly exophytic and without any communication with the main duct. However, IPMNs are frequently multifocal and have a higher risk of recurrence, and enucleation may not allow proper lymph node assessment or ductal margin clearance. Major guideline groups discourage routine enucleation in IPMN due to the risk of missing microscopic malignancy and limited ability to evaluate dysplasia intraoperatively [87].

In *solid pseudopapillary epithelial neoplasms (SPENs)*, enucleation is theoretically feasible for small (<3 cm), well-encapsulated lesions distant from the MPD. However, recent literature (e.g., Wang et al. [89], Zhou et al. [90]) cautions against enucleation in SPENs due to their potential for local invasion, capsular breach, and high rates of postoperative clinically relevant pancreatic fistula (up to 30–40%). Therefore, enucleation in SPEN is only appropriate in exceptional cases, where the lesion is exophytic, away from the duct, and has imaging-confirmed benign behavior, usually in young patients where preserving pancreatic function is paramount [94].

From a technical perspective, enucleation poses a higher risk of pancreatic fistula than standard resections, due to the absence of formal ductal ligation and the proximity of the lesion to the MPD. This is especially relevant in lesions near the head or neck of the pancreas. In high-volume centers, enucleation can be performed safely using laparoscopic or robotic assistance, with careful dissection and sealing of small pancreatic branches. A study by Goh et al. [91] demonstrates that laparoscopic enucleation is associated with shorter hospital stay and preserved endocrine/exocrine function but higher Grade B/C fistula rates compared to formal resection. These findings are supported by other analyses showing increased fistula but acceptable outcomes when performed in specialized centers [88, 92–95].

11.6 AI-Driven Risk Stratification and Surveillance

AI techniques, including deep learning algorithms and radiomics, have shown promise in improving the accuracy of PCN diagnosis and risk assessment [96, 97]. By analyzing imaging data such as CT and MRI scans, AI models can provide more consistent and reliable evaluations of pancreatic cysts, aiding in distinguishing between benign and potentially malignant lesions. This approach helps clinicians make informed decisions regarding the necessity of surgical intervention versus continued surveillance.

One notable development is the use of computational linguistics models to enhance patient identification and follow-up. These models can process radiology reports to detect incidental pancreatic cysts, ensuring that patients receive appropriate surveillance and care [99]. Such systems have demonstrated the potential to reduce disparities in healthcare delivery by automating the identification and management of at-risk individuals.

11.7 Advancements in Imaging and Diagnostic Tools

Recent studies have explored the integration of AI with endoscopic ultrasound (EUS) to improve the differentiation of pancreatic lesions. AI-enhanced EUS has achieved high accuracy in classifying various types of pancreatic cysts and solid lesions, facilitating more precise diagnoses and treatment planning [98].

Additionally, the development of AI algorithms capable of analyzing multi-contrast MRI scans has improved the classification of intraductal papillary mucinous neoplasms (IPMNs). These models combine radiomics and deep learning to enhance the prediction of malignancy risk, supporting clinicians in making evidence-based decisions regarding patient management [100–102]. The integration of AI and ML into the management of PCNs represents a significant advancement in personalized medicine. These technologies offer the potential to improve early detection, risk stratification, and surveillance of pancreatic cysts, ultimately aiming to prevent the progression to pancreatic cancer and enhance patient outcomes [103–106].

11.8 Conclusion

The surgical management of pancreatic cystic neoplasms (PCNs) demands a nuanced, subtype-specific, and patient-centered approach. While *MCNs* warrant resection in all fit patients due to their premalignant potential, *SCNs* are largely benign and best managed conservatively unless symptomatic or diagnostically ambiguous. *IPMNs* require individualized strategies based on ductal involvement, risk features, and evolving guidelines, balancing overtreatment with cancer prevention. *SPENs*, despite occasional vascular involvement, offer excellent outcomes with complete resection, even in complex cases. Emerging tools such as *AI, radiomics, molecular profiling, and liquid biopsy* are reshaping diagnostics and risk stratification, moving toward precision surgery and avoiding unnecessary interventions. Globally, there is a clear shift toward *minimally invasive, organ-preserving techniques*, emphasizing *oncologic adequacy, patient physiology*, and *long-term quality of life.*

References

1. Tanaka M, Fernández-del Castillo C, Adsay V, et al. International consensus guidelines 2012 for the management of IPMN and MCN of the pancreas. Pancreatology. 2012;12(3):183–97.
2. Tanaka M, Fernández-del Castillo C, Kamisawa T, et al. Revisions of international consensus Fukuoka guidelines for the management of IPMN of the pancreas. Pancreatology. 2017;17(5):738–53.
3. Brugge WR, Lewandrowski K, Lee-Lewandrowski E, et al. Diagnosis of pancreatic cystic neoplasms: a report of the cooperative pancreatic cyst study. Gastroenterology. 2004;126(5):1330–6.
4. Elta GH, Enestvedt BK, Sauer BG, Lennon AM. ACG clinical guideline: diagnosis and management of pancreatic cysts. Am J Gastroenterol. 2018;113(4):464–79.
5. Laffan TA, Horton KM, Klein AP, et al. Prevalence of unsuspected pancreatic cysts on MDCT. AJR Am J Roentgenol. 2008;191(3):802–7.
6. Sahora K, Mino-Kenudson M, Brugge W, et al. Branch duct IPMN: does cyst size change predict malignancy? A multicenter study. Ann Surg Oncol. 2013;20(11):3623–30.
7. Allen PJ, D'Angelica M, Gonen M, et al. A selective approach to the resection of cystic lesions of the pancreas: results from 539 consecutive patients. Ann Surg. 2006;244(4):572–82.
8. Fernández-del Castillo C, Targarona J, Thayer SP, et al. Incidental pancreatic cysts: clinicopathologic characteristics and comparison with symptomatic patients. Arch Surg. 2003;138(4):427–34.
9. Furukawa T, Klöppel G, Volkan Adsay N, et al. Classification of types of intraductal papillary-mucinous neoplasm of the pancreas. Ann Surg. 2005;241(1):67–74.
10. Yamaguchi K, Kanemitsu S, Hatori T, et al. Pancreatic carcinoma derived from IPMN. Ann Surg. 2005;242(3):313–21.
11. Kang MJ, Jang JY, Kim SW. Surgical outcomes of branch duct type IPMNs. Ann Surg Oncol. 2011;18(12):3461–8.
12. Sugiyama M, Atomi Y. Secretin-stimulated MRCP in the diagnosis of IPMNs. AJR Am J Roentgenol. 2002;179(1):179–86.
13. Del Chiaro M, Verbeke C, Salvia R, et al. European experts consensus statement on cystic tumours of the pancreas. Dig Liver Dis. 2013;45(9):703–11.
14. Marchegiani G, Andrianello S, Morbin G, et al. IPMN of the pancreas: the Verona experience. Ann Surg. 2015;262(4):792–801.
15. Hackert T, Fritz S, Klauss M, et al. Main-duct IPMN: surgery for high-grade dysplasia. Surgery. 2011;150(5):949–56.
16. Fritz S, Hackert T, Hinz U, et al. Role of serum tumor markers CA19-9 and CEA in the diagnosis of cystic pancreatic lesions. Langenbeck's Arch Surg. 2011;396(5):681–6.
17. Correa-Gallego C, Warshaw AL, Fernandez-Del Castillo C. IPMN of the pancreas and the risk of cancer. Clin Gastroenterol Hepatol. 2010;8(12):957–62.
18. Jang JY, Park T, Lee S, et al. Proposed nomogram predicting risk of malignancy in IPMN. Ann Surg. 2017;266(6):1062–8.
19. Gaujoux S, Brennan MF, Gonen M, et al. Cystic neoplasms of the pancreas: changes in management and outcome. Surgery. 2010;148(4):631–8.
20. Shimizu Y, Yasui M, Nishihara K, et al. Evaluation of mural nodules and septa in pancreatic cystic tumors using MRCP. J Gastroenterol. 2004;39(6):498–506.

21. White R, Winston C, Gonen M, et al. Current management and long-term outcomes of IPMNs. Ann Surg. 2008;248(5):837–46.
22. Crippa S, Salvia R, Warshaw AL, et al. Mucin-producing neoplasms of the pancreas: an appraisal of current knowledge and clinical implications. Surg Clin North Am. 2010;90(2):331–58.
23. Lennon AM, Wolfgang CL, Canto MI, et al. The early detection of pancreatic cancer: what will it take to diagnose and treat curable pancreatic neoplasia? Cancer Res. 2014;74(13):3381–9.
24. Malleo G, Marchegiani G, Borin A, et al. IPMNs with associated invasive carcinoma: role of imaging in surgical decision making. Surg Oncol. 2015;24(2):123–30.
25. Basturk O, Hong SM, Wood LD, et al. A revised classification system and recommendations from the Baltimore consensus meeting for neoplastic precursor lesions in the pancreas. Am J Surg Pathol. 2015;39(12):1730–41.
26. Khashab MA, Shin EJ, Amateau SK, et al. Tumor size and presence of mural nodules correlate with invasive carcinoma in resected branch duct IPMNs. Clin Gastroenterol Hepatol. 2011;9(10):936–41.
27. Springer S, Wang Y, Dal Molin M, et al. A combination of molecular markers and clinical features improve the classification of pancreatic cysts. Gastroenterology. 2015;149(6):1501–10.
28. Allen PJ, Kuk D, Castillo CF, et al. Multi-institutional validation study of the American Gastroenterological Association guidelines for the diagnosis and management of IPMNs. J Am Coll Surg. 2017;224(4):461–9.
29. Ohtsuka T, Fernandez-del Castillo C, Furukawa T, et al. International evidence-based Kyoto guidelines for the management of intraductal papillary mucinous neoplasm of the pancreas. Pancreatology. 2024;24(2):255–70.
30. Elta GH, Appelbaum MI, Ball CG, et al. AGA clinical practice update on management of pancreatic cysts: expert review. Gastroenterology. 2024;166(4):781–92.
31. Oyama H, Tada M, Takagi K, et al. Long-term risk of pancreatic cancer in IPMN patients. Gut. 2022;71(1):123–30.
32. Valsangkar NP, Morales-Oyarvide V, Thayer SP, et al. 851 resected cystic tumors of the pancreas: a 33-year experience at the Massachusetts General Hospital. Surgery. 2012;152(3 Suppl 1):S4–12.
33. Sahora K, Crippa S, Mino-Kenudson M, et al. Multicenter international study of main-duct IPMN: surgery improves survival in patients with high-grade dysplasia. J Gastrointest Surg. 2015;19(5):873–80.
34. Del Chiaro M, Verbeke C, Salvia R, et al. European experts consensus on surveillance of IPMN. Pancreatology. 2013;13(6):539–45.
35. Kimura W, Moriya T, Hirai I, et al. Multicenter study of IPMNs: management and long-term follow-up in Japan. J Hepatobiliary Pancreat Sci. 2010;17(5):770–8.
36. Zhang XM, Mitchell DG, Dohke M, et al. Pancreatic cancer: value of multiphasic contrast-enhanced MR imaging in tumor detection and assessment of resectability. Radiology. 2003;226(3):695–703.
37. Hamada T, Nakai Y, Iwasaki M, et al. Natural history of branch-duct IPMNs: long-term results of a prospective study. Gut. 2025;74(3):542–52.
38. Pitman MB, Deshpande V, Brugge WR. Cytology of pancreatic cystic lesions. Clin Gastroenterol Hepatol. 2008;6(7):691–8.
39. Maker AV, Katabi N, Gonen M, et al. Pancreatic cyst fluid and serum tumor markers predict invasive IPMN. Ann Surg Oncol. 2011;18(1):199–206.
40. Reid MD, Choi H, Balci S, et al. Variation in pathologic diagnosis of pancreatic neoplasms in frozen vs permanent sections. Am J Surg Pathol. 2015;39(6):761–72; Marchegiani G, Mino-Kenudson M, Ferrone CR, et al. Patterns of recurrence after resection of IPMN with invasive carcinoma. Ann Surg Oncol. 2015;22(5):1668–75.
41. Hackert T, Jang JY, Salvia R, Yamaue H, Wolfgang CL. State-of-the-art surgery for IPMN of the pancreas. Surgery. 2021;170(3):581–7.

42. Marchegiani G, Pollini T, Burelli A, Han Y, Jung HS, Kwon W, et al. Surveillance for presumed BD-IPMN of the pancreas: stability, size, and age identify targets for discontinuation. Gastroenterology. 2023;165(5):1016–24.
43. Habib JR, Rompen IF, Javed AA, et al. Outcomes in intraductal papillary mucinous neoplasm-derived pancreatic cancer differ from PanIN-derived pancreatic cancer. J Gastroenterol Hepatol. 2024; https://doi.org/10.1111/jgh.16686.
44. Bassi C, Marchegiani G, Dervenis C, et al. The 2016 update of the ISGPS definition and grading of postoperative pancreatic fistula. Surgery. 2017;161(3):584–91.
45. Postlewait LM, Ethun CG, McInnis MR, et al. Risk factors for recurrence and survival after surgical resection of IPMN. Ann Surg. 2016;263(3):512–9.
46. Balduzzi A, Milanese G, Capurso G, et al. AI-based radiomic model improves malignancy prediction in IPMNs. Radiology. 2023;306(2):e220961.
47. Chakraborty J, Midiri M, Lee E, et al. Deep learning for predicting dysplasia in pancreatic cysts using MRI. J Magn Reson Imaging. 2022;56(4):1289–97.
48. Permuth JB, Choi J, Balarunathan Y, et al. Combining molecular markers with imaging features improves risk prediction in pancreatic cysts. Clin Cancer Res. 2021;27(3):904–915.
49. Permuth JB, Zhang L, Chen DT, et al. Genomic analysis identifies subtypes of intraductal papillary mucinous neoplasms with distinct clinicopathologic features. Ann Surg. 2019;269(6):1051–9.
50. Woodward BD, Singh G, Hanna M, et al. Artificial intelligence for risk stratification of pancreatic cystic lesions: a systematic review and meta-analysis. Pancreatology. 2023;23(1):56–65.
51. Corral JE, Arnold CA, Sandhu DS, et al. Use of artificial intelligence and machine learning for the diagnosis and management of pancreatic cysts: a systematic review. Clin Gastroenterol Hepatol. 2022;20(2):276–288.e4.
52. Permuth JB, Choi J, Balarunathan Y, et al. Combining radiomics with pathology improves survival prediction among patients with resected pancreatic ductal adenocarcinoma. Oncotarget. 2016;7(52):85785–97.
53. Hanania AN, Bantis LE, Feng Z, et al. Quantitative imaging to evaluate malignant potential of IPMNs. Oncotarget. 2016;7(52):85776–84.
54. Thompson LD, Becker RC, Przygodzki RM, Adair CF. Ovarian-type stroma in mucinous cystic neoplasms of the pancreas: a clinicopathologic study of 35 cases. Am J Surg Pathol. 2001;25(5):588–93.
55. Wu J, Jiao Y, Dal Molin M, et al. Whole-exome sequencing of neoplastic cysts of the pancreas reveals recurrent mutations in components of ubiquitin-dependent pathways. Proc Natl Acad Sci USA. 2011;108(52):21188–93.
56. Amato E, Molin MD, Mafficini A, et al. Targeted next-generation sequencing of cancer genes dissects the molecular profiles of intraductal papillary neoplasms of the pancreas. J Pathol. 2014;233(3):217–27.
57. Noë M, Niknafs N, Fischer CG, et al. Genomic characterization of malignant progression in pancreatic mucinous cystic neoplasms. NPJ Precis Oncol. 2018;2:16.
58. Zamboni G, Scarpa A, Bogina G, et al. Mucinous cystic tumors of the pancreas: clinicopathologic features, prognosis, and relationship to other mucinous cystic tumors. Am J Surg Pathol. 1999;23(4):410–22.
59. Edwin B, Sahora K, Crippa S, et al. Minimally invasive distal pancreatectomy for cystic tumors. Surg Endosc. 2021;35(5):2182–9.
60. Warshaw AL, Parangi S. Organ-preserving pancreatic surgery. J Am Coll Surg. 2005;200(2):177–91.
61. Choi JY, Kim MJ, Lee JY, et al. Mucinous cystic neoplasm of the pancreas: CT imaging features and prediction of malignancy. AJR Am J Roentgenol. 2006;187(4):949–55.
62. Overbeek KA, Goudswaard AN, Goudriaan M, et al. Management and outcome of resected mucinous cystic neoplasms: a nationwide cohort study. Br J Surg. 2023;110(7):806–12.
63. Tomasiewicz K, Makohon-Moore AP, Chadalavada K, et al. Circulating tumor DNA analysis as a novel tool for diagnosing high-grade pancreatic cystic neoplasms. Clin Cancer Res. 2022;28(1):106–14.

64. Kim JY, Hong SM. Recent advances in the pathology of mucinous cystic neoplasms of the pancreas. Korean J Pathol. 2014;48(5):307–13.
65. Maker AV, Katabi N, Gonen M, et al. Pancreatic mucinous cystic neoplasms: a single-institution experience of 141 cases. J Gastrointest Surg. 2012;16(4):795–802.
66. Takahashi H, et al. Frozen section diagnosis during pancreatic surgery. J Hepatobiliary Pancreat Sci. 2020;27(1):4–10.
67. Yamaguchi K, et al. Japanese consensus guidelines 2023 for the management of pancreatic cystic neoplasms. J Hepatobiliary Pancreat Sci. 2023;30(2):181–203.
68. Mino-Kenudson M. Diagnostic implications of pancreatic intraepithelial neoplasia and IPMN. Semin Diagn Pathol. 2014;31(6):443–54.
69. Bassi C, Salvia R, Butturini G, et al. Surgical treatment of pancreatic cystic neoplasms. HPB (Oxford). 2006;8(5):315–21.
70. Takahashi H, Nakagohri T, Konishi M, et al. Utility of intraoperative frozen section diagnosis in determining the surgical margin of pancreatic cancer. J Hepatobiliary Pancreat Sci. 2020;27(1):4–10.
71. He J, Cameron JL, Ahuja N, et al. Is it necessary to perform frozen section evaluation of pancreatic neck margins during resection for cystic neoplasms? Ann Surg. 2013;257(3):463–9.
72. Bassi C, Salvia R, Butturini G, et al. Management of pancreatic cystic lesions: the Verona experience. Surg Oncol Clin N Am. 2010;19(2):263–74.
73. Wang X, Zhang Y, Sun L, et al. Surgical outcomes and vascular involvement in solid pseudopapillary neoplasms: a multicenter analysis. Front Oncol. 2024;14:1223119.
74. Lu H, Li Y, Zhao W, et al. Predictive value of Ki-67 and tumor size in assessing SPEN aggressiveness. BMC Cancer. 2024;24(1):212.
75. Yang F, Jin C, Long J, et al. Surgical management of solid pseudopapillary tumor of the pancreas: aggressive or less? Ann Surg Oncol. 2016;23(2):513–9.
76. Hackert T, Schulz HU, Hinz U, et al. Solid pseudopapillary tumors of the pancreas: specific surgical management and long-term outcome. Eur J Surg Oncol. 2011;37(7):567–73.
77. Zhou Y, Gao S, Li L, et al. Central pancreatectomy: indications and postoperative outcomes. Ann Surg. 2015;261(3):693–700.
78. Zhou Y, Yang G, Cui Y, et al. Enucleation versus resection for pancreatic neoplasms: a meta-analysis. Surgery. 2011;149(6):823–36.
79. Wang W, Zhang L, Han B, et al. Role of enucleation in management of SPEN: a 10-year single center review. World J Gastrointest Surg. 2022;14(8):826–34.
80. Machado MC, da Cunha JE, Bacchella T, et al. Intraoperative rupture of pancreatic SPEN and risk of peritoneal dissemination: an institutional analysis. HPB (Oxford). 2020;22(1):90–6.
81. Martin RC, Klimstra DS, Brennan MF, et al. Solid pseudopapillary tumors of the pancreas: a surgical enigma? Ann Surg Oncol. 2012;19(2):547–54.
82. Ohtsuka T, et al. Japanese guidelines for the management of pancreatic solid pseudopapillary neoplasms (SPENs). Pancreatology 2024;24(2):101–114.
83. Bassi C, Salvia R, Butturini G, et al. Surgical management of pancreatic cystic tumors: the Verona perspective. Surg Oncol Clin N Am. 2010;19(2):263–74.
84. Schmid RM, Friess H, Kleeff J. Pancreatic neoplasms: Heidelberg approach to follow-up and management. Digestion. 2010;82(4):248–55.
85. El-Hayek KM, Brown N, O'Rourke C, et al. Enucleation of pancreatic neoplasms: is it worthwhile? Surg Endosc. 2013;27(5):1420–5.
86. Vege SS, Ziring B, Jain R, et al. AGA guideline on the diagnosis and management of asymptomatic neoplastic pancreatic cysts. Gastroenterology. 2015;148(4):819–22.
87. Crippa S, Bassi C, Salvia R, et al. Enucleation of pancreatic neoplasms. Br J Surg. 2007;94(10):1254–9.
88. Wang X, Zhang J, Wu J, et al. Enucleation versus resection for SPENs: a retrospective study and meta-analysis. World J Surg. 2022;46(2):343–51.
89. Zhou Y, Gao S, Zhang T, et al. Enucleation versus standard resection for SPENs: a meta-analysis. Surgery. 2011;149(4):471–80.

90. Goh BKP, Tan YM, Chung YFA, et al. Laparoscopic versus open enucleation for pancreatic tumors. J Gastrointest Surg. 2010;14(4):649–55.
91. Hackert T, Fritz S, Klauss M, et al. Enucleation in pancreatic surgery: indications and outcome. Ann Surg. 2011;254(6):1027–34.
92. Del Chiaro M, Verbeke C, Kartalis N, et al. Minimally invasive enucleation of pancreatic neoplasms: international multicenter study. Surgery. 2015;158(6):1574–80.
93. Law JK, Ahmed A, Singh VK, et al. Solid pseudopapillary neoplasms: a systematic review. Pancreas. 2014;43(3):331–7.
94. Heger U, Sun H, Hinz U, et al. Resection outcomes in cystic pancreatic lesions. Br J Surg. 2014;101(5):512–20.
95. Corral JE, Hussein S, Kandel P, et al. Deep learning analysis of pancreatic cyst fluid cytology and histology. Gastrointest Endosc. 2021;93(6):1334–1342.e1.
96. Qureshi A, Khalvati F, Bandali E, et al. Radiomics classification of pancreatic cysts using MRI. Clin Radiol. 2021;76(6):445.e19–27.
97. Huang P, Sun J, Wang W, et al. AI-assisted EUS for pancreatic neoplasms: multicenter study. EBioMedicine. 2022;75:103762.
98. Diaz M, Newton A, Cohen M, et al. NLP to detect incidental pancreatic cysts in radiology reports. NPJ Digit Med. 2023;6(1):82.
99. Balduzzi A, Pistillo MP, Malleo G, et al. AI model with radiomics and deep learning for IPMN malignancy prediction. Pancreatology. 2023;23(6):580–9.
100. Choi J, Hwang JH, Kim JE, et al. AI-based risk stratification for pancreatic cysts: multicenter study. Radiology. 2024;310(1):e230348.
101. Xie Y, Lu L, Kulkarni AV, et al. Radiomics and ML for risk in branch duct IPMN. Ann Surg Oncol. 2022;29(8):4913–22.
102. Nasief H, Zheng C, Schott D, et al. ML model for early mortality in pancreatic cancer. Front Oncol. 2019;9:874.
103. Kurita Y, Kawamoto S, Siripongsakun S, et al. Deep learning for survival prediction post-resection in pancreatic cancer. Radiology. 2021;301(1):194–203.
104. Fujikawa T, Yoshida M, Toya Y, et al. Future directions for AI in pancreatic cystic neoplasms. World J Gastroenterol. 2023;29(21):3222–36.
105. Nasief H, Zheng C, Schott D, et al. Predicting mortality in pancreatic cancer using radiomics. Front Oncol. 2019;9:874.
106. Kurita Y, Kawamoto S, Siripongsakun S, et al. DL-based survival prediction model for pancreatic cancer. Radiology. 2021;301(1):194–203.

Emerging Technologies in Pancreatic Cyst Diagnosis

12

Saurabh Dawra, Ravi Kumar Sharma, and Romika Dawra

Abstract

Pancreatic cystic lesions (PCLs) are emerging as a common incidental finding, fueled by the routine use of imaging in aging populations. Differentiating benign from premalignant or malignant cysts remain a major challenge, as conventional imaging and cytology provide limited sensitivity and specificity.

We reviewed emerging diagnostic modalities including radiomics, contrast-enhanced harmonic endoscopic ultrasound (CH-EUS), confocal laser endomicroscopy (CLE), EUS-guided microforceps biopsy, and cyst fluid biomarker analysis. Evidence from multicenter trials, validation studies, and meta-analyses was synthesized to evaluate diagnostic performance, reproducibility, and limitations.

Current first-line tools—cross-sectional imaging and EUS-FNA cytology—are limited (EUS morphology sensitivity ~50%; cytology ~60%; cyst fluid CEA >192 ng/mL, sensitivity 58%, specificity 87%). Radiomics models integrating CT/MRI features with clinical data achieved 76–92% accuracy for cyst subtype classification and malignant risk stratification, though external validation is lacking. CH-EUS improved mural nodule detection (sensitivity up to 97%, specificity 75%), outperforming CT (77%) and MRI (79%). Needle-based CLE provided real-time histology-like imaging; multicenter trials reported >90% sensitivity and specificity for mucinous vs. nonmucinous cysts, with accuracy superior to cyst fluid CEA. Interobserver agreement varied (κ 0.66–0.82), but deep learning

S. Dawra (✉)
Department of Gastroenterology, Command Hospital, Udhampur, India

R. K. Sharma
Department of Biotechnology, Chandigarh University, Mohali, Punjab, India

R. Dawra
Department of Microbiology, Dinanath Mangeshkar Hospital & Research Center, Pune, India

R. K. Sharma et al. (eds.), *Differential Diagnosis and Management of Pancreatic Cystic Lesions*, https://doi.org/10.1007/978-981-92-0654-4_12

networks applied to CLE videos achieved >90% classification accuracy. EUS-guided microforceps biopsy showed pooled sensitivity of 76.6% and specificity of 98.9%. Cyst fluid biomarkers demonstrated promise: glucose <50 mg/dL (93% sensitivity, 89% specificity), GNAS/KRAS mutations (90% sensitivity, 100% specificity), and combined molecular panels (88%/98% for advanced neoplasia). DNA methylation, miRNA panels, and glycoproteomics further enhanced risk stratification but remain investigational.

Emerging technologies are reshaping PCL diagnostics. Radiomics, CH-EUS, CLE, microforceps biopsy, and molecular biomarkers provide complementary strengths. Their integration into standardized algorithms, supported by multicenter validation, will be essential to optimize patient outcomes.

Keywords

Pancreatic cyst · Pancreatic neoplasms · Endosonography · Biopsy · Fine-needle · Confocal microscopy · Radiomics · Biomarkers · Tumor · DNA mutational analysis · Intraductal mucinous neoplasm · Mucinous cystic neoplasm · Serous cystadenoma · Solid pseudopapillary neoplasms

12.1 Introduction

Pancreatic cystic lesions (PCLs) are increasing being diagnosed owing to an ever-increasing use of imaging modalities in an aging population. It is estimated that 2.4–13.5% of all patients who undergo abdominal imaging may harbor incidentally detected PCLs [1]. This has brought forth an increasing necessity to differentiate benign, low risk lesions from high-risk, malignant ones. The most lethal form is the pancreatic cancer, notorious for its aggressive behavior and rapid progression. Thus, our ability to identify precursor neoplasm in PCLs offers a window of opportunity for early diagnosis and intervention.

Traditionally, cross-sectional imaging, endoscopic ultrasound (EUS), and biomarkers have been employed often in combination, to achieve a possible diagnosis with variable sensitivity and specificity. A 1.5 or 3 Tesla magnetic resonance pancreatography (MRCP) can differentiate benign from malignant pancreatic cysts in 55%–76% of the cases, while it is only 40%–50% accurate in diagnosing the specific type of cysts [2]. A contrast-enhanced computerized tomography (CECT) abdomen has comparable sensitivity to identify a benign lesion from a malignant one but often suffers from lack of specificity in differentiating the type of cyst [3].

There are several emerging technologies that are poised to revolutionize diagnosis and management of PCLs. This chapter aims to highlight these newer techniques with a critical review of the available literature, their advantages as well as limitations.

12.2 Radiomics

Radiomics aims to convert the hidden information stored in standard-of-care digital images acquired through various modalities like ultrasound (USG), computerized imaging tomography (CT), magnetic resonance imaging (MRI), and positron emission tomography (PET) to high-quality data.

12.2.1 Process of Radiomics

The combination of stored images with lesion-specific molecular data using next-generation sequencing technologies (NGS) and high-throughput arrays provides high-quality computer-aided diagnosis [4]. Radiomics offers distinct advantages; it utilizes standard radiographic images, using readily available software. Lesion segmentation defines the boundaries of a suspected lesion, followed by creation of 3D model utilizing all the voxels in the region of interest (ROI). Asymmetry, sharpness, entropy, and grayscale variation of textures are recorded. Fractal analysis subsequently quantifies nonrepetitive and repetitive patterns. Finally, patient-specific characteristics along with selected radiomic metrics are added to a model using the machine learning approach [5]. Radiomics scores over "deep learning" as it provides highly interpretable data using a smaller sample size and less reliability on hardware equipment [6]. Flowchart below summarizes a simplified view of this complex process.

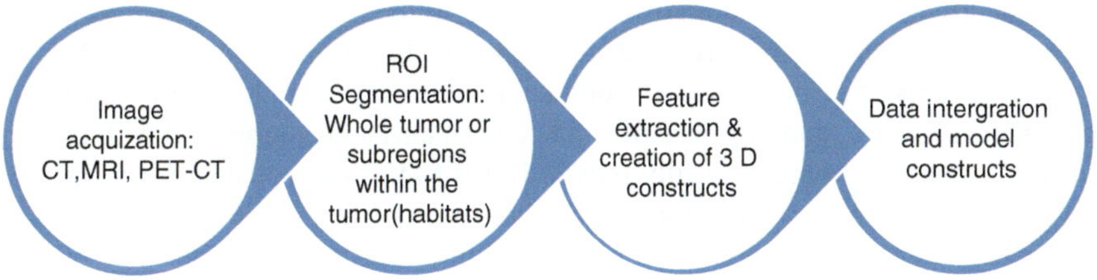

12.2.2 Radiomics in PCLs

In one of the first studies on the subject, Dimitriev et al. used patient-specific demographic features, namely age and gender, pancreatic lesion-related imaging features, i.e., location, shape, and intensity, and subjected this information to random forest classifier and convolutional neural network. The authors proposed an accuracy of 84% in predicting common PCLs: intraductal mucinous neoplasm (IPMN), mucinous cystic neoplasm (MCN), serous cystadenoma (SCA), and solid pseudopapillary neoplasm (SPN) [7]. To avoid an overdiagnosis, a preoperative predictive model was proposed by Wei et al. The aim was to differentiate SCA from other PCLs. They used 17 image-specific intensity and texture features, combined it with 05 guideline-derived features, namely gender, location of lesion, size, moment difference, and mean rectangular fitting factor, and subjected these statistically significant features toward building a diagnostic model with the help of "support vector machine (SVM)" and "least absolute shrinkage and selection operator (LASSO)" machine learning tools. Their proposed model had a predicted accuracy of 83% among 60 patients included in the validation cohort and 76% in the cross-validation cohort [8]. Chen et al. have also used LASSO and logistic regression to identify radiomic features aimed to differentiate SCA from other mucin-producing PCLs (MCN, IPMN). Interestingly, they have utilized radiomic features of triple-phase CT scan (venous phase, late arterial phase, and plain CT) in addition to clinical features (number of cysts) to construct a model with a higher predictive value than those employing radiomic features of a single-phase or dual-phase CT [9]. Fang et al. proposed a nomogram built using MRI T2-weighted imaging features (T2W) in combination with clinical features (tumor location, its size and shape, gender, and history of pancreatitis). This particular nomogram differentiates SCA from MCN with an AUC of 0.93 and 0.86 in training and validation cohorts, respectively [10].

Among all the PCLs, IPMN has the highest malignant potential. Surgical resection is the treatment of choice for main-duct IPMN (MD-IPMN) and mixed-type IPMN (MT-IPMN) owing to their higher risk of malignant transformation (38–68%). Branch-duct IPMN (BD-IPMN) on the other hand requires further characterization to determine features predictive of higher grades of dysplasia [11, 12]. Thus, preoperative risk assessment of the malignant potential is a key decision-making step. Cui et al. have used the size of the main pancreatic duct (MPD), carbohydrate antigen 19-9 (CA 19-9), and MRI radiomic features using logistic regression analysis and LASSO to build a preoperative predictive model for BD- IPMN with AUC of 0.903 and 0.884 in training and external validation cohort, respectively [13]. Tobalay et al. have used CT radiomic features to differentiate benign from malignant IPMN [14].

Chakraborty et al. have used five clinical features (age, gender, presence of pain abdomen, cyst size, and presence of solid component) and combined it with presurgical CT images of pathologically proven BD-IPMNs analyzed using support vector machine tool and random forest classifier to propose a model with an AUC of 0.81 in differentiating malignant IPMNs from low-risk ones and a negative predictive value of 90% [15].

Bootstrapping Repeat Lasso with Random selections (BLR) is a feature selection algorithm that increases the stability and reduces errors of selection with the help of repeat bootstrapping. The selected 436 radiomic features and 9 clinical features were used to differentiate malignant from benign lesions using SVM with an AUC of 0.92 and 0.83 in independent and cross-training cohort, respectively [8].

Permuth et al. combined CT radiomic features of diagnosed IPMN patients to analyzed micro-ribonucleic acid (mi RNA) data via logistic regression analysis. Their model has a predictive accuracy of 92% in low-grade IPMNs from invasive IPMNs upon principal component analyses and cross-validation [16].

SPN is a solid cystic tumor of low malignant potential which often presents with well-defined margins and heterogeneous changes after enhancement on imaging. Surgical resection is the recommended treatment for SPN, which commonly affects young females [1, 17]. Around 14.2% of all SPNs are known to have aggressive behavior [18]. Huang et al. have proposed four different predictive models for preoperative assessment of SPNs using two-dimensional (2D) arterial, 2D venous, three-dimensional (3D) arterial, and 3D venous models. 3D arterial model with AUC of 0.914 was better than all other predictive models. The combined arteriovenous model performed even better (AUC: 0.918) [19]. Liag et al. have used T1-weighted (T1W), T2W, diffusion-weighted (DW), and contrast-enhanced T1W images to construct a log-combined model that integrates models based on each of these sequences and clinical features to predict the preoperative risk of aggressive behavior with an AUC of 0.81 and a sensitivity and specificity of 0.75 and 0.78, respectively [20]. Table 12.1 summarizes the studies evaluating the role of radiomics in PCLs.

12.2.3 Limitations of Radiomics

Use of radiomics in the differential diagnosis of PCLs, however, has its fair share of limitations, the most notable being the lack of standardization. Different researchers

Table 12.1 Studies evaluating the role of radiomics in PCLs

Author (Reference)	No. of patients	Imaging modality used	Model building	Results
Dimitreiv et al. [7]	134	CT	Random Forest	84% accurate to predict common PCLs
Wei et al. [8]	260	CT	SVM & LASSO	83% accuracy to predict SCA in validation cohort and 76% in cross-validation cohort
Chen et al. [9]	89	CT	LASSO	96% accurate to differentiate SCA from MCNs in training cohort and 81% in validation cohort
Cuie et al. [13]	222	MRI	LASSO	90.3% accurate to predict BD-IPMN in training cohort and 88.4% in validation cohort
Tobaly et al. [14]	296	CT	Logistic regression	Accuracy of 84% in training cohort and 71% in validation cohort to differentiate benign vs. malignant IPMN
Chakraborty et al. [15]	103	CT	Random Forrest classifier	81% accurate to predict high-risk from low-risk IPMN
Permuth et al. [16]	38	CT	Logistic regression	Accuracy 92% to differentiate benign from malignant IPMN, sensitivity (83%), specificity (89%)
Liang et al. [20]	111	MRI	Logistic regression	Accuracy 77% to differentiate invasive from noninvasive SPN, sensitivity (75%), specificity (78%)

have used varied methods for image acquisition, feature extraction, and statistical analyses. The published studies till date have not validated their results against an independent external dataset. "Overfitting" or extraction of more features than the number of samples makes these features redundant. More often creating "complex constructs" from medical image-derived data proves difficult to derive inference [5].

12.3 Contrast-Enhanced Harmonic EUS (CH-EUS)

EUS is an established imaging modality for the diagnosis and surveillance of PCLs. It assesses the cyst architecture and high-risk features. For surveillance of cysts >2 cm, the Fukuoka guidelines recommend alternating use of MRI and EUS [21]. Conventional B mode EUS (B-EUS) has limited ability to assess the solid component of PCLs. Use of Doppler EUS can detect large blood vessels within the solid component but is hampered by the lack of sensitivity to pick up parenchymal perfusion [22]. From the first described use of carbon dioxide microbubbles under angiography by Kato et al. in 1995 to the first use of intravenous contrast agent in 1998, the use of contrast in EUS has gradually evolved to contrast harmonic method [23–25]. CH-EUS aims to improve the quantitative and qualitative assessment of PCLs by a better visualization of fine blood flow in the tissues and vasculature. Better contrast resolution and reduction of "blooming artifacts" are noteworthy advantages. It is a better modality to differentiate mural nodule from mucus presence within a cyst as it demonstrates the blood flow in the target lesion.

12.3.1 CH-EUS for Differentiating Neoplastic Pancreatic Cysts from Pseudocyst (PC)

Kamata et al. retrospectively analyzed data of 70 patients who underwent CH-EUS, B- EUS, and subsequent surgical resection. CH-EUS had similar sensitivity as B-EUS to pick up mural nodule (97%) but was more specific (75% vs. 40% respectively). The authors have reported that mural nodule height ≥4 mm on CH-EUS is indicative of malignancy (Odd's ratio: 56.0) [26]. Fusaroli et al. studied 76 patients and documented "hyperenhancing" pattern in SCA and MCNs while "hypoenhancement" in PC [27]. Zhong et al. have reported that the accuracy of CH-EUS to differentiate PCLs was 92.3% vs. 76.9% for CT, CH-EUS vs. MRI was 93.0 5 vs. 78.9% and CH-EUS vs. B-EUS was 92.7% vs. 84.2%, respectively [28].

12.3.2 CH-EUS for Diagnosis of Mural Nodule and Differentiating Pancreatic Adenocarcinoma from Other Solid Pancreatic Lesions

Ohno et al. studied CH-EUS in 166 patients of BD-IPMNs who underwent surgical resection. They documented the presence of mural nodule that involved the MPD or secondarily involved the MPD. CH-EUS was able to document the involvement of MPD with a sensitivity, specificity, and accuracy of 83.5%, 87.0%, and 84.9%, respectively [29]. Ishikawa et al. have studied the enhancement pattern of pancreatic solid lesions (hypoechoic, hyperechoic, and isoechoic vs. the surrounding pancreatic parenchyma). Images obtained at 20, 40, and 60 s were used for assessment. Those with pancreatic adenocarcinoma had hypovascular pattern after 20s and 40s of contrast injection. This pattern had a sensitivity, specificity, and diagnostic accuracy of 83.1%, 86.8%, and 84.3%, respectively to differentiate adenocarcinoma from other sold lesions [30]. Yamashita et al. enrolled 115 patients, all of whom underwent CECT, B-EUS, CH-EUS, and surgical resection. CH-EUS picked up mural nodule in 92% cases, while B-EUS and CECT had a reported accuracy of 83% and 72%, respectively. For malignant IPMN, these modalities exhibited the following diagnostic accuracy: CH = EUS (75%), B-EUS (73%), and CECT (63%) [31].

12.4 Confocal Laser Endomicroscopy (CLE)

EUS-guided fine-needle aspiration cytology (EUS FNA) is the recommended diagnostic modality for high-risk PCLs [1] [21, 32, 33]. EUS has a sensitivity of 50% to detect high-risk morphological changes within PCLs, while EUS-guided cytology is 60% sensitive to guide decision-making about operability or surveillance of PCLs. The presence of high carcinoembryonic antigen (CEA) >800 ng/mL is highly specific (98%) but only 48% sensitive to pick up mucinous cysts [34]. CLE is an endoscopic imaging technique that utilizes laser beam to obtain real-time images of tissues and microvasculature. Needle-based CLE (nCLE) allows microscopic imaging during a EUS-FNA and aims to improve the differential diagnosis of various PCLs [35]. Konda et al. were the first to document the feasibility of nCLE during EUS-FNA procedure for PCLs [36]. Subsequently, Giovannini et al. attempted to provide image interpretation criteria and proposed a diagnostic criterion for predicting malignant potential in PCLs using -guided nCLE [37]. Several multicenter trials have documented the efficacy of nCLE for the differential diagnosis of PCLs [35].

12.4.1 Technique

The technique involves a CLE miniprobe compatible with the operating channel of 19 G EUS-FNA needle. The miniprobe provides 325 μm field of view and a resolution of 3.5 μm [38]. Once the EUS-FNA needle is prepared, the stylet is removed and the miniprobe is inserted through the locking device. It is advanced till the distal end is visible. The miniprobe is then retracted into the needle, and this assembly is then inserted into the working channel of EUS scope. Once a cyst puncture is achieved, the miniprobe is advanced till it touches the opposite cyst wall. 2.5 mL of 10% fluorescein is injected for fluorescent imaging. Real-type images capturing the cyst wall and microvasculature are obtained for up to 6 min. Pancreatic cyst fluid can thereafter be aspirated for cytology and biochemical analysis [35, 38].

12.4.2 Diagnostic Criteria for nCLE

Napoleon et al., in their study conducted across three centers (CNTACT), have reviewed 31 patients with a single documented PCL. The study involved combination of nCLE with EUS-FNA. The final diagnosis was established on histopathological examination of a resected specimen or a committee consensus. nCLE images were reviewed by six investigators, and the presence of superficial vascular pattern which corresponded to "dense and subepithelial capillary vascularization" was identified as a diagnostic criterion for SCA with sensitivity, specificity, positive, and negative predictive values of 69%, 100%, 100%, and 82%, respectively, with good interobserver agreement ($\kappa = 0.77$) [39]. In their subsequent study (CONTACT 1), Napoleon et al. included 31 patients and described nCLE criteria for other PCLs as follows: "thick gray lines for MCN", "field of bright particles" for PC, "papillary projections with a white center and a darker epithelial border" for IPMN. They were able to achieve a conclusive diagnosis in 74% of patients. This study, which was validated by four external observers, demonstrated 100% specificity for establishing diagnosis of non mucinous cysts and >90% for mucinous cysts [40]. The CONTACT 2 study recruited 78 patients of PCLs who had a reference diagnosis. nCLE provided a conclusive diagnosis in 91% of cases. The diagnostic accuracy of nCLE was compared with the cyst fluid CEA and EUS morphology. nCLE had a sensitivity and specificity of >95% for SCN, MCN, and premalignant PCLs. nCLE had better diagnostic accuracy than EUS in differentiating benign vs. malignant PCLs and performed better than CEA in differentiating mucinous from nonmucinous cysts [41]. Kadayifci et al. were able to acquire images using nCLE in 18 out of 20 patients. They could document predefined structures with a diagnostic accuracy of 80% and sensitivity and specificity of 66% and 100%, respectively, for those with mucinous cysts. However, such structural identification of characteristic features was not seen in those with nonmucinous cysts [42]. Keane et al. analyzed 56 patients with PCLs. nCLE was able to achieve a final diagnosis (assesses on imaging, cytology, and multidisciplinary team review) in 77% of cases, while cytology could achieve the same in 66% of cases [43].

12.4.3 Interobserver Agreement (IOA) and Interobserver Reliability (IOR)

In a majority of these studies, IOA varies, and there is definite paucity of data on IOR. Napoleon et al. retrospectively performed the validation of results included in CONTACT 1 study. Four external reviewers blinded to the diagnosis participated. A conclusive result was obtained in 74% of patients with "substantial" IOA [40]. Krishna et al. performed a validation study on retrospectively collected data of 49 patients who underwent nCLE over a period of 30 months. Six observers who were nCLE-naïve and blinded to the diagnosis participated. IOA was analyzed in two phases. In the first phase, there was substantial IOA for differentiating mucinous from nonmucinous lesions ($\kappa = 0.67$, 95% CI:0.57–0.77). In the second phase which was done after a 2-week "wash-out" phase, the image interpretation of the three previously described patterns (fern-like vascularity, bright particles on dark background, and presence of epithelial bands) improved, while IOA for the diagnosis of mucinous PCLs remained "substantial" ($\kappa = 0.66$, 95% CI: 0.56–0.76). The IOR was also "substantial" for establishing a diagnosis of mucinous PCL ($\kappa = 0.78$) [44]. In contrast to these studies, Karia et al. have assessed IOA agreement involving six interventional endoscopists using six variables (presence of vessels, villi, acinar patter, reticular pattern, clumps, and debris). The overall IOA for PCL diagnosis was low. The k values ranged from 0.04 for vessels to 0.22 for dark clumps [45]. Machicado et al. have studied data set comprising 76 patients of PCLs from three prospective studies. A panel of 13 experts blinded to the diagnosis reviewed the data (presented as video library) in two phases, each separated by a 2-week "wash-out" phase. They have reported "almost perfect" IOA ($\kappa = 0.42$, 95% CI: 0.77–0.87) in differentiating mucinous from nonmucinous PCLs and similar IOR ($\kappa = 0.82$, 95%CI: 0.78–0.85) [46].

12.4.4 Deep Learning Network (DLN) Using CLE for Diagnosis of PCLs

Recent research utilizing DLN for the diagnosis of PCLs has shown promising results. These networks are particularly useful for image and video analyses. Angelina et al. have used ResNet-50 and ResNet-101 DLN for PCL classification. They incorporated data of 50 pancreatic CLE training videos and 18 test videos. RestNet-50 and RestNet-101 could correctly identify 08 and 17 out of 18 test videos, respectively [47].

12.4.5 Adverse Events and Limitations

Post-procedure pancreatitis, intracystic bleeding, cyst infection, and transient abdominal pain are the common adverse events [41, 48, 49]. Acute pancreatitis (AP) is the most common reported adverse event in approximately 3% of cases [44, 48]. It has been postulated that the adverse events have a reciprocal co-relation with the endoscopists' expertise. All reported cases of AP have been associated with a transgastric needle approach and are usually mild [3]. nCLE has an associated learning curve. This starts with device familiarization, generation, and interpretation of images specific to a particular type of PCL. In addition, nCLE is hampered by its inability to study deeper layers of the cyst wall, especially in those with solid components or mural nodules [3].

12.5 EUS-Guided Microforceps Biopsy

Moray microbiopsy forceps is a "through-the-needle" forceps with a sheath diameter of 0.8 mm and jaw opening width of 4.3 mm. After the puncture of pancreatic cyst, the forceps is introduced via a 19 G EUS-FNA needle. This is of particular benefit in PCLs with a mural nodule. Among the initial studies, involving 28 patients, Kovacevic et al. have reported a technical success rate of 85.7%, and a definite histopathological diagnosis in 19 patients was achieved [50]. Multiple other studies have demonstrated the feasibility and technical success of achieving a definite diagnosis.

Meta-analyses of the published studies have shown technical success of tissue acquisition, diagnostic yield, and diagnostic accuracy. The most recent meta-analyses by Gopakumar et al. have included 11 studies with 575 patients. EUS guided through the needle forceps had a pooled sensitivity and specificity of 76.6% and 98.9%, respectively, to differentiate neoplastic from a non-neoplastic lesion It had a pooled diagnostic odd's ratio of 41.34 (95% CI:17.42–98.08) in diagnosing a malignant from a nonmalignant PCL [51].

Table 12.2 describes the recent published meta-analyses evaluating the role of EUS-guided microforceps biopsy in the diagnosis of PCLs.

12.6 Differentiating Epithelial Subtypes of IPMN

IPMNs have been subclassified into four histological subtypes, namely, gastric foveolar, intestinal, oncocytic, and pancreatobiliary. This classification is based on immunohistochemical characterization of mucin containing glycoproteins and papillary proliferation in the resected specimens [56]. This differentiation has prognostic significance as invasive oncocytic and colloid carcinoma derived from intestinal subtype has a better prognosis than tubular carcinoma derived from gastric subtype [57, 58]. Single-operator pancreatoscopy has been used to differentiate these subtypes preoperatively. Hibi et al. have reported 79% agreement between the histological specimen and cytological examination of pancreatic juice obtained on pancreatoscopy. Hara et al. have performed mucin histochemical analysis of pancreatic juice obtained from 36 patients who subsequently underwent surgical resection of IPMN, with 89% concordance between mucin histochemical staining and the histopathological subtype [59].

12.7 Cyst Fluid Biomarkers

Detection of mutations and metabolic changes in the pancreatic cyst fluid, serum, or on pancreatic biopsy are novel tools in the differentiation of PCLs. Cyst fluid CEA at a cutoff value >192 ng/mL is 58% sensitive and 87% specific to detect mucinous PCLs. Cyst fluid glucose at a cutoff value <50 ng/dL exhibits 93% sensitivity and 89% specificity for the same. However, neither of these is useful to detect invasive

Table 12.2 Recent published meta-analyses evaluating the role of EUS-guided microforceps biopsy in the diagnosis of PCLs

Author	Number of studies included	Number of patients	Technical success	Diagnostic yield	Histological accuracy	Adverse Events	Sensitivity/Specificity of diagnosis of Mucinous cyst
Tacelli et al. [52]	09	454	98.5%	69.5%	86.7%	8.6%	88.6%/69.5%
Westerveld et al. [53]	08	426	98.2%	72.5%	Sub group analysis : 82.3 % for specific cyst diagnosis	07%	90.1%/94%
Rift et al. [54]	10	99	98.2%				86%/95%
Balaban et al. [55]	09	463	98.5%	88.2%	68.6%	9.7%	

carcinoma or high-grade dysplasia [60, 61]. There are promising technologies involving molecular analysis on the horizon involving cyst fluid biomarkers for the differentiation of PCLs.

12.7.1 Molecular Analysis

Molecular analysis involves next-generation sequencing (NGS) to detect deoxyribonucleic acid (DNA) from the cyst fluid. The process involves reading the DNA sequence at each fragment and identification of genetic variations to understand their clinical significance. Mucinous cysts have been documented to have mutations involving "mitogen-activated protein kinase (MAPK)" gene, "guanine nucleotide-binding protein (GNAS)" ± "Kirsten rat sarcoma viral oncogene homolog (KRAS)" gene with a sensitivity and specificity of 90% and 100%, respectively [62, 63]. Genetic alterations in "phosphatidylinositol-4,5-bisphonate 3- kinase catalytic subunit alpha (PIK3CA)", "Mothers against decapentaplegic homolog 4 (SMAD 4)", "cyclin-dependent kinase inhibitor 2A(CDKN2A)," and "tumor protein 53(TP53)" can detect neoplasia with a sensitivity of 10%, 09%, 11%, and 42%, respectively, and specificity of 97%, 98%, 97%, and 95%, respectively [64]. The study by Pannicia et al. that included 1933 PCLs has shown that for the detection of advanced neoplasia, combining GNAS/MAPK and TP53/SMAD-4/ "mechanist target of rapamycin kinase (MTOR)"/"catenin beta 1(CTNNB1)" improves the sensitivity and specificity to 88% and 98%, respectively [62]. Cyst fluid molecular analysis that detects low-frequency mutations in TP53, PIK3CA, and "Phosphatase and Tensin Homolog deleted on chromosome 10 (PTEN)" has been shown to occur prior to histological transformation to high-grade dysplasia [65]. Fugikura et al. have documented high prevalence of hotspot mutations in previously unreported "Kruppel-like factor 4 (KLF4)" gene [66]. Although molecular analysis offers great promise, it is not a reliable standalone diagnostic modality.

12.7.2 DNA Methylation

DNA methylation patterns in cyst fluid have been used for distinguishing high-grade IPMNs from low-grade ones. Cysteine dioxygenase gene 1(CDO1) promoter hypermethylation using "TaqMan quantitative methylation-specific polymerase chain reaction" has been found to be specific for IPMN and, in fact, may accumulate as the tumor undergoes adenoma–carcinoma progression [67]. BCL2/adenovirus E1B 19-k Da-interacting protein 3(BNIP3) is a protein involved in the regulation of apoptosis and autophagy. Gene-regulating BNIP3 undergoes selective methylation in high-grade IMN and may serve as a promising biomarker [68].

12.7.3 Micro-Ribonucleic Acid (miRNA) Analysis

miRNA expression in pancreatic fluid is a promising biomarker to detect malignant transformation in IPMNs. Shirakami et al. performed miRNA analysis using a highly sensitive DNA chip on cyst fluid obtained during the surgical resection of IPMNs. A combination of six miRNAs (miR 711, miR6126, miR6798, miR6780, miR3679-5p, miR6879-5p, and miR6798-5p) was highly enriched in patients with IPM carcinoma vs. those with IPM adenoma [69].

12.7.4 Glycoprotein Analysis

Alteration in protein glycosylation is an important component of the molecular process of carcinogenesis. Detection of cancer-specific glycoproteins is an area of active research. Cui et al. used mass spectrometry-based glycoproteomic analysis on pancreatic cyst fluid and have identified "N-glycosylated phosphorylase kinase regulatory subunit beta (PHKB)", "Carcinoembryonic antigen-related cell adhesion molecule 5(CEACAM5)", and "ATPase H+ transporting V0 subunit a4 (ATP6V0A4)" as potential biomarkers for the detection of malignant PCLs [13].

12.8 Artificial Intelligence (AI)-Based Algorithms

Yusuke Kurita et al. have attempted to utilize AI using deep learning to construct an algorithm to differentiate benign from malignant PCLs. This algorithm utilizes anatomical factors like location and type of cyst, its association with MPD in addition to cyst fluid cytology, cyst fluid amylase, CEA, CA 19.9, and carbohydrate antigen 125 (CA 125). They have included 85 patients who underwent pancreatic cyst fluid analysis following either surgical resection or EUS aspiration. Their AI-based algorithm was 91.9% sensitive and 92.9% specific to differentiate malignant from benign PCLs. Moreover, AI exhibited higher sensitivity than CEA (60.9%, $p = 0.021$) as well as cyst fluid cytology (47.8%, $p = 0.001$) [70].

12.9 Conclusion

An accurate and thorough evaluation of PCL is particularly important given the risk of malignant transformation. The ongoing research in the field of imaging, tissue acquisition, an array of biomarkers, and the emerging role of AI provides valuable opportunities for health care providers to improve patient outcomes and enhanced treatment modalities. This also provides an impetus for further research and encourages innovation.

References

1. Elta GH, Enestvedt BK, Sauer BG, Lennon AM. ACG clinical guideline: diagnosis and management of pancreatic cysts. Am J Gastroenterol. 2018;113(4):464–79. https://doi.org/10.1038/ajg.2018.14. Epub 2018 Feb 27. PMID: 29485131.
2. Lee LS. Updates in diagnosis and management of pancreatic cysts. World J Gastroenterol. 2021;27(34):5700–14. https://doi.org/10.3748/wjg.v27.i34.5700. PMID: 34629795; PMCID: PMC8473602.Lee LS.
3. Singh RR, Gopakumar H, Sharma NR. Diagnosis and management of pancreatic cysts: a comprehensive review of the literature. Diagnostics (Basel). 2023;13(3):550. https://doi.org/10.3390/diagnostics13030550. PMID: 36766654; PMCID: PMC9914101.
4. Antonelli L, et al. Integrating imaging and omics data: a review. Biomed Signal Process Control. 2019;52:264–80. https://doi.org/10.1016/j.bspc.2019.04.032.
5. Dalal V, Carmicheal J, Dhaliwal A, Jain M, Kaur S, Batra SK. Radiomics in stratification of pancreatic cystic lesions: machine learning in action. Cancer Lett. 2020;469:228–37. https://doi.org/10.1016/j.canlet.2019.10.023. Epub 2019 Oct 17. PMID: 31629933; PMCID: PMC6927395.
6. Mao KZ, Ma C, Song B. Radiomics advances in the evaluation of pancreatic cystic neoplasms. Heliyon. 2024;10(3):e25535. https://doi.org/10.1016/j.heliyon.2024.e25535. PMID: 38333791; PMCID: PMC10850586.
7. Dmitriev K, Kaufman AE, Javed AA, Hruban RH, Fishman EK, Lennon AM, Saltz JH. Classification of pancreatic cysts in computed tomography images using a random forest and convolutional neural network ensemble. Med Image Comput Comput Assist Interv. 2017;10435:150–8. https://doi.org/10.1007/978-3-319-66179-7_18. Epub 2017 Sep 4. PMID: 29881827; PMCID: PMC5987215.
8. Wei R, Lin K, Yan W, Guo Y, Wang Y, Li J, Zhu J. Computer-aided diagnosis of pancreas serous cystic neoplasms: a Radiomics method on preoperative MDCT images. Technol Cancer Res Treat. 2019;18:1533033818824339. https://doi.org/10.1177/1533033818824339. PMID: 30803366; PMCID: PMC6374001.
9. Chen S, Ren S, Guo K, Daniels MJ, Wang Z, Chen R. Preoperative differentiation of serous cystic neoplasms from mucin-producing pancreatic cystic neoplasms using a CT-based radiomics nomogram. Abdom Radiol (NY). 2021;46(6):2637–46. https://doi.org/10.1007/s00261-021-02954-8. Epub 2021 Feb 8. PMID: 33558952.
10. Fang X, Zhang Q, Liu F, Li J, Wang T, Cao K, et al. T2-weighted image Radiomics nomogram to predict pancreatic serous and mucinous cystic neoplasms. Acad Radiol. 2023;30(8):1562–71. https://doi.org/10.1016/j.acra.2022.10.008. Epub 2022 Nov 12. PMID: 36379815.
11. Pulvirenti A, Margonis GA, Morales-Oyarvide V, McIntyre CA, Lawrence SA, Goldman DA, et al. Intraductal papillary mucinous neoplasms: have IAP consensus guidelines changed our approach? Results from a multi-institutional study. Ann Surg. 2021;274(6):e980–7. https://doi.org/10.1097/SLA.0000000000003703. PMID: 31804389; PMCID: PMC8503800.
12. Stark A, Donahue TR, Reber HA, Hines OJ. Pancreatic cyst disease: a review. JAMA. 2016;315(17):1882–93. https://doi.org/10.1001/jama.2016.4690. PMID: 27139061.
13. Cui S, Tang T, Su Q, Wang Y, Shu Z, Yang W, Gong X, et al. Radiomic nomogram based on MRI to predict grade of branching type intraductal papillary mucinous neoplasms of the pancreas: a multicenter study. Cancer Imaging. 2021;21(1):26. https://doi.org/10.1186/s40644-021-00395-6. PMID: 33750453; PMCID: PMC7942000.
14. Tobaly D, Santinha J, Sartoris R, Dioguardi Burgio M, Matos C, Cros J, et al. CT-based Radiomics analysis to predict malignancy in patients with intraductal papillary mucinous neoplasm (IPMN) of the pancreas. Cancers (Basel). 2020;12(11):3089. https://doi.org/10.3390/cancers12113089. PMID: 33114028; PMCID: PMC7690711.
15. Chakraborty J, Midya A, Gazit L, Attiyeh M, Langdon-Embry L, Allen PJ, et al. CT radiomics to predict high-risk intraductal papillary mucinous neoplasms of the pancreas. Med Phys.

2018;45(11):5019–29. https://doi.org/10.1002/mp.13159. Epub 2018 Sep 27. PMID: 30176047; PMCID: PMC8050835.

16. Permuth JB, Choi J, Balarunathan Y, Kim J, Chen DT, Chen L, Florida pancreas collaborative, et al. Combining Radiomic features with a miRNA classifier may improve prediction of malignant pathology for pancreatic intraductal papillary mucinous neoplasms. Oncotarget. 2016;7(52):85785–97. https://doi.org/10.18632/oncotarget.11768. PMID: 27589689; PMCID: PMC5349874.
17. Ardeshna DR, Cao T, Rodgers B, Onongaya C, Jones D, Chen W, et al. Recent advances in the diagnostic evaluation of pancreatic cystic lesions. World J Gastroenterol. 2022;28(6):624–34. https://doi.org/10.3748/wjg.v28.i6.624. PMID: 35317424; PMCID: PMC8900547.
18. Yu P, Cheng X, Du Y, Yang L, Xu Z, Yin W, Zhong Z, et al. Solid pseudopapillary neoplasms of the pancreas: a 19-year multicenter experience in China. J Gastrointest Surg. 2015;19(8):1433–40. https://doi.org/10.1007/s11605-015-2862-8. Epub 2015 May 23. PMID: 26001371.
19. Huang WP, Liu SY, Han YJ, Li LM, Liang P, Gao JB. Development of CT-based imaging signature for preoperative prediction of invasive behavior in pancreatic solid pseudopapillary neoplasm. Front Oncol. 2021;11:677814. https://doi.org/10.3389/fonc.2021.677814. PMID: 34079766; PMCID: PMC8166224.
20. Liang X, He W, Huang C, Feng Z, Guan X, Liu Y, et al. Preoperative prediction of invasive behavior of pancreatic solid pseudopapillary neoplasm by MRI-based multiparametric radiomics models. Abdom Radiol (NY). 2022;47(11):3782–91. https://doi.org/10.1007/s00261-022-03639-6. Epub 2022 Aug 17. PMID: 35976419.
21. Tanaka M, Fernández-Del Castillo C, Kamisawa T, Jang JY, Levy P, Ohtsuka T, et al. Revisions of international consensus Fukuoka guidelines for the management of IPMN of the pancreas. Pancreatology. 2017;17(5):738–53. https://doi.org/10.1016/j.pan.2017.07.007. Epub 2017 Jul 13. PMID: 28735806.
22. Hickman K, Sadler TJ, Zhang TT, Boninsegna E, Majcher V, Godfrey E. Pancreatic cystic lesions and the role of contrast enhanced endoscopic ultrasound. Clin Radiol. 2022;77(6):418–27. https://doi.org/10.1016/j.crad.2022.02.017. Epub 2022 Apr 3. PMID: 35387743.
23. Kato T, Tsukamoto Y, Naitoh Y, Hirooka Y, Furukawa T, Hayakawa T. Ultrasonographic and endoscopic ultrasonographic angiography in pancreatic mass lesions. Acta Radiol. 1995;36(4):381–7. PMID: 7619616.
24. Hirooka Y, Goto H, Ito A, Hayakawa S, Watanabe Y, Ishiguro Y, et al. Contrast-enhanced endoscopic ultrasonography in pancreatic diseases: a preliminary study. Am J Gastroenterol. 1998;93(4):632–5. https://doi.org/10.1111/j.1572-0241.1998.179_b.x. PMID: 9576461.
25. Kitano M, Yamashita Y, Kamata K, Ang TL, Imazu H, Ohno E, Working group for the International Consensus Guidelines for Contrast-Enhanced Harmonic Endoscopic Ultrasound, et al. The Asian Federation of Societies for ultrasound in medicine and biology (AFSUMB) guidelines for contrast-enhanced endoscopic ultrasound. Ultrasound Med Biol. 2021;47(6):1433–47. https://doi.org/10.1016/j.ultrasmedbio.2021.01.030. Epub 2021 Feb 27. PMID: 33653627.
26. Kamata K, Kitano M, Omoto S, Kadosaka K, Miyata T, Yamao K, et al. Contrast-enhanced harmonic endoscopic ultrasonography for differential diagnosis of pancreatic cysts. Endoscopy. 2016;48(1):35–41. https://doi.org/10.1055/s-0034-1393564. Epub 2015 Nov 25. PMID: 26605974.
27. Fusaroli P, Serrani M, De Giorgio R, D'Ercole MC, Ceroni L, Lisotti A, et al. Contrast harmonic-endoscopic ultrasound is useful to identify neoplastic features of pancreatic cysts (with videos). Pancreas. 2016;45(2):265–8. https://doi.org/10.1097/MPA.0000000000000441. PMID: 26474428.
28. Zhong L, Chai N, Linghu E, Li H, Yang J, Tang P. A prospective study on contrast-enhanced endoscopic ultrasound for differential diagnosis of pancreatic cystic neoplasms. Dig Dis Sci. 2019;64(12):3616–22. https://doi.org/10.1007/s10620-019-05718-z. Epub 2019 Jul 9. PMID: 31290040.

29. Ohno E, Kawashima H, Ishikawa T, Iida T, Suzuki H, Uetsuki K, et al. Can contrast-enhanced harmonic endoscopic ultrasonography accurately diagnose main pancreatic duct involvement in intraductal papillary mucinous neoplasms? Pancreatology. 2020;20(5):887–94. https://doi.org/10.1016/j.pan.2020.06.004. Epub 2020 Jun 11. PMID: 32651080.
30. Ishikawa T, Hirooka Y, Kawashima H, Ohno E, Hashizume K, Funasaka K, et al. Multiphase evaluation of contrast-enhanced endoscopic ultrasonography in the diagnosis of pancreatic solid lesions. Pancreatology. 2018;18(3):291–7. https://doi.org/10.1016/j.pan.2018.02.002. Epub 2018 Feb 9. PMID: 29449151.
31. Yamashita Y, Kawaji Y, Shimokawa T, Yamazaki H, Tamura T, Hatamaru K, et al. Usefulness of contrast-enhanced harmonic endoscopic ultrasonography for diagnosis of malignancy in Intraductal papillary mucinous neoplasm. Diagnostics (Basel). 2022;12(9):2141. https://doi.org/10.3390/diagnostics12092141. PMID: 36140542; PMCID: PMC9497750.
32. European Study Group on Cystic Tumours of the Pancreas. European evidence-based guidelines on pancreatic cystic neoplasms. Gut. 2018;67(5):789–804. https://doi.org/10.1136/gutjnl-2018-316027. Epub 2018 Mar 24. PMID: 29574408; PMCID: PMC5890653.
33. Vege SS, Ziring B, Jain R, Moayyedi P, Clinical Guidelines Committee, American Gastroenterology Association. American gastroenterological association institute guideline on the diagnosis and management of asymptomatic neoplastic pancreatic cysts. Gastroenterology. 2015;148(4):819–22. quize12–3. https://doi.org/10.1053/j.gastro.2015.01.015. PMID: 25805375.
34. Scheiman JM, Hwang JH, Moayyedi P. American gastroenterological association technical review on the diagnosis and management of asymptomatic neoplastic pancreatic cysts. Gastroenterology. 2015;148(4):824–48. e22. https://doi.org/10.1053/j.gastro.2015.01.014. PMID: 25805376.
35. Napoleon B, Krishna SG, Marco B, Carr-Locke D, Chang KJ, Ginès À, et al. Confocal endomicroscopy for evaluation of pancreatic cystic lesions: a systematic review and international Delphi consensus report. Endosc Int Open. 2020;8(11):E1566–81. https://doi.org/10.1055/a-1229-4156. Epub 2020 Oct 22. PMID: 33140012; PMCID: PMC7581463.
36. Konda VJ, Aslanian HR, Wallace MB, Siddiqui UD, Hart J, Waxman I. First assessment of needle-based confocal laser endomicroscopy during EUS-FNA procedures of the pancreas (with videos). Gastrointest Endosc. 2011;74(5):1049–60. https://doi.org/10.1016/j.gie.2011.07.018. Epub 2011 Sep 15. PMID: 21924718.
37. Giovannini M, Caillol F, Poizat F, Bories E, Pesenti C, Monges G, et al. Feasibility of intratumoral confocal microscopy under endoscopic ultrasound guidance. Endosc Ultrasound. 2012;1(2):80–3. https://doi.org/10.7178/eus.02.005. PMID: 24949342; PMCID: PMC4062216.
38. Wu CCH, Lim SJM, Tan DMY. Endoscopic ultrasound-guided needle-based confocal laser endomicroscopy for pancreatic cystic lesions: current status and future prospects. Clin Endosc. 2024;57(4):434–45. https://doi.org/10.5946/ce.2023.157. Epub 2024 Jul 8. PMID: 38978396; PMCID: PMC11294861.
39. Napoléon B, Lemaistre AI, Pujol B, Caillol F, Lucidarme D, Bourdariat R, et al. A novel approach to the diagnosis of pancreatic serous cystadenoma: needle-based confocal laser endomicroscopy. Endoscopy. 2015;47(1):26–32. https://doi.org/10.1055/s-0034-1390693. Epub 2014 Oct 17. PMID: 25325684.
40. Napoleon B, Lemaistre AI, Pujol B, Caillol F, Lucidarme D, Bourdariat R, et al. In vivo characterization of pancreatic cystic lesions by needle-based confocal laser endomicroscopy (nCLE): proposition of a comprehensive nCLE classification confirmed by an external retrospective evaluation. Surg Endosc. 2016;30(6):2603–12. https://doi.org/10.1007/s00464-015-4510-5. Epub 2015 Oct 1. PMID: 26428198.
41. Napoleon B, Palazzo M, Lemaistre AI, Caillol F, Palazzo L, Aubert A, et al. Needle-based confocal laser endomicroscopy of pancreatic cystic lesions: a prospective multicenter validation study in patients with definite diagnosis. Endoscopy. 2019;51(9):825–35. https://doi.org/10.1055/a-0732-5356. Epub 2018 Oct 22. PMID: 30347425.

42. Kadayifci A, Atar M, Basar O, Forcione DG, Brugge WR. Needle-based confocal laser Endomicroscopy for evaluation of cystic neoplasms of the pancreas. Dig Dis Sci. 2017;62(5):1346–53. https://doi.org/10.1007/s10620-017-4521-2. Epub 2017 Mar 9. PMID: 28281172.
43. Keane MG, Wehnert N, Perez-Machado M, Fusai GK, Thorburn D, Oppong KW, et al. A prospective trial of CONfocal endomicroscopy in CYSTic lesions of the pancreas: CONCYST-01. Endosc Int Open. 2019;7(9):E1117–22. https://doi.org/10.1055/a-0957-2976. Epub 2019 Aug 29. PMID: 31475228; PMCID: PMC6715431.
44. Krishna SG, Swanson B, Hart PA, El-Dika S, Walker JP, McCarthy ST, et al. Validation of diagnostic characteristics of needle based confocal laser endomicroscopy in differentiation of pancreatic cystic lesions. Endosc Int Open. 2016;4(11):E1124–35. https://doi.org/10.1055/s-0042-116491. Epub 2016 Sep 30. PMID: 27853737; PMCID: PMC5110338.
45. Karia K, Waxman I, Konda VJ, Gress FG, Sethi A, Siddiqui UD, Sharaiha RZ, et al. Needle-based confocal endomicroscopy for pancreatic cysts: the current agreement in interpretation. Gastrointest Endosc. 2016;83(5):924–7. https://doi.org/10.1016/j.gie.2015.08.080. Epub 2015 Sep 14. PMID: 26382051.
46. Machicado JD, Napoleon B, Lennon AM, El-Dika S, Pereira SP, Tan D, et al. Accuracy and agreement of a large panel of endosonographers for endomicroscopy-guided virtual biopsy of pancreatic cystic lesions. Pancreatology. 2022;22(7):994–1002. https://doi.org/10.1016/j.pan.2022.08.012. Epub 2022 Aug 31. PMID: 36089484; PMCID: PMC10548449
47. Lee TC, Angelina CL, Kongkam P, et al. Deep-learning-enabled computer-aided diagnosis in the classification of pancreatic cystic lesions on confocal laser endomicroscopy. Diagnostics (Basel, Switzerland). 2023;13(7):1289. https://doi.org/10.3390/diagnostics13071289. PMID: 37046507; PMCID: PMC10093377.
48. Konda VJ, Meining A, Jamil LH, Giovannini M, Hwang JH, Wallace MB, et al. A pilot study of in vivo identification of pancreatic cystic neoplasms with needle-based confocal laser endomicroscopy under endosonographic guidance. Endoscopy. 2013;45(12):1006–13. https://doi.org/10.1055/s-0033-1344714. Epub 2013 Oct 25. PMID: 24163192.
49. Keegan MJ, et al. Needle-based confocal laser endomicroscopy findings in 101 consecutive undifferentiated pancreatic cysts: does routine use of cytopathology change management? Endoscopy. 2019;51:S43.
50. Kovacevic B, Karstensen JG, Havre RF, Pham KD, Giovannini M, Dabizzi E, et al. Initial experience with EUS-guided microbiopsy forceps in diagnosing pancreatic cystic lesions: a multicenter feasibility study (with video). Endosc Ultrasound. 2018;7(6):383–8. https://doi.org/10.4103/eus.eus_16_18. PMID: 30168479; PMCID: PMC6289018.
51. Gopakumar H, Puli SR. Value of endoscopic ultrasound-guided through-the-needle biopsy in pancreatic cystic lesions. A systematic review and meta-analysis. J Gastrointest Cancer. 2024;55(1):15–25. https://doi.org/10.1007/s12029-023-00949-w. Epub 2023 Jun 21. PMID: 37341913.
52. Tacelli M, Celsa C, Magro B, Barchiesi M, Barresi L, Capurso G, et al. Diagnostic performance of endoscopic ultrasound through-the-needle microforceps biopsy of pancreatic cystic lesions: systematic review with meta-analysis. Dig Endosc. 2020;32(7):1018–30. https://doi.org/10.1111/den.13626. Epub 2020 Feb 26. PMID: 31912580.
53. Westerveld DR, Ponniah SA, Draganov PV, Yang D. Diagnostic yield of EUS-guided through-the-needle microforceps biopsy versus EUS-FNA of pancreatic cystic lesions: a systematic review and meta-analysis. Endosc Int Open. 2020;8(5):E656–67. https://doi.org/10.1055/a-1119-6543. Epub 2020 Apr 17. PMID: 32355885; PMCID: PMC7164999.
54. Rift CV, et al. Diagnostic accuracy of EUS-guided through-the-needle-biopsies and simultaneously obtained fine needle aspiration for cytology from pancreatic cysts: a systematic review and meta-analysis. Pathol Res Pract. 2021;220:153368.
55. Balaban VD, Cazacu IM, Pinte L, Jinga M, Bhutani MS, Saftoiu A. EUS-through-the-needle microbiopsy forceps in pancreatic cystic lesions: a systematic review. Endosc Ultrasound. 2021;10(1):19–24. https://doi.org/10.4103/eus.eus_23_20. PMID: 32611848; P.

56. Furukawa T, Klöppel G, Volkan Adsay N, Albores-Saavedra J, Fukushima N, Horii A, et al. Classification of types of intraductal papillary-mucinous neoplasm of the pancreas: a consensus study. Virchows Arch. 2005;447(5):794–9. https://doi.org/10.1007/s00428-005-0039-7. Epub 2005 Aug 9. PMID: 16088402.MCID: PMC7980686
57. Nakata K, Ohuchida K, Aishima S, Sadakari Y, Kayashima T, Miyasaka Y, et al. Invasive carcinoma derived from intestinal-type intraductal papillary mucinous neoplasm is associated with minimal invasion, colloid carcinoma, and less invasive behavior, leading to a better prognosis. Pancreas. 2011;40(4):581–7. https://doi.org/10.1097/MPA.0b013e318214fa86. PMID: 21499213.
58. Mino-Kenudson M, Fernández-del Castillo C, Baba Y, Valsangkar NP, Liss AS, Hsu M, et al. Prognosis of invasive intraductal papillary mucinous neoplasm depends on histological and precursor epithelial subtypes. Gut. 2011;60(12):1712–20. https://doi.org/10.1136/gut.2010.232272. Epub 2011 Apr 20. PMID: 21508421; PMCID: PMC3806085
59. Carroll NZ, Reyes B, Vázquez L. Intraductal papillary mucinous neoplasms of the pancreas: challenges and new insights [Internet]. In: Challenges in pancreatic pathology. INTECH; 2017. Available from: https://doi.org/10.5772/6649.
60. Ohtsuka T, Fernandez-Del Castillo C, Furukawa T, Hijioka S, Jang JY, Lennon AM, et al. International evidence-based Kyoto guidelines for the management of intraductal papillary mucinous neoplasm of the pancreas. Pancreatology. 2024;24(2):255–70. https://doi.org/10.1016/j.pan.2023.12.009. Epub 2023 Dec 28. PMID: 38182527.
61. Ngamruengphong S, Lennon AM. Analysis of pancreatic cyst fluid. Surg Pathol Clin. 2016;9(4):677–84. https://doi.org/10.1016/j.path.2016.05.010. PMID: 27926366; PMCID: PMC5145907.
62. Paniccia A, Polanco PM, Boone BA, Wald AI, McGrath K, Brand RE, Khalid A, et al. Prospective, multi-institutional, real-time next-generation sequencing of pancreatic cyst fluid reveals diverse genomic alterations that improve the clinical management of pancreatic cysts. Gastroenterology. 2023;164(1):117–33.e7. https://doi.org/10.1053/j.gastro.2022.09.028. Epub 2022 Oct 6. PMID: 36209796; PMCID: PMC9844531.
63. Pflüger MJ, Jamouss KT, Afghani E, Lim SJ, Rodriguez Franco S, Mayo H, et al. Predictive ability of pancreatic cyst fluid biomarkers: a systematic review and meta-analysis. Pancreatology. 2023;23(7):868–77. https://doi.org/10.1016/j.pan.2023.05.005. Epub 2023 May 15. PMID: 37230894.
64. Springer S, Masica DL, Dal Molin M, Douville C, Thoburn CJ, Afsari B, Li L, et al. A multimodality test to guide the management of patients with a pancreatic cyst. Sci Transl Med. 2019;11(501):eaav4772. https://doi.org/10.1126/scitranslmed.aav4772. PMID: 31316009; PMCID: PMC7859881.
65. Singhi AD, McGrath K, Brand RE, Khalid A, Zeh HJ, Chennat JS, et al. Preoperative next-generation sequencing of pancreatic cyst fluid is highly accurate in cyst classification and detection of advanced neoplasia. Gut. 2018;67(12):2131–41. https://doi.org/10.1136/gutjnl-2016-313586. Epub 2017 Sep 28. PMID: 28970292; PMCID: PMC6241612.
66. Fujikura K, Hosoda W, Felsenstein M, Song Q, Reiter JG, Zheng L, et al. Multiregion whole-exome sequencing of intraductal papillary mucinous neoplasms reveals frequent somatic *KLF4* mutations predominantly in low-grade regions. Gut. 2021;70(5):928–39. https://doi.org/10.1136/gutjnl-2020-321217. Epub 2020 Oct 7. PMID: 33028669; PMCID: PMC8262510
67. Fujiyama Y, Kumamoto Y, Nishizawa N, Nakamoto S, Harada H, Yokota K, et al. Promoter DNA Hypermethylation of the cysteine dioxygenase 1 (CDO1) gene in Intraductal papillary mucinous neoplasm (IPMN). Ann Surg Oncol. 2020;27(10):4007–16. https://doi.org/10.1245/s10434-020-08291-2. Epub 2020 Mar 6. PMID: 32144623.
68. Hong SM, Omura N, Vincent A, Li A, Knight S, Yu J, et al. Genome-wide CpG island profiling of intraductal papillary mucinous neoplasms of the pancreas. Clin Cancer Res. 2012;18(3):700–12. https://doi.org/10.1158/1078-0432.CCR-11-1718. Epub 2011 Dec 15. PMID: 22173550; PMCID: PMC3271174.
69. Shirakami Y, Iwashita T, Uemura S, Imai H, Murase K, Shimizu M. Micro-RNA analysis of pancreatic cyst fluid for diagnosing malignant transformation of Intraductal papillary muci-

nous neoplasm by comparing Intraductal papillary mucinous adenoma and carcinoma. J Clin Med. 2021;10(11):2249. https://doi.org/10.3390/jcm10112249. PMID: 34067335; PMCID: PMC8196884.

70. Kurita Y, Kuwahara T, Hara K, Mizuno N, Okuno N, Matsumoto S, et al. Diagnostic ability of artificial intelligence using deep learning analysis of cyst fluid in differentiating malignant from benign pancreatic cystic lesions. Sci Rep. 2019;9(1):6893. https://doi.org/10.1038/s41598-019-43314-3. PMID: 31053726; PMCID: PMC6499768.

Genetics of Pancreatic Cystic Tumors

13

Ravi Kumar Sharma, Alpa Singh, Surinder Singh Rana, and Navnit Kumar Mishra

Abstract

Pancreatic cystic tumors (PCTs) are a heterogeneous group of pancreatic neoplasms with variable malignant potential. Advances in imaging and molecular genetics have improved their detection and characterization. This chapter explores the genetic and molecular mechanisms underlying major PCTs, including intraductal papillary mucinous neoplasms (IPMNs), mucinous cystic neoplasms (MCNs), serous cystic neoplasms (SCNs), and solid pseudopapillary neoplasms (SPENs). Each form of PCT is characterized by specific genetic mutations that drive its development and determine its clinical course such as KRAS and GNAS in IPMNs, KRAS, RNF43, TP53, and SMAD4 in MCNs, VHL in SCNs, and CTNNB1 in SPENs. Familial syndromes such as Von Hippel–Lindau (VHL), Peutz-Jeghers (PJS), Lynch, FAMMM, and BRCA1/2-related syndromes contribute to inherited susceptibility to PCTs.

The molecular pathogenesis of these tumors involves sequential genetic events-early oncogenic activation, intermediate tumor suppressor loss, and late-stage invasive transformation. Genetic testing using next-generation sequencing (NGS) and liquid biopsy of cyst fluid enhances diagnostic precision, enabling differentiation between benign and malignant cysts. Biomarkers such as KRAS, GNAS, TP53, and SMAD4 have diagnostic and prognostic

R. K. Sharma (✉) · A. Singh
Department of Biotechnology, Chandigarh University, Mohali, Punjab, India

S. S. Rana
Department of Gastroenterology, Postgraduate Institute of Medical education and Research, Chandigarh, India

N. K. Mishra
School of Biosciences and Technology, Galgotia University, Greator Noida, Uttar Pradesh, India

R. K. Sharma et al. (eds.), *Differential Diagnosis and Management of Pancreatic Cystic Lesions*, https://doi.org/10.1007/978-981-92-0654-4_13

significance. Emerging multi-omics and AI-based approaches are transforming early detection and targeted therapy strategies. Integrating molecular genetics into clinical management promises improved outcomes through personalized medicine and early intervention in malignant progression of pancreatic cystic neoplasms.

Keywords

Genetics · Point Mutation · *KRAS* · *GNAS* · *TP53* · *VHL* · Missense mutation

13.1 Introduction

13.1.1 Overview of Pancreatic Cystic Tumors (PCTs)

Pancreatic cysts are a type of cystic lesions observed within the pancreas. Pancreatic cystic tumors (PCTs) represent 2–10% of all pancreatic lesions and can range from benign to malignant [1]. PCTs are distinguished as either mucinous or nonmucinous cystic neoplasms [2]. The most common types of PCTs are intraductal mucinous neoplasms (IPMNs), mucinous cystic neoplasms (MCNs), and serous cystic neoplasms (SCNs), which account for over 90% of cases [3, 4]. The rarer forms of PCTs include intraductal tubular neoplasms (ITPNs), acinar cell cystadenoma (ACA), cystic pancreatic endocrine neoplasm (CPEN), and solid pseudopapillary tumor (SPT) [4].

In the early 1980s, researchers noted that some MCNs in the pancreas were not connected to the pancreatic duct system [5]. In 1996, the World Health Organization (WHO) distinguished between IPMNs and MCNs, emphasizing the presence of ovarian stroma in MCNs [4]. As a result, MCNs and IPMNs are now recognized as two distinct malignant tumors, each with unique biological, pathological, and prognostic characteristics.

13.1.2 Importance of Genetics in Understanding PCTs

Genetic advancements are becoming increasingly important in understanding PCTs. They play a significant role in diagnosis, identifying risk factors, and shaping treatment approaches [6]. Given the breadth of PCTs, it is essential to evaluate their underlying genetic characteristics to distinguish benign from malignant or potentially malignant tumors [7]. Genetic identification can help to differentiate between various forms of PCTs. Certain genetic alterations are associated with an increased risk of malignant progression and can serve as biomarkers for the early diagnosis of malignancies in PCTs [8].

13.1.3 Multi-OMICS Study of Pancreatic Cysts

Integration of OMICS study in pancreatic cysts has revealed the constituting biomarkers present in cystic fluid [9]. These biomarkers could be the potential targets for characterizing pancreatic cysts [10]. Further, they can be mapped to physiological pathways for drug developments. The advancement in multi-Omics techniques from genomics to Kyoto Encyclopedia of Genes and Genomes (KEGG) metabolic pathways has identified the RNA transcripts linked to upregulation and downregulation of significant genes. The inclusion of multi-Omics in the context of PCT utilizes the combination of bimolecular analytical techniques. These techniques are differential gene expression and gene enrichment analysis from the genomics and transcriptomics data. The proteomics and metabolomics data from the pancreatic cystic fluids precisely find the metabolite profiles and identify the molecule driving the cystic progression. Moreover, the recent advancement in spatial transcriptomics in combination with bioinformatics tools has precisely and efficiently identified the gene expression profile and their spatial location in the pancreatic cysts [11]. These recent research findings on pancreatic cysts have identified the spatiotemporal-resolved biomarkers responsible for the malignant transformation of IPMNs significantly utilizing deep learning method on spatial transcriptomics data.

13.2 Classification of PCTs

13.2.1 Intraductal Papillary Mucinous Neoplasm (IPMN)

IPMN is a cystic neoplasm that affects the pancreatic duct [12]. It is classified into two categories based on the section of the ductal system from which it originated: main-duct IPMN and branch-duct IPMN [13]. Some tumors exhibit features of both types and are referred to as mixed PMNs. These tumors are characterized by intraluminal papillary growth, which dilates the adjacent areas of the affected duct [13]. IPMNs are more commonly found in the head of the pancreas, though they can also develop in the body and tail [14]. They are more frequently observed in men than in women, with an average age of diagnosis ranging from 64 to 67 years [15]. Symptoms typically include recurrent pancreatitis, stomach discomfort, jaundice, and weight loss due to ductal obstruction. These tumors often display a variety of genetic abnormalities across different pancreatic lesions [16].

13.2.1.1 Genetic Alternations in IPMNs

IPMNs of the pancreas represent precursor lesions that can progress to one of the most lethal forms of pancreatic cancer, pancreatic ductal adenocarcinoma (PDAC) [17]. This progression is often driven by a series of genetic alterations in major genes, including KRAS, GNAS, and RNF43 [18, 19]. Understanding the mechanisms underlying this transition to malignancy is essential for developing strategies to detect and treat PC at an early stage.

KRAS Mutation

The Kirsten-ras sarcoma viral oncogene homolog (KRAS) gene is located on the short arm of chromosome 12p [20]. Mutations in the KRAS gene are reported in 38.2% to 100% of cases and occasionally occur at codon 13 [19, 21]. There is no significant difference in the prevalence of KRAS mutation across various grades of dysplasia: 87% in low-grade dysplasia, 90.2% in intermediate dysplasia, and 70.7% in high-grade dysplasia [22].

GNAS Mutation

The guanine nucleotide-binding protein alpha-stimulating (GNAS) gene is an oncogene located on the long arm of chromosome 20 (20q13.3) [23]. Mutations in GNAS are detected in 61% of IPMN cases and are more prevalent in advanced lesions [24]: 19% in low-grade dysplasia, 23% in intermediate-grade dysplasia, and 58% in high-grade dysplasia [25]. Histological subtypes also differ in GNAS mutation rates: 100% in the intestinal type, 71% in the pancreatobiliary type, and 51% in the gastric type [26].

13.2.1.2 RNF 43 Mutations

The Ring Finger Protein 43 (RNF43) gene plays a crucial role in regulating the Wnt signaling pathway, which governs cell growth, proliferation, and differentiation [27]. RNF43 encodes a ubiquitin E3 in truncating loss-of-function alterations, impairing its ability to inhibit Wnt signaling [28]. This unrestrained signaling promotes abnormal cell growth, increasing the risk of malignant transformation in IPMNs. RNF43 mutations are a hallmark of IPMNs, particularly in the gastric and intestinal subtypes [29].

13.2.2 Mucinous Cystic Neoplasm (MCN)

MCN is characterized by a unique mesenchymal component, referred to as "ovarian type stroma," which surrounds the cyst [30]. Unlike IPMN, MCN primarily affects younger individuals and is more commonly observed in women, although it is relatively rare in men [31].

MCN typically presents as a single, multilocular cyst filled with mucin and enclosed by a thick fibrotic capsule [32]. It is predominantly located in the body or tail of the pancreas and does not communicate with the pancreatic duct system [30, 33].

13.2.2.1 Genetic Alternations in MCN

The genetic alterations associated with MCNs are critical to understanding their behavior, growth, and potential transformation into PDAC. Several mutations and chromosomal abnormalities have been identified in MCNs, contributing to their progression toward malignancy. Main genetic mutations include KRAS, RNF43, TP53, and SMAD4 [19, 34, 35].

KRAS Mutation

KRAS mutations, particularly at codon 12, are among the most frequent in MCNs [19, 36]. These mutations lead to amino acid substitutions that result in the continuous activation of the KRAS protein, driving downstream signaling pathways such as MAPK (Mitogen-Activated Protein Kinase) and PI3K/AKT [37]. These pathways promote cellular proliferation, survival, and invasion [38]. While KRAS mutations alone are insufficient to drive malignancy, they often coexist with other genetic alterations such as TP53 or SMAD4 mutations [39], which facilitate the transition from low-grade dysplasia to high-grade dysplasia and eventually to invasive PC [40].

TP53 Mutation

The TP53 tumor suppressor gene plays a pivotal role in maintaining genomic stability [41]. Mutations in TP53, frequently seen in various cancers, often involve missense mutations that alter the amino acids in the DNA-binding domain of the p53 protein, impairing its ability to activate target genes [42]. Loss of heterozygosity (LOH) at the TP53 locus is also common, further compromising p53 function [43]. These mutations are generally absent in the early stage of MCNs but become more frequent as the neoplasms progress to high-grade dysplasia or invasive carcinoma [44]. TP53 mutations are markers of poor prognosis, associated with more aggressive lesions and a higher risk of progression to PDAC [45].

RNF43 Mutations

RNF43, another tumor suppressor gene, encodes an E3 ubiquitin ligase that negatively regulates the Wnt/b-catenin signaling pathway, which is critical for cell proliferation and differentiation [46]. RNF43 mutations disrupt this regulatory function, leading to unrestrained Wnt signaling, increased cellular proliferation, and neoplastic progression [47].

RNF43 is frequently observed in MCNs and linked to the formation and growth of cystic lesions by improper folding of E3 ubiquitin ligase [48]. As a tumor suppressor, RNF43 promotes the degradation of frizzled receptors, essential components of the Wnt signaling pathway [49]. When RNF43 is mutated, this degradation process is disrupted, resulting in persistent Wnt signaling and a growth advantage for the neoplastic cells [49].

RNF43 mutations are agonist to KRAS mutations, intensifying the transformation of PCT to neoplastic MCNs and enhancing the progression to dysplasia or invasive carcinoma [50]. These mutations also have diagnostic value, helping to differentiate MCNs from other PCTs. Additionally, they provide insights into the biological behavior of MCNs, including their malignant potential [51].

Loss of Chromosome 3p

The deleterious mutation of chromosome 3 at the short-arm terminal is observed in various cancers, including MCNs of the pancreas [52]. This deletion leads to the inactivation of several tumor suppressor genes located on chromosome 3p, contributing to neoplastic transformation in MCNs [53].

The short arm of chromosome 3 (3p) houses key tumor suppressor genes, such asPBRM1 (Polybromo 1), SETD2, and VHL (Von Hippel–Lindau) [54]. When the genetic material from this region is lost, the functional activity of these tumor suppressors is diminished. This reduces their ability to regulate cell growth and maintain normal cellular processes, fostering a predisposition to tumor development [53].

The loss of chromosome 3p can occur relatively early in the progression of MCNs [53]. This genetic event sets the stage for additional oncogenic changes, such as mutations in KRAS or TP53, which are commonly associated with MCNs and are critical drivers of malignancy [55].

Detecting the loss of chromosome 3p through genetic testing can serve as a diagnostic marker to differentiate MCNs from other PCTs [56]. Additionally, this alteration, in conjunction with other mutations, provides valuable insights into the neoplasm's biological behavior and its potential for aggressive progression. Identifying chromosome 3p loss may also help in risk stratification and inform treatment strategies. Understanding chromosome 3p loss enhances our ability to classify and manage MCNs, particularly those at higher risk of malignant transformation [53].

13.2.3 Serous Cystic Neoplasm (SCN)

Histology of SCN is characterized by epithelial cells with uniformly abundant glycogen and rounded nuclei containing homogeneous chromatin [57]. These cells are associated with a prominent microvascular meshwork within the epithelium [58]. SCNs are predominantly located in the body or tail of the pancreas and account for approximately 24–30% of all PCTs [1].

Females are more prone to SCNs at their average age of 62 years, and their prevalence increases with advancing age. However, most patients with SCNs are asymptomatic [59].The occurrences are typically nonspecific, with symptoms including abdominal pain, pancreatic biliary complications, or diabetes mellitus [60].

13.2.3.1 Genetic Alternations in SCN

Pancreatic SCNs are typically benign with a low risk of progression to malignancy [61]. However, specific genetic alterations drive their formation and provide valuable insights into their development and behavior. SCNs are primarily associated with VHL gene mutations and loss of chromosome 3p [62], both critical factors in their formation and growth. These genetic changes disrupt hypoxia pathways, contributing to cyst formation [63]. The genetic profile of SCNs is distinct from other PCTs, with a comparatively insignificant frequency or absence of oncogenic mutations such as TP53 or KRAS [64]. This aligns with their non-aggressive nature.

VHL Mutations

The Von Hippel–Lindau (VHL) gene locus is 3p25 and is significantly prone to mutations often observed in SCNs [62, 65]. The function of VHL is to suppress the tumor by regulating the homoeostatic oxygen level through its interaction to a dimeric protein named as hypoxia-inducible factors (HIFs) [66]. Normally, the VHL protein helps target HIFs for degradation under normoxic (normal oxygen) conditions, maintaining a balance in cell growth and angiogenesis [66].

In SCNs, the deleterious mutations of the VHL gene locus 3p25 result in a loss of its regulatory function. The loss of regulatory function within the VHL gene also occurs through point mutations [62]. VHL gene loses its heterozygosity by completely losing one allele, which is often accompanied by mutation in its remaining alleles. This hypermethylation in the promoter region suppresses the VHL expression [67].

This causes deficiency in VHL protein synthesis, eventually leading to cyst formation by impaired HIF regulation [68]. The presence of VHL mutations or 3p loss serves as a molecular hallmark, aiding in the diagnosis of SCNs and distinguishing them from other PCTs, which typically lack VHL mutations [69]. Molecular testing for VHL alterations can help to confirm SCNs [70].

Lack of KRAS, TP53, and GNAS Mutations

SCNs exhibit a distinct genetic variation as compared to other PCTs. One of the unique variations is the lack of genetic mutations in the GNAS, TP53, and KRAS genes than that of MCNs and SCNs [55]. This absence highlights a fundamental difference in their molecular pathogenesis and is consistent with SCNs' benign nature and low malignant potential. The absence of TP53 mutations in SCNs indicates that they do not undergo genetic alterations typically associated with high-grade dysplasia or malignant transformation [71]. This aligns with their noninvasive and low-grade characteristics, differentiating them from more aggressive cysts. GNAS mutations, often observed in IPMNs, are not present in SCNs [72]. This suggests that cAMP signaling, a pathway influenced by GNAS, is not significant in the development of SCNs. This further reinforces their distinct biological behavior.

13.2.4 Solid Pseudo-Papillary Tumor (SPT)

SPTs are considered low-grade malignant tumors [73]. They are characterized by diminished cohesive extracellular matrix organizing the epithelial cells. Biopsy reveals that they are characterized by poorly cohesive, monomorphic epithelial cells forming coagulated pseudo-papillary lumps [74]. SPENs can occur in any region of the pancreas and account for 1–2% of all PCTs [75].

These tumors are predominately observed in young women, with an average age of diagnosis around 28 years [76]. Patients with abdominal pain experience discomfort; however, most SPENs are detected incidentally during imaging studies conducted for unrelated reasons [77].

13.2.4.1 Genetic Alternations in SPENs

These tumors are defined by specific genetic alterations that differentiate them from other PCTs. Unlike other pancreatic neoplasms, SPENs do not typically have genetic mutations in CDKN2A, TP53, SMAD4, and KRAS genes [55]. This absence of genetic mutations in major oncogenes and tumor suppressor genes observed in PDAC or mucinous neoplasms suggests that SPENs follow a tumorigenic pathway. This unique genetic profile aligns with the indolent behavior of SPENs, as they do not progress through the aggressive genetic trajectories typical of other pancreatic malignancies [44].

CTNNB1 Mutations

Mutations in the CTNNB1 gene are the hallmark of SPENs, present in over 90% of cases [78]. The CTNNB1 gene encodes β-catenin associated with Wnt signaling and cell proliferation pathway by regulating cell adhesion and transcriptional activity [79]. The genetic alterations in the CTNNB1 gene corresponds to mutated β-catenin protein, leading to its accumulation in the nucleus. This accumulation activity targets downstream genes involved in cell proliferation and survival [80].

This mutation takes place in the exon 3 region of the CTNNB1 gene, which is essential for β-catenin degradation. The resulting stabilization of β-catenin and hyperactivation of the Wnt pathway contribute to tumorigenesis [81].

While CTNNB1 mutations are the most consistent genetic feature of SPENs, recent studies have explored additional potential genetic alterations, such as changes in genes involved in cell cycle regulation. For instance, mutations in TSC2 and PTEN, which play roles in cell growth and signaling pathways, have been reported, although these are less frequent and not as well characterized as CTNNB1 mutations [82].

SPENs exhibit a high degree of genomic stability, lacking the significant chromosomal aberrations and genomic instability typical of more aggressive pancreatic cancers like PDAC. This stability underscores their low-grade nature and supports their tendency toward localized growth rather than metastatic spread [83].

13.3 Familial Syndromes and PCTs

13.3.1 Von Hippel–Lindau (VHL) Syndrome

VHL syndrome is a hereditary mutation in the gene located on chromosome 3 specifically at cytoband 3p25–26, which is a tumor suppressor gene. Historically, the name of this syndrome is from Eugen von Hippel and Arvind Lindau. They first revealed the characteristic mutations and its pathology [63, 84]. While up to 20% of newly diagnosed cases result from de novo mutations, VHL syndrome is typically inherited as an autosomal dominant disorder with nearly complete penetrance [62].

VHL syndrome is characterized by the mutations at the cytoband 3p25–26 region causing malignant, benign tumors and cysts in the diverse organs and tissues [63]. Most prevalent organs are central nervous system (CNS) and ophthalmic retinal hemangioblastomas, adrenal gland pheochromocytomas, endolymphatic cysts, neuroendocrine tumors in pancreas, and renal cell carcinoma [85].

13.3.1.1 Association with SCN

VHL syndrome is strongly linked with the progression of SCNs observed in the pathophysiology of pancreatic tissues. SCNs are generally benign cystic tumors that are a recognized manifestation of this genetic disorder [64].

SCNs in VHL patients are typically detected incidentally during imaging studies performed as part of routine surveillance. They are characterized by microcystic or macrocystic structures filled with digestive pancreatic enzymes predominantly containing glycogen molecules in the epithelial cells. These lesions may present as single or multiple cystic formations within the pancreas and are nonfunctional, meaning they do not produce hormones [64].

Although SCNs are typically benign, they can increase in size over time [86]. In some cases, this growth may lead to abdominal discomfort or compression of adjacent structures. Despite these potential complications, SCNs in the context of VHL syndrome usually remain non-aggressive and are managed conservatively unless symptomatic [64].

13.3.2 Peutz–Jeghers Syndrome

Peutz–Jeghers Syndrome (PJS) is a hereditary genetic disorder that causes benign gastrointestinal polyps and colored spots on the mucous and cutaneous membranes [87]. It is an autosomal dominant hereditary genetic disorder. Precisely, an allelic mutation in the tumor suppressor STK11 gene is sufficient to cause tumours [88].

Peutz–Jeghers syndrome is commonly associated with STK11 gene (also named as LKB1) mutations located on the chromosome region 19p13.3 [87]. STK11 is a tumor suppressor gene that encodes a serine/threonine kinase protein. The function of the gene is to regulate the cell growth, its polarity, and metabolic processes. Mutations in STK11 disrupt its tumor suppressor function, leading to uncontrolled cell growth, which results in the formation of polyps on the mucous lining of the gastrointestinal tract. The symptoms also include cutaneous pigmentation [87].

13.3.2.1 Association with IPMN

PJS is associated with various gastrointestinal and extra-gastrointestinal cancers, including those of the pancreas [87]. One of the pancreatic conditions linked to PJS is the development of IPMNs [89].

Persons with PJS have significantly increased risk of transforming to pancreatic neoplasms, including IPMNs and pancreatic adenocarcinoma [89]. The STK11 mutation causes neoplastic pancreatic cysts like IPMNs by losing the tumor suppressing activity. The loss of STK11's tumor-suppressive capabilities predisposes individuals with PJS to abnormal cellular growth in the pancreas, highlighting the connection between the syndrome and the increased risk of pancreatic neoplasms [87, 89].

13.3.3 Familial Pancreatic Cancer Syndromes

Familial pancreatic cancer (FPC) syndromes refer to inherited genetic disorders that elevate the risk of developing pancreatic cancer within families [90]. These syndromes are associated with mutations in specific genes that influence cellular growth, repair, and regulation, thereby contributing to the development of pancreatic cancer [91]. Some of the unique familial syndromes linked to an enhanced likelihood of pancreatic cancers are as follows:

13.3.3.1 Hereditary Inflammation of the Pancreas (Pancreatitis, PRSS1 Mutation)

The PRSS1 (Protease serine 1) gene is implicated in hereditary pancreatitis, a condition marked by recurrent episodes of acute pancreatitis that typically begin in childhood or early adulthood and may progress to chronic pancreatitis [92].

Persons with hereditary inflammation of the pancreas (pancreatitis) have significant risk of developing pancreatic cancer in their life, with estimates ranging from 25 to 40% [93]. The K23R amino acid point mutations in the PRSS1 gene causes the uncontrolled production of trypsinogen, an enzyme precursor [94]. This aberrant activation leads to self-digestion of pancreatic tissue, causing inflammation and tissue damage. Over time, the persistent damage and inflammation increase the likelihood of malignant transformation, contributing to the elevated cancer risk associated with this condition [95].

13.3.3.2 Familial Atypical Multiple Mole Melanoma (FAMMM) Syndrome

The gene involved in FAMMM syndrome is CDKN2A located at chromosome 9 band p21.3 [96]. The CDKN2A gene encodes two unique cell cycle proteins that regulate two critical cell cycle RB1 and p53 pathways. This syndrome causes many abnormal moles and enhances the risk of melanoma [96].

Individuals with CDKN2A mutations are also susceptible to advancing pancreatic cancer, with the risk estimated to be 17–25% [97]. Cyclin-dependent kinase inhibitor 2A (p16) is also a tumor suppressor gene that significantly regulates the cell cycle [98]. Mutations in the gene can disrupt normal cell control, leading to uncontrolled cell growth. This dysregulation contributes to the development of both melanoma and pancreatic tumors [96, 97].

13.3.3.3 Hereditary Breast and Ovarian Cancer Syndrome (BRCA1/BRCA2 Mutations)

BRCA1 and BRCA2 genes encode proteins which repair the damaged DNA [99]. Point mutations of both genes cause ovarian and breast cancers; they are also associated with enhanced risk of pancreatic cancer [99].

Individuals with BRCA2 mutations are susceptible to pancreatic cancer of approximately 5–10%. However, mutations in BRCA1 confer a lower but still elevated risk [100]. Both BRCA1 and BRCA2 genes encode proteins significant in DNA nick repair through the process of homologous recombination [101]. Mutations in these genes impair DNA repair mechanisms, leading to genomic instability and a heightened likelihood of developing pancreatic and other cancers [102].

13.3.3.4 Lynch Syndrome

The Lynch syndrome is associated with the PMS2, MSH6, EPCAM, MLH1, and MSH2 genes [103]. An individual with Lynch syndrome is susceptible to endometrial, colorectal, and gastrointestinal cancers, including pancreatic cancers [104].

Persons with Lynch syndrome have approximately 5–10% risk of developing pancreatic cancer [105]. Mutations in the mismatch repair (MMR) genes cause microsatellite instability (MSI), which is characterized by errors in DNA replication. This instability significantly increases the likelihood of malignant transformation in various tissues, including the pancreas [105].

13.3.3.5 Peutz–Jeghers Syndrome (PJS)

The hereditary mutation in STK11 (LKB1) gene is associated with Peutz–Jeghers syndrome [106]. PJS is characterized by distinctive gastrointestinal hamartomatous polyps and mucocutaneous pigmentation, similar to the symptoms of VHL syndrome [107]. These hamartomatous polyps are disorganized tissue characterized by autosomal dominant inheritance. Individuals with PJS have a relatively higher susceptibility estimated to be of 11–36% for processing pancreatic cancer [108]. This syndrome is linked to STK11 tumor suppressor gene that is involved in synchronizing and coordinating the cell metabolism growth and polarity [109]. Therefore any mutations in the STK11 gene causes unregulated cell proliferation, which increases the risk of pancreatic neoplasms and other malignancies [110].

13.3.3.6 Von Hippel–Lindau (VHL) Syndrome

The VHL gene is responsible for VHL syndrome [111]. This syndrome forms renal cell carcinoma, hemangioblastomas, and pancreatic cystic neoplasms [112]. Individuals with VHL mutations have an increased risk of developing pancreatic cystic neoplasms, such as serous cyst adenomas, although the risk of pancreatic ductal adenocarcinoma is less clearly defined [113]. The physiology of the VHL gene is linked to progressing angiogenesis and cell growth. Genetic alterations in this gene can lead to dysregulation of these processes, contributing to tumorigenesis in multiple organs, including the pancreas [114].

13.4 Molecular Pathogenesis of PCT

The progression from IPMN to PDAC involves a series of molecular alterations and histological changes, reflecting the transition from benign to malignant states [115]. This process can be categorized into distinct stages.

13.4.1 Initiation Stage: Early Genetic Alterations

Among the earliest and most frequent genetic alterations in IPMN, KRAS mutation is found in approximately 70–90% of cases [29]. These mutations activate signaling pathways that drive cell proliferation, laying the groundwork for subsequent genetic changes [55].

Particularly prevalent in the intestinal subtype of IPMNs, GNAS mutations result in the continuous activation of the Gs alpha subunit, contributing to mucin overproduction and cyst formation [116].

RNF43, a tumor suppressor gene, is frequently mutated in IPMNs [18]. Loss-of-function mutations in RNF43 dysregulate cell growth through the Wnt signaling pathway, facilitating neoplastic progression [28].

13.4.2 Progression Stage: Intermediate Genetic Changes

The progression of IPMN is due to the deactivation of the tumor suppressor gene P16/CDKN2A. The metabolic processes of this gene include cell cycle regulation [117]. This deactivation signifies a critical transition toward more dysplastic changes. The SMAD4 gene regulates the production of TGF-beta cytokine. The loss of this gene in IPMN advances to dysplasia, and invasive carcinoma becomes increasingly common. This loss serves as a hallmark of the progression from IPMN to invasive pancreatic ductal adenocarcinoma [118].

13.4.3 Invasive Stage: Late Genetic Alterations and Full Malignant Transformation

A critical step in the progression to PDAC is the inactivation of the TP53 gene [45]. Loss of function in this gene impairs the ability of cells to undergo apoptosis in response to DNA damage, allowing cells to become fully malignant [45].

Structural alterations, such as the loss of 18q (where SMAD4 resides) and 17p (where TP53 is located) chromosomal regions, occur as IPMN evolves into PDAC [119]. The epigenetic factors, such as histone modification and DNA methylation, are primarily involved in gene expression and drive the transition from IPMN to PDAC [120].

13.4.4 Histological Transformation: Changes in Cellular Architecture

IPMNs start as low-grade lesions inside the pancreatic ducts, characterized by thick mucus production. Over time, the lesions can progress to high-grade dysplasia, where abnormal cellular architecture and nuclear atypia become more pronounced

[121]. When the invasive component develops, it penetrates the pancreatic stroma and resembles PDAC histologically, featuring poorly differentiated and highly aggressive tumor cells [122].

13.5 Genetic Testing and Clinical Implications

13.5.1 Importance of Genetic Profiling for Risk Assessment

Genetic profiling allows for the early detection of mutations that are indicative of a high likelihood of progression to malignancy [123]. Mutations in genes such as KRAS, GNAS, and TP53 are often associated with more aggressive cystic neoplasms, such as IPMNs, that may transform into PDAC [34]. Identifying the likelihood mutations can help distinguish potentially dangerous tissue or organ lesions that require either surgical intervention or chemotherapy which reduces the peril of unnecessary surgeries [123].

Genetic profiling helps in differentiating subtypes of PCTs based on their molecular signatures. For instance, GNAS mutations are more commonly associated with IPMN [72], while VHL gene alterations are indicative of SCN [113]. This information aids in tailoring surveillance and treatment strategies specific to the type of cyst. Early detection and management of high-risk PCTs through genetic profiling can improve patient prognosis and survival rates. This assures timely intervention in the progression to pancreatic neoplasm of the tumors in cases where there is a significant risk of progression to pancreatic cancer, which is often diagnosed at the advanced stage having piteous prognosis [64].

13.5.2 Genetic Biomarkers for Diagnosis and Prognosis

Genetic biomarkers are indispensable for accurately diagnosing PCTs and assessing their risk of malignancy. They provide clinicians with crucial information for differentiating between benign and potentially cancerous lesions, enabling more precise risk stratification and management [124].

Genetic biomarkers such as the presence of a KRAS mutation can indicate a higher risk of progression to invasive PDAC [125, 126]. However, GNAS mutations are useful in identifying lesions with the potential for neoplastic progression, especially when found alongside other mutations like TP53 or SMAD4 [39]. However, TP53 mutation can be a critical marker for determining the need for more aggressive surgical intervention [127]. Detection of VHL mutations is useful for identifying low-risk lesions that may only require monitoring [70]. While RNF43 mutations are associated with cyst formation, they are not necessarily indicative of an increased risk for invasive cancer [128].

13.5.3 Use of Liquid Biopsies and Next-Generation Sequencing

The advancement of liquid biopsies and ultra-high-throughput sequencing (NGS) has improved the diagnosis, risk assessment, and clinical treatment of PCTs [129]. These advanced techniques offer less invasive and more precise approaches for detecting genetic alterations and monitoring disease progression [129, 130].

The detection of circulating biomarkers in biofluids such as blood, serum, pancreatic cyst fluid, or urine by liquid biopsy provides real time molecular profiling of PCTs. These biomarkers are RNA, exosomes, circulating tumor DNA, cell-free DNA, and several proteins present in the biofluids [131]. In the context of PCTs, the cyst fluid is mainly analyzed by microscopic biopsy. The sample is obtained through endoscopic ultrasound-guided fine-needle aspiration (EUS-FNA), which provides the genetic as well as the biopolymer profile of a cyst [132].

NGS is a high-throughput sequencing technology that enables simultaneous biochemical analysis of several genetic mutations across a large number of genes. It can be applied to DNA from the cyst fluid obtained through EUS-FNA or cfDNA (cell-free DNA) from blood samples. NGS can help distinguish different types of pancreatic cystic neoplasms by identifying mutation patterns that are specific to certain cysts [133].

13.6 Emerging Research and Future Directions

13.6.1 Identification of Novel Genetic Mutations

Genetic studies of PCTs have increasingly focused on identifying novel genetic mutations that can be the potential biomarkers which help in diagnosis, risk assessment, and assuring the significant intervention. Some of the emerging genetic mutations being studied in PCTs involve NRAS mutations that could serve as alternative diagnostic markers in cases where KRAS mutations are absent, providing additional insights into the pathogenesis of certain MCN and IPMN [134]. Since CTNNB1 mutations are not common in other PCTs, their presence could be a distinguishing feature for diagnosing SPNs [135]. They might also offer new therapeutic targets for treatment. The SMAD4 status can help in determining the aggressiveness of certain pancreatic cystic tumors and may be used as a prognostic marker [136]. Ongoing research is exploring the role of RNF43 as a potential therapeutic target, as its mutation may render cells more dependent on Wnt signaling, which could be exploited with targeted therapies [137]. Studies suggest that GATA6 mutations could interact with other known mutations like KRAS and TP53, potentially contributing to the tumor's malignant potential [138]. It is also being investigated for its role in drug resistance. Many of these novel genetic mutations are currently under study for their roles in tumorigenesis, their potential to serve as early diagnostic markers, and their implications for personalized treatment approaches [139].

13.6.2 Implications for Targeted Therapies and Personalized Medicine

The detailed insights about the genetic profile of PCTs have significant implications in targeted therapies and personalized medicine. With the identification of key genetic mutations and pathways associated with different types of pancreatic cystic neoplasms, it is now possible to tailor treatment strategies more precisely [139]. Several genetic disorders associated to PCTs, such as mutations in the PIK3CA, RNF43, GNAS, and KRAS genes, are involved in key signaling pathways like the MAPK, Wnt/β-catenin, and PI3K/AKT metabolic pathways [55]. Understanding these mutations enables the development of therapies targeting specific pathways.

13.6.3 Role of Genetics in Early Detection of Malignant Progression

Genetics have a unique importance in the early detection of malignant progression in PCTs, offering insights into which cysts are likely to remain benign and eventually progress to pancreatic cancer. Genetic analysis of these tumors helps in assessing the risk of malignancy, guiding clinical decision-making, and enabling timely intervention. Certain genetic mutations are strongly associated with the progression of PCTs into malignant forms like PDAC. By analyzing the presence or absence of these high-risk mutations, clinicians can better stratify patients into those who need closer surveillance and those who may not require immediate intervention. Genetic analysis complements traditional imaging and cytology, improving the accuracy of diagnosing pancreatic cystic neoplasms. This helps to prevent overtreatment of neoplastic lesions while ensuring early intervention and treatment for those with a higher risk of malignancy [117, 140].

13.7 Conclusion/Future Direction

This can be concluded that most of the syndromes associated with mutually exclusive genes potentially aggravate PCTs. PCTs are a heterogeneous group of lesions, each characterized by distinct genetic alterations that influence their potential for malignancy. The detailed insights of the aforementioned genetic alternations are requisites for accurate and early diagnosis of the severity in PCTs. Ongoing research is needed to discover additional mutations that contribute to the progression of benign cystic lesions to invasive carcinoma. Exploration of epigenetic physiochemical changes, such as methylated cytosine nucleotide in DNA altering the histone, could further elucidate metabolic mechanisms driving malignancy in PCTs. Research on liquid biopsy assay by enhancing specificity and sensitivity would be essential for early detection of malignancy and assessing treatment response in patients with pancreatic cystic neoplasms. Further studies should focus on the feasibility and cost-effectiveness of integrating NGS into routine clinical care for PCTs.

References

1. Jabłońska B, Gudz A, Hinborch T, Bujała B, Biskup K, Mrowiec S. Pancreatic cystic tumors: a single-center observational study. Medicina (B Aires). 2023;59(2):241.
2. Ardeshna DR, et al. Recent advances in the diagnostic evaluation of pancreatic cystic lesions. World J Gastroenterol. 2022;28(6):624.
3. Klotz R, Hackert T, Büchler MW. Natural history of cystic neoplasms: IPMN, MCN, SCN, and SPN. In: The pancreas: an integrated textbook of basic science, medicine, and surgery; 2023. p. 666–73.
4. Xiao S-Y, Ye Z. Pancreatic cystic tumors: an update. J Pancreatol. 2018;1(1):2–18.
5. Milanetto AC, et al. Simple mucinous cyst: another potential cancer precursor in the pancreas? Case report with molecular characterization and systematic review of the literature. Virchows Arch. 2021;479:179–89.
6. Raman A, Lennon AM. Cyst fluid biomarkers-diagnosis and prediction of malignancy for cystic lesions of the pancreas. Visc Med. 2018;34(3):178–81.
7. Makohon-Moore A, Iacobuzio-Donahue CA. Pancreatic cancer biology and genetics from an evolutionary perspective. Nat Rev Cancer. 2016;16(9):553–65.
8. Carmicheal J, et al. Elevating pancreatic cystic lesion stratification: current and future pancreatic cancer biomarker (s). Biochim Biophys Acta (BBA). 2020;1873(1):188318.
9. Kane LE, et al. Multi-omic biomarker panel in pancreatic cyst fluid and serum predicts patients at a high risk of pancreatic cancer development. Sci Rep. 2025;15(1):129.
10. Kane LE, Mellotte GS, Conlon KC, Ryan BM, Maher SG. Multi-omic biomarkers as potential tools for the characterisation of pancreatic cystic lesions and cancer: innovative patient data integration. Cancers (Basel). 2021;13(4):769.
11. Agostini A, et al. Identification of spatially-resolved markers of malignant transformation in Intraductal Papillary Mucinous Neoplasms. Nat Commun. 2024;15(1):2764.
12. Hecht EM, et al. Intraductal papillary mucinous neoplasm (IPMN) of the pancreas: recommendations for Standardized Imaging and Reporting from the Society of Abdominal Radiology IPMN disease focused panel. Abdom Radiol. 2021;46:1586–606.
13. Jabłońska B, Szmigiel Pawełand Mrowiec S. Pancreatic intraductal papillary mucinous neoplasms: current diagnosis and management. World J Gastrointest Oncol. 2021;13(12):1880.
14. Zhou H, et al. Threshold of main pancreatic duct for malignancy in intraductal papillary mucinous neoplasm at head-neck and body-tail. BMC Gastroenterol. 2022;22(1):473.
15. Castellano-Megías VM, Ibarrola-de Andrés C, López-Alonso G, Colina-Ruizdelgado F. Pathological features and diagnosis of intraductal papillary mucinous neoplasm of the pancreas. World J Gastrointest Oncol. 2014;6(9):311.
16. Dumlu EG, Karakoç D, Özdemir A. Intraductal papillary mucinous neoplasm of the pancreas: current perspectives. Int Surg. 2015;100(6):1060–8.
17. Ren B, Liu X, Suriawinata AA. Pancreatic ductal adenocarcinoma and its precursor lesions: histopathology, cytopathology, and molecular pathology. Am J Pathol. 2019;189(1):9–21.
18. Lee J-H, Kim Y, Choi J-W, Kim Y-S. KRAS, GNAS, and RNF43 mutations in intraductal papillary mucinous neoplasm of the pancreas: a meta-analysis. Springerplus. 2016;5:1–12.
19. Sharma RK, et al. Lower cyst fluid carcinoembryonic antigen cutoff is helpful in the differential diagnosis of mucinous versus non-mucinous pancreatic cysts. Indian J Gastroenterol. 2022;41(4):397–404.
20. Weiss RA. A perspective on the early days of RAS research. Cancer Metastasis Rev. 2020;39(4):1023–8.
21. Chubarov AS, Oscorbin IP, Filipenko ML, Lomzov AA, Pyshnyi DV. Allele-specific PCR for KRAS mutation detection using phosphoryl guanidine modified primers. Diagnostics. 2020;10(11):872.
22. Tulla KA, Maker AV. Can we better predict the biologic behavior of incidental IPMN? A comprehensive analysis of molecular diagnostics and biomarkers in intraductal papillary mucinous neoplasms of the pancreas. Langenbeck's Arch Surg. 2018;403:151–94.

23. Tufano M, Ciofi D, Amendolea A, Stagi S. Auxological and endocrinological features in children with McCune albright syndrome: a review. Front Endocrinol (Lausanne). 2020;11:522.
24. Kadayifci A, et al. Value of adding GNAS testing to pancreatic cyst fluid KRAS and carcinoembryonic antigen analysis for the diagnosis of intraductal papillary mucinous neoplasms. Dig Endosc. 2017;29(1):111–7.
25. Mas L, Lupinacci RM, Cros J, Bachet J-B, Coulet F, Svrcek M. Intraductal papillary mucinous carcinoma versus conventional pancreatic ductal adenocarcinoma: a comprehensive review of clinical-pathological features, outcomes, and molecular insights. Int J Mol Sci. 2021;22(13):6756.
26. Shimizu T, et al. Pancreatobiliary-type intraductal papillary mucinous neoplasm of the pancreas may have 2 subtypes with distinct clinicopathologic and genetic features. Hum Pathol. 2019;91:26–35.
27. Radaszkiewicz T. The role of RING finger proteins in Wnt signalling. Masarykova univerzita; 2020.
28. Bugter JM, Fenderico N, Maurice MM. Mutations and mechanisms of WNT pathway tumour suppressors in cancer. Nat Rev Cancer. 2021;21(1):5–21.
29. Furukawa T. Mechanisms of development and progression of pancreatic neoplasms. Pathol Int. 2022;72(11):529–40.
30. Xie W, Liang H, Guo Y, Xiao S-Y. Update on mucinous cystic neoplasm of the pancreas: a narrative review. J Pancreatol. 2021;4(03):115–21.
31. Fogliati A, et al. Implications of pregnancy on MCN of the pancreas: a multicentric case-control study. Pancreatology. 2024;24:747.
32. Lee MH, et al. Mucin-producing cystic hepatobiliary neoplasms: updated nomenclature and clinical, pathologic, and imaging features. Radiographics. 2021;41(6):1592–610.
33. Zhou W, et al. Pancreatic mucinous cystic neoplasm communicating with main pancreatic duct: an unrecognized presentation of pancreatic mucinous neoplasm? Anticancer Res. 2017;37(12):7017–21.
34. Raut P, Nimmakayala RK, Batra SK, Ponnusamy MP. Clinical and molecular attributes and evaluation of pancreatic cystic neoplasm. Biochim Biophys Acta (BBA). 2023;1878(1):188851.
35. Wartenberg M, Karamitopoulou-Diamantis E. Mucinous cystic neoplasm (MCN) and MCN with associated invasive component. In: Pathology of the pancreas. Springer; 2022. p. 140–4.
36. McCarty TR, Paleti S, Rustagi T. Molecular analysis of EUS-acquired pancreatic cyst fluid for KRAS and GNAS mutations for diagnosis of intraductal papillary mucinous neoplasia and mucinous cystic lesions: a systematic review and meta-analysis. Gastrointest Endosc. 2021;93(5):1019–33.
37. Ferreira A, Pereira F, Reis C, Oliveira MJ, Sousa MJ, Preto A. Crucial role of oncogenic KRAS mutations in apoptosis and autophagy regulation: therapeutic implications. Cells. 2022;11(14):2183.
38. Mondal K, Posa MK, Shenoy RP, Roychoudhury S. KRAS mutation subtypes and their association with other driver mutations in oncogenic pathways. Cells. 2024;13(14):1221.
39. Voutsadakis IA, Digklia A. Pancreatic adenocarcinomas without KRAS, TP53, CDKN2A and SMAD4 mutations and CDKN2A/CDKN2B copy number alterations: a review of the genomic landscape to unveil therapeutic avenues. Chinese Clin Oncol. 2023;12(1):2.
40. Jasar D, Filipovski V, Kubelka-Sabit K. Clinicopathological and histomorphological association in K-ras mutated colorectal cancer. Virchows Arch. 2022;481:1–364.
41. Aubrey BJ, Strasser A, Kelly GL. Tumor-suppressor functions of the TP53 pathway. Cold Spring Harb Perspect Med. 2016;6(5):a026062.
42. Wang H, Guo M, Wei H, Chen Y. Targeting p53 pathways: mechanisms, structures, and advances in therapy. Signal Transduct Target Ther. 2023;8(1):92.
43. Zhang L, Abro B, Campbell A, Ding Y. TP53 mutations in myeloid neoplasms: implications for accurate laboratory detection, diagnosis, and treatment. Lab Med. 2024;55(6):686–99.
44. Rishi A, Goggins M, Wood LD, Hruban RH. Pathological and molecular evaluation of pancreatic neoplasms. Semin Oncol. 2015;42(1):28–39.

45. Stefanoudakis D, Frountzas M, Schizas D, Michalopoulos NV, Drakaki A, Toutouzas KG. Significance of TP53, CDKN2A, SMAD4 and KRAS in pancreatic cancer. Curr Issues Mol Biol. 2024;46(4):2827–44.
46. Ng V, et al. Ubiquitylation in canonical Wnt signaling. 2021.
47. Zhong Z, Virshup DM. Recurrent mutations in tumor suppressor FBXW7 bypass Wnt/$β$-catenin addiction in cancer. Sci Adv. 2024;10(14):eadk1031.
48. Sakihama K, et al. RNF43 as a predictor of malignant transformation of pancreatic mucinous cystic neoplasm. Virchows Arch. 2022;480(6):1189–99.
49. Farnhammer F, Colozza G, Kim J. RNF43 and ZNRF3 in Wnt signaling-a master regulator at the membrane. Int J Stem Cells. 2023;16(4):376.
50. Noë M, et al. Genomic characterization of malignant progression in neoplastic pancreatic cysts. Nat Commun. 2020;11(1):4085.
51. Chidambaram S, Kawka M, Gall TMH, Cunningham D, Jiao LR. Can we predict the progression of premalignant pancreatic cystic tumors to ductal adenocarcinoma? Future Oncol. 2022;18(23):2605–12.
52. Springer S, et al. A combination of molecular markers and clinical features improve the classification of pancreatic cysts. Gastroenterology. 2015;149(6):1501–10.
53. Inoue K, Fry EA. Haploinsufficient tumor suppressor genes. Adv Med Biol. 2017;118:83.
54. Bihr S, et al. Expression and mutation patterns of PBRM1, BAP1 and SETD2 mirror specific evolutionary subtypes in clear cell renal cell carcinoma. Neoplasia. 2019;21(2):247–56.
55. Visani M, et al. Molecular alterations in pancreatic tumors. World J Gastroenterol. 2021;27(21):2710.
56. Liu Z, Zhang S. Molecular markers contribute to the clinical diagnosis for pancreatic cystic neoplasms. Chin Med J. 2020;133(7):847–52.
57. Sanchez-Matamoros Martin I, Bellido-Luque J, Tuñón JMC, Nogales Muñoz A. Pancreatic cystic neoplasms: serous cystadenoma, mucinous cystadenoma. In: Recent innovations in surgical procedures of pancreatic neoplasms. Springer; 2023. p. 13–21.
58. Basturk O, Askan G. Benign tumors and tumorlike lesions of the pancreas. Surg Pathol Clin. 2016;9(4):619–41.
59. Brugge WR. Diagnosis and management of cystic lesions of the pancreas. J Gastrointest Oncol. 2015;6(4):375.
60. Jais B, et al. Serous cystic neoplasm of the pancreas: a multinational study of 2622 patients under the auspices of the International Association of Pancreatology and European Pancreatic Club (European Study Group on Cystic Tumors of the Pancreas). Gut. 2016;65(2):305–12.
61. Karoumpalis I, Christodoulou DK. Cystic lesions of the pancreas. Ann Gastroenterol Q. 2016;29(2):155.
62. Varshney N, Kebede AA, Owusu-Dapaah H, Lather J, Kaushik M, Bhullar JS. A review of Von Hippel-Lindau syndrome. J Kidney Cancer VHL. 2017;4(3):20.
63. Gläsker S, Vergauwen E, Koch CA, Kutikov A, Vortmeyer AO. Von Hippel-Lindau disease: current challenges and future prospects. Onco Targets Ther. 2020;Volume 13:5669–90.
64. Charville GW, Kao C-S. Serous neoplasms of the pancreas: a comprehensive review. Arch Pathol Lab Med. 2018;142(9):1134–40.
65. Büscheck F, et al. Prevalence and clinical significance of VHL mutations and 3p25 deletions in renal tumor subtypes. Oncotarget. 2020;11(3):237.
66. Yang G, Shi R, Zhang Q. Hypoxia and oxygen-sensing signaling in gene regulation and cancer progression. Int J Mol Sci. 2020;21(21):8162.
67. Papadopoulos N, Hruban RH. Molecular mechanisms of cystic neoplasia. In: The pancreas: an integrated textbook of basic science, medicine, and surgery; 2023. p. 630–7.
68. Schödel J, et al. Hypoxia, hypoxia-inducible transcription factors, and renal cancer. Eur Urol. 2016;69(4):646–57.
69. Wu Y. Multi-omics investigation of tumor heterogeneity, oncogenic signaling, and treatment response in human cancers. St. Louis: Washington University; 2022.
70. Binderup MLM, et al. von Hippel-Lindau disease: updated guideline for diagnosis and surveillance. Eur J Med Genet. 2022;65(8):104538.

71. Laquière AE, et al. Genomic profile concordance between pancreatic cyst fluid and neoplastic tissue. World J Gastroenterol. 2019;25(36):5530.
72. Hata T, et al. GNAS mutation detection in circulating cell-free DNA is a specific predictor for intraductal papillary mucinous neoplasms of the pancreas, especially for intestinal subtype. Sci Rep. 2020;10(1):17761.
73. Paluri RK, John TA, Anastasopoulou C, Babiker HM. Solid Pseudopapillary epithelial neoplasm (SPEN) of the pancreas. In: StatPearls [Internet]. StatPearls Publishing; 2024.
74. Fuentes EJ, Beltrán ML, Contreras KJ, Vásquez BM, Ábrego P. Solid pseudopapillary tumor of the pancreas, an unusual neoplasm.
75. Dubey IB, Gupta S, Paruthy S, Bhandari V. Solid pseudopapillary epithelial neoplasm of the pancreas: a case report. J Med Sci Res. 2022;5(3):34.
76. La Rosa S, Bongiovanni M. Pancreatic solid pseudopapillary neoplasm: key pathologic and genetic features. Arch Pathol Lab Med. 2020;144(7):829–37.
77. Omiyale AO. Solid pseudopapillary neoplasm of the pancreas. World J Hepatol. 2021;13(8):896.
78. Lu X, Chen H, Zhang T. Solid pseudopapillary neoplasm (SPN) of the pancreas: current understanding on its malignant potential and management. Discov Oncol. 2024;15(1):77.
79. Song P, et al. Wnt/$β$-catenin signaling pathway in carcinogenesis and cancer therapy. J Hematol Oncol. 2024;17(1):46.
80. Kim G, et al. Nuclear $β$-catenin localization and mutation of the CTNNB1 gene: a context-dependent association. Mod Pathol. 2018;31(10):1553–9.
81. Zhang Y, Wang X. Targeting the Wnt/$β$-catenin signaling pathway in cancer. J Hematol Oncol. 2020;13(1):165.
82. Groenewald W, Lund AH, Gay DM. The role of WNT pathway mutations in cancer development and an overview of therapeutic options. Cells. 2023;12(7):990.
83. Mostafa ME, Erbarut-Seven I, Pehlivanoglu B, Adsay V. Pathologic classification of 'pancreatic cancers': current concepts and challenges. Chinese Clin Oncol. 2018;6(6):59.
84. Ricketts CJ, et al. A germline 1; 3 translocation disrupting the VHL gene: a novel genetic cause for von Hippel-Lindau. J Med Genet. 2022;59(1):18–22.
85. Cicchetti R, et al. Advances in molecular mechanisms of kidney disease: integrating renal tumorigenesis of hereditary cancer syndrome. Int J Mol Sci. 2024;25(16):9060.
86. Farrell JJ. Prevalence, diagnosis and management of pancreatic cystic neoplasms: current status and future directions. Gut Liver. 2015;9(5):571.
87. Amru RL, Dhok A. Peutz-Jeghers syndrome: a comprehensive review of genetics, clinical features, and management approaches. Cureus. 2024;16(4):e58887.
88. Klimkowski S, et al. Peutz--jeghers syndrome and the role of imaging: Pathophysiology, diagnosis, and associated cancers. Cancers (Basel). 2021;13(20):5121.
89. Liu Q, et al. Intraductal oncocytic papillary neoplasm arising in Peutz-Jeghers Syndrome bile duct: a unique case report. Diagn Pathol. 2022;17(1):96.
90. Llach J, Carballal S, Moreira L. Familial pancreatic cancer: current perspectives. Cancer Manag Res. 2020;Volume 12:743–58.
91. Kasuga A, et al. Molecular features and clinical management of hereditary pancreatic cancer syndromes and familial pancreatic cancer. Int J Mol Sci. 2022;23(3):1205.
92. Shelton CA. Hereditary pancreatitis: a prototype of chronic pancreatitis to characterize variable genomic elements that impact disease features and family dynamics. University of Pittsburgh; 2019.
93. Klatte DCF, Wallace MB, Löhr M, Bruno MJ, van Leerdam ME. Hereditary pancreatic cancer. Best Pract Res Clin Gastroenterol. 2022;58:101783.
94. Hegyi E, Sahin-Tóth M. Genetic risk in chronic pancreatitis: the trypsin-dependent pathway. Dig Dis Sci. 2017;62(7):1692–701.
95. Klein AP. Pancreatic cancer epidemiology: understanding the role of lifestyle and inherited risk factors. Nat Rev Gastroenterol Hepatol. 2021;18(7):493–502.

96. Yeap I, Becker T, Azimi F, Kernohan M. The management of hereditary melanoma, FAMMM syndrome and germline CDKN2A mutations: a narrative review. Australas J Plast Surg. 2022;5(2):12–22.
97. Leof ER, Zhu X, Rabe KG, McCormick JB, Petersen GM, Breitkopf CR. Pancreatic cancer and melanoma related perceptions and behaviors following disclosure of CDKN2A variant status as a research result. Genet Med. 2019;21(11):2468–77.
98. Chen Y, et al. CDKN2A (p16INK4A) affects the anti-tumor effect of CDK inhibitor in somatotroph adenomas. Int J Mol Med. 2021;47(2):500–10.
99. Petrucelli N, Daly MB, Pal T. BRCA1-and BRCA2-associated hereditary breast and ovarian cancer. 2022.
100. Lai E, et al. BRCA-mutant pancreatic ductal adenocarcinoma. Br J Cancer. 2021;125(10):1321–32.
101. Prakash R, Zhang Y, Feng W, Jasin M. Homologous recombination and human health: the roles of BRCA1, BRCA2, and associated proteins. Cold Spring Harb Perspect Biol. 2015;7(4):a016600.
102. Krais JJ, Johnson N. BRCA1 mutations in cancer: coordinating deficiencies in homologous recombination with tumorigenesis. Cancer Res. 2020;80(21):4601–9.
103. Li X, Liu G, Wu W. Recent advances in Lynch syndrome. Exp Hematol Oncol. 2021;10(1):37.
104. Bujanda L, Herreros-Villanueva M. Pancreatic cancer in lynch syndrome patients. J Cancer. 2017;8(18):3667.
105. Schöniger S, Rüschoff J. Mismatch repair deficiency and microsatellite instability. Encyclopedia. 2022;2(3):1559–76.
106. Altamish M, et al. Role of the serine/threonine kinase 11 (STK11) or liver kinase B1 (LKB1) gene in Peutz-Jeghers syndrome. Crit Rev Eukaryot Gene Expr. 2020;30(3):245.
107. Gorji L, Albrecht P. Hamartomatous polyps: diagnosis, surveillance, and management. World J Gastroenterol. 2023;29(8):1304.
108. Corral JE, Mareth KF, Riegert-Johnson DL, Das A, Wallace MB. Diagnostic yield from screening asymptomatic individuals at high risk for pancreatic cancer: a meta-analysis of cohort studies. Clin Gastroenterol Hepatol. 2019;17(1):41–53.
109. Kang J, Gallucci S, Pan J, Oakhill JS, Sanij E. The role of STK11/LKB1 in cancer biology: implications for ovarian tumorigenesis and progression. Front Cell Dev Biol. 2024;12:1449543.
110. Grant TJ, Hua K, Singh A. Molecular pathogenesis of pancreatic cancer. Prog Mol Biol Transl Sci. 2016;144:241–75.
111. Nielsen SM, et al. Von Hippel-Lindau disease: genetics and role of genetic counseling in a multiple neoplasia syndrome. J Clin Oncol. 2016;34(18):2172–81.
112. Coco D, Leanza S. Von Hippel-Lindau syndrome: medical syndrome or surgical syndrome? A surgical perspective. J Kidney Cancer VHL. 2022;9(1):27.
113. Laks S, et al. Management recommendations for pancreatic manifestations of von Hippel--Lindau disease. Cancer. 2022;128(3):435–46.
114. Gómez-Virgilio L, et al. Genetics, pathophysiology, and current challenges in Von Hippel--Lindau disease therapeutics. Diagnostics. 2024;14(17):1909.
115. Szymoński K, Milian-Ciesielska K, Lipiec E, Adamek D. Current pathology model of pancreatic cancer. Cancers (Basel). 2022;14(9):2321.
116. Oni TE. Development of novel early detection and therapeutic strategies in pancreatic cancer. State University of New York at Stony Brook; 2020.
117. Sikdar N, Saha G, Dutta A, Ghosh S, Shrikhande SV, Banerjee S. Genetic alterations of periampullary and pancreatic ductal adenocarcinoma: an overview. Curr Genomics. 2018;19(6):444–63.
118. Xia R, et al. The utility of molecular studies on pancreatic cystic lesions: a comprehensive review. Hum Pathol Reports. 2024;36:300741.
119. Prado MM. MicroRNAs as bile-based biomarkers for pancreatic and biliary-tract cancers. London: Imperial College; 2019.

120. Shockley KE, B. To, Chen W, Lozanski G, Cruz-Monserrate Z, Krishna SG. The role of genetic, metabolic, inflammatory, and immunologic mediators in the progression of intraductal papillary mucinous neoplasms to pancreatic adenocarcinoma. Cancers (Basel). 2023;15(6):1722.
121. Pagliari D, et al. Uptodate in the assessment and management of intraductal papillary mucinous neoplasms of the pancreas. Eur Rev Med Pharmacol Sci. 2017;21(12):2858–74.
122. Haque F. Biological function and clinical implication of coagulation proteins during malignant transformation of pancreatic cells. University of York; 2023.
123. Kamps R, et al. Next-generation sequencing in oncology: genetic diagnosis, risk prediction and cancer classification. Int J Mol Sci. 2017;18(2):308.
124. Ideno N, Mori Y, Nakamura M, Ohtsuka T. Early detection of pancreatic cancer: role of biomarkers in pancreatic fluid samples. Diagnostics. 2020;10(12):1056.
125. Giannis D, Moris D, Barbas AS. Diagnostic, predictive and prognostic molecular biomarkers in pancreatic cancer: an overview for clinicians. Cancers (Basel). 2021;13(5):1071.
126. Sharma RK, Chhabra P, Rana SS. Pancreatic cystic lesions: aiding in the early diagnosis of pancreatic cancer. Front Gastroenterol, Frontiers Media SA. 2024;2:1355275.
127. van der Sijde F, et al. Circulating TP53 mutations are associated with early tumor progression and poor survival in pancreatic cancer patients treated with FOLFIRINOX. Ther Adv Med Oncol. 2021;13:17588359211033704.
128. Sethi V, Giri B, Saluja A, Dudeja V. Insights into the pathogenesis of pancreatic cystic neoplasms. Dig Dis Sci. 2017;62:1778–86.
129. Kaczor-Urbanowicz KE, et al. Reviews on current liquid biopsy for detection and management of pancreatic cancers. Pancreas. 2020;49(9):1141–52.
130. Paniccia A, et al. Prospective, multi-institutional, real-time next-generation sequencing of pancreatic cyst fluid reveals diverse genomic alterations that improve the clinical management of pancreatic cysts. Gastroenterology. 2023;164(1):117–33.
131. Wang K, Wang X, Pan Q, Zhao B. Liquid biopsy techniques and pancreatic cancer: diagnosis, monitoring, and evaluation. Mol Cancer. 2023;22(1):167.
132. Zhao Y, et al. Application of endoscopic ultrasound-guided-fine needle aspiration combined with cyst fluid analysis for the diagnosis of mediastinal cystic lesions. Thorac Cancer. 2019;10(2):156–62.
133. Satam H, et al. Next-generation sequencing technology: current trends and advancements. Biology (Basel). 2023;12(7):997.
134. Badheeb M, et al. Pancreatic tumorigenesis: precursors, genetic risk factors and screening. Curr Oncol. 2022;29(11):8693–719.
135. Rodriguez-Matta E, Hemmerich A, Starr J, Mody K, Severson EA, Colon-Otero G. Molecular genetic changes in solid pseudopapillary neoplasms (SPN) of the pancreas. Acta Oncol (Madr). 2020;59(9):1024–7.
136. Ahmed S, Bradshaw A-D, Gera S, Dewan MZ, Xu R. The TGF-$β$/Smad4 signaling pathway in pancreatic carcinogenesis and its clinical significance. J Clin Med. 2017;6(1):5.
137. Yu J, et al. The functional landscape of patient-derived RNF43 mutations predicts sensitivity to Wnt inhibition. Cancer Res. 2020;80(24):5619–32.
138. Yang J-I, et al. GATA6 amplification is associated with improved survival of TP53-mutated pancreatic cancer. medRxiv. 2023:2003–23.
139. Chang JC, Kundranda M. Novel diagnostic and predictive biomarkers in pancreatic adenocarcinoma. Int J Mol Sci. 2017;18(3):667.
140. Patel S. Management of pancreatic cancer, an issue of surgical clinics, E-Book, vol. 104, no. 5. Elsevier Health Sciences; 2024.

Role of Artificial Intelligence in Pancreatic Cyst Diagnosis

14

Gaurav Mahajan, Hardeep Kaur, Srinu Deshidi, and Surinder Singh Rana

Abstract

Pancreatic cystic lesions have become increasingly prevalent and diagnostically challenging due to their diverse characteristics and potential for malignant transformation in certain cases. Accurate risk stratification is crucial for optimizing surveillance and intervention strategies. However, conventional diagnostic modalities, such as radiologic interpretation, endoscopic assessment, and cyst fluid analysis, often yield ambiguous or discordant findings. Artificial Intelligence (AI) has emerged as a key innovation capable of addressing these limitations through advanced computational analysis of complex, high-dimensional data. Contemporary AI models, including deep convolutional neural networks and multimodal machine learning architectures, demonstrate significant improvements in cyst detection, automated segmentation, and ability to differentiate between nonmucinous and mucinous lesions across computed tomography (CT), magnetic resonance imaging (MRI), and endoscopic ultrasound (EUS) imaging. Radiomic and pathologic feature extraction, when integrated with clinical, biochemical, and molecular signatures, further enhances predictive accuracy for

G. Mahajan (✉)
Department of Gastroenterology, Indian Naval Hospital Ship Asvini, Colaba, Mumbai, Maharashtra, India

H. Kaur
Department of Pediatrics, Indian Naval Hospital Ship Asvini, Colaba, Mumbai, Maharashtra, India

S. Deshidi
Department of Gastroenterology, Jagruth Multispeciality Hospital, Khammam, Telangana, India

S. S. Rana
Department of Gastroenterology, Postgraduate Institute of Medical Education and Research, Chandigarh, India

R. K. Sharma et al. (eds.), *Differential Diagnosis and Management of Pancreatic Cystic Lesions*, https://doi.org/10.1007/978-981-92-0654-4_14

dysplasia grading and malignancy risk assessment. Notably, AI-enabled decision support systems have the potential to reduce observer variability, refine guideline-based management algorithms, and minimize unnecessary surgical resections. However, the translation of AI into routine clinical practice is constrained by limitations in dataset heterogeneity, reproducibility, external validation, and algorithm interpretability. Ethical concerns—including data governance, model transparency, and potential biases—emphasize the necessity of rigorous methodological standards and regulatory oversight. This chapter synthesizes extant evidence, evaluates emerging AI methodologies, and outlines critical challenges and future directions. Collectively, AI is poised to transform the diagnostic paradigm for pancreatic cysts, advancing precision medicine and enhancing patient outcomes through more reliable, data-driven risk assessment.

Keywords

Artificial intelligence · Pancreatic cystic lesions · IPMN · Pancreatic cancer · Artificial neural networks · Machine learning · Deep learning

14.1 Introduction

Pancreatic cancers, which often go undetected due to the absence of early symptoms, typically manifest after they have spread or become incurable. Approximately 80–85% of these cancers are diagnosed at an advanced stage [1]. Early diagnosis and surgical resection are the primary avenues for improving pancreatic cancer survival. This is underscored by relatively high five-year overall survival rates observed among individuals diagnosed with stage 0 and 1A pancreatic ductal adenocarcinoma (PDAC), which stand at 85.8% and 68.7%, respectively [2].

Nearly 20% of PDAC originates as pancreatic cystic lesions (PCLs), with intraductal papillary mucinous neoplasms (IPMNs) being the most common type [3]. IPMNs, comprising approximately half of all PCLs, are characterized by their papillary architecture. Histologically, IPMNs have the potential to progress to high-grade dysplasia and subsequently develop into pancreatic cancer [4]. IPMNs are categorized based on their anatomical location. The most common type is branch-duct (BD) IPMNs, characterized by a cyst that communicates with the primary pancreatic duct [3]. Main-duct (MD) IPMNs are defined as dilation of the primary pancreatic duct without any other obstructive factors. Mixed IPMNs show features of both BD-IPMNs and MD-IPMNs. Mucinous cystic neoplasms (MCNs), another type of mucinous cyst, also pose a risk of malignancy.

Nonmucinous pancreatic cysts include solid pseudopapillary neoplasms or SPNs and cystic neuroendocrine tumors, which are less aggressive than PDAC. Serous cystadenomas and lymphoepithelial cysts constitute benign nonmucinous cysts. The risk of malignant transformation in serous cystadenomas is <0.1% [5].

Approximately 13% of abdominal radiological examinations done in asymptomatic individuals can identify a pancreatic cyst, and this rate of cyst identification increases with age. This can cause a diagnostic dilemma in differentiating benign and malignant cysts [6]. The present standard of care for risk stratification of PCLs involves cyst fluid analysis using EUS-guided fine-needle aspiration and measuring carcinoembryonic antigen, amylase, and glucose levels as well as cytological analysis. However, these methods can help identify high-grade dysplasia or adenocarcinoma in only up to 65 to 75% of patients [7]. Certain advanced centers may offer innovative diagnostic procedures that incorporate cystic fluid next-generation sequencing or NGS analysis, EUS-guided through-the-needle biopsy, and EUS-guided needle-based confocal laser endomicroscopy. These can provide clinicians with a comprehensive range of information.

Considering the challenges and risks associated with pancreatic surgery, innovative diagnostic models, such as utilizing machine learning (ML) and artificial intelligence (AI), are gaining popularity to enhance the risk stratification of PCLs.

14.2 Scope of Artificial Intelligence

AI has found applications in various fields, including medicine, where it is increasingly being utilized in disease detection and diagnosis. Recently, AI has demonstrated its versatility in the assessment of gastroenterological conditions by utilizing endoscopic lesion identification, analyzing inflammatory lesions on imaging modalities, and assessing liver fibrosis [8]. Notably, in 2021, the FDA granted approval to an AI assistance tool that aids endoscopists in identifying concerning lesions during colonoscopies [9].

AI operates through various stages, including machine learning (ML) and deep learning (DL). ML utilizes mathematical algorithms to analyze input data and predict output values without explicit programming [10]. However, ML requires training with datasets that encompass both input and output data. Artificial neural networks (ANNs) are AI-based computing algorithms that emulate the functionality of human neurons. Every ANN consists of an input layer and an output layer with intervening hidden layers, which weigh data characteristics and input from other neurons to determine the output [8, 10, 11]. DL comprises multiple ANNs, thereby enabling complex processing and automatic detection of relevant features within the input data. Many DL algorithms have been extensively used and applied to various medical specialties with convoluted neural networks (CNNs) recently demonstrating superior performance over trained doctors in identifying pathology within specific photographs [12, 13].

Recent advancements in AI have been utilized for the detection, classification, and diagnosis of PCLs. AI provides clinicians with modalities to process deeper layers of data pertaining to PCLs that are beyond human perception. The integration of AI with diagnostic modalities for PCL, such as digital pathomics, radiomics, and genomics, holds the potential for enhanced risk stratification of these rather difficult-to-diagnose lesions.

14.3 Foundations of Artificial Intelligence in Pancreatic Diseases

Artificial intelligence encompasses a range of computational techniques that enable pattern recognition and predictive modeling. Machine learning algorithms utilize structured data, while deep learning models, particularly CNNs, are highly effective in image analysis.

In pancreatic cyst diagnosis, AI can be applied to:

- Lesion detection and segmentation
- Cyst classification
- Malignancy prediction
- Multimodal data integration

The transition toward multimodal AI systems (Fig. 14.1) represents a major advancement, allowing integration of imaging, pathology, and molecular data to improve diagnostic accuracy.

The various domains where AI has demonstrated assistive role in PCL diagnosis include cross-sectional imaging, EUS, radiomics, pathomics, and genomics (Table 14.1).

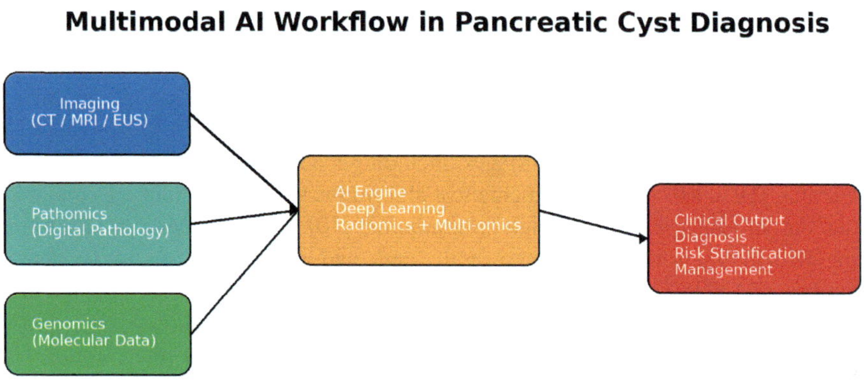

Fig. 14.1 Multimodel AI workflow in pancreatic cyst diagnosis

Table 14.1 Applications of AI in pancreatic cyst diagnosis

Domain	AI application	Clinical benefit
Imaging (CT/MRI)	Detection, classification	Improved accuracy
EUS	Real-time analysis	Reduced operator variability
Radiomics	Feature extraction	Noninvasive diagnosis
Pathomics	Histology analysis	Reduced subjectivity
Genomics	Mutation analysis	Precision medicine

14.3.1 Artificial Intelligence in Cross-Sectional Imaging

Cross-sectional imaging remains the cornerstone of pancreatic cyst evaluation. However, interpretation is often subjective and influenced by radiologist experience. AI has significantly improved both the detection and characterization of pancreatic cystic lesions. Deep learning models trained on CT images can automatically identify pancreatic cysts and classify them based on morphological features such as size, wall thickness, septations, and enhancement patterns. These models have demonstrated diagnostic accuracies comparable to expert radiologists and, in some cases, superior performance in differentiating mucinous from nonmucinous cysts [14–16].

MRI-based AI models offer additional advantages due to superior soft tissue contrast and the ability to assess ductal communication. AI algorithms applied to MR cholangiopancreatography (MRCP) sequences can accurately identify communication with the main pancreatic duct, a key feature in diagnosing IPMNs. In addition, AI models have shown high accuracy in predicting high-grade dysplasia and invasive carcinoma in IPMNs, often outperforming guideline-based criteria [15].

Automated segmentation is another important application. Certain AI algorithms can delineate cyst boundaries with high precision, enabling the accurate measurement of cyst volume and morphological features. This reduces interobserver variability and facilitates longitudinal monitoring. Volumetric analysis provides a more comprehensive assessment of cyst progression compared to traditional linear measurements [16].

Recent developments include time-series AI models that incorporate longitudinal imaging data to detect dynamic changes associated with malignant transformation. This represents a significant advancement in surveillance strategies.

14.3.2 Radiomics: Quantitative Imaging and Predictive Modeling

Radiomics refers to the computational transformation of medical imaging data into a large set of quantitative descriptors that capture underlying tissue heterogeneity and structural complexity [17–19]. These parameters encompass first-order intensity metrics, higher-order texture features, morphological attributes, and advanced wavelet-derived signatures. In pancreatic cystic lesions, radiomics has demonstrated significant potential in differentiating cyst subtypes and predicting malignant potential. Texture analysis, for example, can identify subtle differences in internal architecture between mucinous and nonmucinous cysts. Frameworks leveraging radiomic signatures have demonstrated robust diagnostic performance, frequently achieving high discriminatory capability in differentiating cyst subtypes [19].

Radiomics-based models have also been shown to predict histopathological features such as dysplasia grade and invasive carcinoma. Texture analysis of pancreatic pathology has shown good predictiveness in defining the PNET histotype. Radiomics may represent a supportive tool in diagnostic imaging for the differential diagnosis with PDAC [20]. The integration of radiomics with clinical and laboratory data further enhances predictive performance. These clinical-radiomic models provide robust risk stratification and are particularly useful in indeterminate cases. Radiomics also serves as a bridge to radiogenomics, linking imaging features with underlying genetic alterations [18]. Despite these advances, challenges remain in standardization and reproducibility. Variability in imaging protocols and feature extraction methods can affect the model performance.

14.3.3 Artificial Intelligence in Endoscopic Ultrasound

EUS has emerged as a cornerstone modality in the evaluation of pancreatic cystic lesions due to its ability to provide high-resolution, real-time imaging and facilitate tissue acquisition. Unlike cross-sectional imaging, EUS enables detailed assessment of internal cyst architecture, mural nodules, septations, and vascular patterns. However, its diagnostic accuracy remains highly operator-dependent, with significant interobserver variability, particularly in differentiating mucinous from nonmucinous cysts and identifying features suggestive of malignancy. AI has been increasingly integrated into EUS to address these limitations, offering the potential to standardize interpretation, enhance diagnostic accuracy, and improve procedural outcomes. The various AI applications in endoscopic ultrasound are represented vitally in Fig. 14.2.

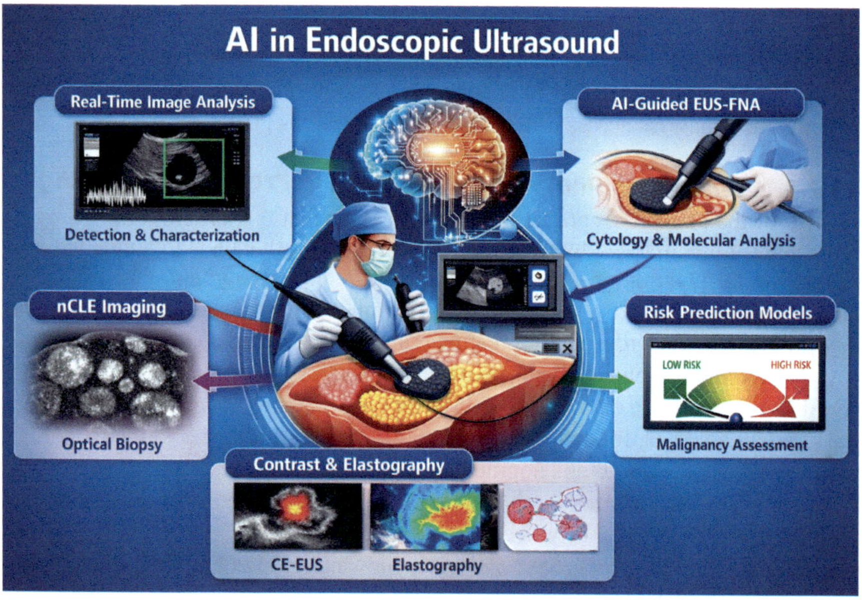

Fig. 14.2 Role of artificial intelligence in endoscopic ultrasound for pancreatic cyst diagnosis. The figure was generated with the assistance of an artificial intelligence tool and subsequently reviewed and edited by the authors

14.3.3.1 AI-Assisted Image Analysis in EUS

The application of deep learning algorithms, particularly CNNs, to EUS imaging has enabled automated detection and characterization of pancreatic lesions. These models are trained on large datasets of annotated EUS images and video sequences, allowing them to recognize complex patterns associated with different cyst types.

AI-assisted EUS systems can identify key morphological features such as mural nodules, cyst wall irregularities, and septations with high accuracy. In several studies, AI models have demonstrated diagnostic performance comparable to expert endosonographers, with sensitivities and specificities exceeding 85–90% for differentiating benign from malignant lesions [21, 22]. Furthermore, AI reduces intra- and interobserver variability, thereby improving consistency in interpretation.

An important advantage of AI in EUS is its ability to analyze video data in real time. Unlike static imaging, EUS generates dynamic sequences, and AI models can process multiple frames simultaneously to improve lesion detection. This is particularly useful for identifying subtle features such as small mural nodules or focal wall thickening that may be missed during routine examination.

14.3.3.2 AI in Risk Stratification and Malignancy Prediction

Risk stratification of pancreatic cysts is a critical component of clinical decision-making. Traditional criteria rely on morphological features and cyst fluid markers, which often lack specificity. AI models have been developed to integrate multiple EUS-derived features, including size, echogenicity, vascularity, and structural complexity, to predict the malignant potential.

ML algorithms combining EUS imaging features with clinical parameters have demonstrated improved predictive accuracy compared to conventional guideline-based approaches. AI models can identify subtle patterns associated with high-grade dysplasia and early invasive carcinoma, enabling earlier intervention.

Additionally, AI can generate quantitative risk scores that assist clinicians in decision-making. These scores provide an objective assessment of malignancy risk, reducing reliance on subjective interpretation, and potentially improving adherence to management guidelines.

14.3.3.3 AI-Guided EUS-FNA and Cyst Fluid Analysis

EUS-guided FNA remains a key diagnostic tool for pancreatic cyst evaluation, allowing the analysis of cyst fluid for cytology, biochemical markers, and molecular alterations. However, its diagnostic yield is limited by sampling error and variability in interpretation.

AI can be applied to optimize EUS-FNA in several ways. Real-time image analysis can guide needle placement by identifying the most representative regions within a cyst, such as areas with mural nodules or solid components. This targeted approach reduces false-negative results and improves diagnostic accuracy. Furthermore, AI algorithms have been developed to analyze cyst fluid data, including CEA levels, cytology, and molecular markers. By integrating these parameters, AI models can more accurately classify cysts and predict malignancy compared to individual markers alone [22].

Recent advances also include AI-assisted cytology, where DL models analyze digitized cytology slides to detect malignant cells. This approach enhances sensitivity, particularly in samples with low cellularity, and reduces interobserver variability among pathologists.

14.3.3.4 Needle-Based Confocal Laser Endomicroscopy (nCLE) and AI

nCLE represents a significant innovation in EUS-guided diagnostics, allowing in vivo microscopic visualization of cyst epithelium. This technique provides real-time histology-like images, enabling differentiation between cyst types based on characteristic patterns. AI has further enhanced the utility of nCLE by enabling automated pattern recognition. DL models trained on nCLE images can accurately classify cysts as mucinous or nonmucinous and identify features suggestive of malignancy. This "optical biopsy" approach has demonstrated high diagnostic accuracy and may reduce the need for repeated sampling [23].The integration of AI with nCLE also improves workflow efficiency by providing immediate diagnostic feedback during the procedure, allowing clinicians to make real-time decisions regarding management.

14.3.3.5 Contrast-Enhanced EUS and Elastography

Contrast-enhanced EUS (CE-EUS) and elastography provide functional information that complements structural imaging. CE-EUS assesses vascularity, which is particularly useful in identifying malignant features such as hyper-enhancing mural nodules. Elastography evaluates tissue stiffness, which may correlate with fibrosis or malignancy. AI enhances the analysis of these modalities by providing quantitative assessment of vascular patterns and stiffness measurements. ML models can integrate these parameters with conventional imaging features to improve lesion characterization.

14.3.4 Pathomics: Artificial Intelligence in Histopathology

Pathomics refers to the application of AI to digital pathology. The transition to digital pathology has enabled the application of DL algorithms for detailed analysis of histological architecture and cellular morphology. AI algorithms can detect dysplasia and malignancy by analyzing features such as nuclear atypia, mitotic activity, and glandular architecture. This improves diagnostic accuracy and reduces interobserver variability [15, 24].

In cytology, AI enhances the detection of malignant cells in samples obtained via EUS-FNA. This is particularly valuable in PCLs, where cytological sensitivity is often limited. AI-driven spatial analysis provides insights into tumor progression and may identify novel biomarkers. Pathomics can be integrated with radiomics and genomics to create comprehensive diagnostic models, further improving predictive accuracy.

14.3.5 Genomics and Multi-omics Integration

Molecular analysis has become an essential component of pancreatic cyst evaluation. Mutations in genes such as KRAS and GNAS are associated with mucinous cysts, while TP53 and SMAD4 alterations are linked to malignant transformation [25, 26]. Multi-omics approaches incorporate proteomics, metabolomics, and lipidomics, providing a comprehensive understanding of cyst biology. AI-driven integration of these datasets enhances predictive accuracy and identifies novel biomarkers [27].

14.4 Limitations and Challenges

Despite its promise, AI in pancreatic cyst diagnosis faces several challenges. Many studies are retrospective and single-center, limiting generalizability. Lack of standardized imaging protocols and data preprocessing methods affects reproducibility. The black-box nature of DL models raises concerns about interpretability and trust. Integration into clinical workflows requires infrastructure, training, and cost investment. Ethical considerations, including data privacy and algorithmic bias, must also be addressed.

14.5 Future Directions

Future developments should focus on multimodal AI systems integrating imaging, pathology, and genomics. Real-time AI applications in EUS will enhance procedural accuracy. Explainable AI will improve transparency and clinical adoption. Large multicenter prospective studies are needed to validate AI models and establish their clinical utility. Integration into clinical guidelines will mark the transition toward data-driven precision medicine.

14.6 Conclusion

Artificial intelligence represents a paradigm shift in pancreatic cyst diagnosis. By integrating multimodal data, AI-driven analytical models enhance diagnostic precision while simultaneously minimizing observer-dependent variability. Continued research and validation will be essential for widespread clinical adoption.

Bibliography

1. Siegel RL, Miller KD, Jemal A. Cancer statistics, 2020. CA Cancer J Clin. 2020;70(1):7–30. https://doi.org/10.3322/caac.21590.
2. Sagami R, Sato T, Mizukami K, et al. Diagnostic strategy for early pancreatic cancer. Diagnostics (Basel). 2022;12(2):377. https://doi.org/10.3390/diagnostics12020377.

3. Tanaka M, Fernández-del Castillo C, Kamisawa T, et al. Fukuoka guidelines for IPMN management. Pancreatology. 2017;17(5):738–53. https://doi.org/10.1016/j.pan.2017.07.007.
4. Andrejevic-Blant S, Kosmahl M, Sipos B, Klöppel G. IPMN: evolving pathological entity. Virchows Arch. 2007;451(5):863–9. https://doi.org/10.1007/s00428-007-0512-6.
5. Jais B, Rebours V, Malleo G, et al. Serous cystic neoplasms: multinational study. Gut. 2016;65(2):305–12. https://doi.org/10.1136/gutjnl-2015-309638.
6. Zerboni G, Signoretti M, Crippa S, et al. Prevalence of incidental pancreatic cysts. Pancreatology. 2019;19(1):2–9. https://doi.org/10.1016/j.pan.2018.11.014.
7. Scheiman JM, Hwang JH, Moayyedi P. AGA technical review on pancreatic cysts. Gastroenterology. 2015;148(4):824–48. https://doi.org/10.1053/j.gastro.2015.01.014.
8. Le Berre C, Sandborn WJ, Aridhi S, et al. AI in gastroenterology and hepatology. Gastroenterology. 2020;158(1):76–94. https://doi.org/10.1053/j.gastro.2019.08.058.
9. Koh FH, Ladlad J, Teo EK, et al. Real-time AI endoscopy improves detection. Surg Endosc. 2023;37(1):165–71. https://doi.org/10.1007/s00464-022-09470-w.
10. Yang YJ, Bang CS. AI applications in gastroenterology. World J Gastroenterol. 2019;25(14):1666–83. https://doi.org/10.3748/wjg.v25.i14.1666.
11. Rajkomar A, Dean J, Kohane I. Machine learning in medicine. N Engl J Med. 2019;380(14):1347–58. https://doi.org/10.1056/NEJMra1814259.
12. Brinker TJ, Hekler A, Enk AH, et al. Deep learning vs dermatologists. Eur J Cancer. 2019;113:47–54. https://doi.org/10.1016/j.ejca.2019.04.001.
13. Hekler A, Utikal JS, Enk AH, et al. AI vs pathologists in histology. Eur J Cancer. 2019;118:91–6. https://doi.org/10.1016/j.ejca.2019.06.012.
14. LeCun Y, Bengio Y, Hinton G. Deep learning. Nature. 2015;521:436–44. https://doi.org/10.1038/nature14539.
15. Esteva A, Robicquet A, Ramsundar B, et al. Deep learning in healthcare. Nat Med. 2019;25:24–9. https://doi.org/10.1038/s41591-018-0316-z.
16. Erickson BJ, Korfiatis P, Akkus Z, et al. Machine learning in medical imaging. Radiographics. 2017;37(2):505–15. https://doi.org/10.1148/rg.2017160130.
17. Gillies RJ, Kinahan PE, Hricak H. Radiomics: images are data. Radiology. 2016;278(2):563–77. https://doi.org/10.1148/radiol.2015151169.
18. Aerts HJWL, Velazquez ER, Leijenaar RTH, et al. Radiomics and tumor phenotype. Nat Commun. 2014;5:4006. https://doi.org/10.1038/ncomms5006.
19. Zhang L, Diao B, Fan Z, Zhan H. Radiomics for differentiating pancreatic mucinous cystic neoplasm from serous cystic neoplasm: systematic review and meta-analysis. Acad Radiol. 2025;32(5):2679–88. https://doi.org/10.1016/j.acra.2024.11.047.
20. De Robertis R, Mascarin B, Bardhi E, et al. Radiomics in pancreatic tumor diagnosis. Eur J Radiol Open. 2025;14:100651. https://doi.org/10.1016/j.ejro.2025.100651.
21. Bang JY, Săftoiu A, Udrіştoiu A, et al. AI for real-time EUS pancreatic detection. Endoscopy. 2026;58(3):223–32. https://doi.org/10.1055/a-2701-6530.
22. Kuwahara T, et al. Deep learning in EUS diagnosis. Endoscopy. 2023;55(3):242–9.
23. Napoleon B, et al. nCLE in pancreatic cysts. Endoscopy. 2019;51(9):825–35. https://doi.org/10.1055/a-0952-3652.
24. Topol EJ. High-performance medicine. Nat Med. 2019;25:44–56. https://doi.org/10.1038/s41591-018-0300-1.
25. Springer S, Masica DL, Dal Molin M, et al. Molecular markers in pancreatic cysts. Sci Transl Med. 2019;11(501):eaav4772. https://doi.org/10.1126/scitranslmed.aav4772.
26. Singhi AD, Nikiforova MN, Chennat J, et al. Cyst fluid genetic analysis. Gastroenterology. 2014;146(5):1361–9. https://doi.org/10.1053/j.gastro.2014.01.007.
27. Kane LE, Mellotte GS, Conlon KC, et al. Multi-omics biomarkers in pancreatic cysts. Cancers (Basel). 2021;13(4):769. https://doi.org/10.3390/cancers13040769.

Ablative Therapies for Pancreatic Cystic Neoplasms

15

Krithi Krishna Koduri, Jahangeer Basha,
and Sundeep Lakhtakia

Abstract

Pancreatic cystic neoplasms (PCNs) are increasingly detected incidentally with the widespread use of cross-sectional imaging. While many cysts are benign, mucinous lesions such as intraductal papillary mucinous neoplasms and mucinous cystic neoplasms carry a significant risk of malignant transformation, creating management dilemmas. Surgical resection, though curative, is associated with substantial morbidity, mortality, and long-term metabolic consequences, particularly in elderly or comorbid patients. Surveillance alone offers no therapeutic benefit and carries psychological and resource burdens. Endoscopic ultrasound (EUS)-guided ablative therapies have emerged as minimally invasive alternatives aimed at eradicating premalignant cyst epithelium while preserving pancreatic parenchyma. This chapter reviews the rationale, patient selection, technical considerations, efficacy, and safety of available EUS-guided modalities, including ethanol ablation, ethanol-based and alcohol-free chemotherapeutic injection, lauromacrogol sclerosis, and radiofrequency ablation. Among these, ethanol combined with paclitaxel and alcohol-free chemotherapeutic ablation demonstrates the highest cyst resolution rates with acceptable safety profiles.

Keywords

Cyst ablation · EUS · PCN · Radiofrequency ablation

K. K. Koduri · J. Basha · S. Lakhtakia (✉)
Department of Gastroenterology, AIG Hospitals, Gachibowli, Hyderabad, India

R. K. Sharma et al. (eds.), *Differential Diagnosis and Management of Pancreatic Cystic Lesions*, https://doi.org/10.1007/978-981-92-0654-4_15

15.1 Introduction

Pancreatic cystic neoplasms (PCNs) are increasingly being incidentally detected, mainly due to advances in cross-sectional imaging (computed tomography (CT)) and magnetic resonance imaging (MRI) along with their increased usage. The prevalence of pancreatic cyst is estimated to be around 2% in the general population, and it rises significantly with age, reaching up to 38% in individuals over 80 years [1–3].

Based on the cyst fluid characteristics, PCNs are typically classified as *mucinous* (includes intraductal papillary mucinous neoplasm (IPMNs, mucinous cystic neoplasms (MCNs)) and *nonmucinous* (serous cystic neoplasm (SCN) and solid pseudopapillary neoplasms (SPNs)), and other tumors such as cystic pancreatic neuroendocrine tumors (NETs).

The management of PCNs often poses a clinical challenge due to their varied malignant potential. Mucinous lesions carry a significant risk of malignancy, around 20–25% for MCNs and 40–90% for IPMNs [4–7]. The current management strategies, that vary from surgical resection to surveillance and often pose clinical dilemmas. This is mainly due to the morbidity associated with surgery on one side and the anxiety and resource burden linked to indefinite surveillance on the other side. Consequently, minimally invasive approaches such as EUS-guided ablative therapies have emerged as promising alternatives [8].

15.2 Rationale for Ablative Therapies

Surgical resection offers curative therapy but carries a substantial risk of complications. Surgical morbidity ranges from 20 to 40%, and reported mortality rates are up to 2–3% [9–11]. Endoscopic ablative therapies provide a middle ground or an opportunity for treating patients, especially elderly, who may not be the ideal surgical candidates, and for whom guidelines suggest cessation of screening itself. These minimally invasive procedures, performed under EUS guidance, enable direct targeting of cystic lesions. The primary objective is to ablate the epithelial lining of the cyst, thereby eliminating the source of neoplastic transformation while preserving surrounding pancreatic tissue.

Surgery versus ablative therapy At present, the existing guidelines have not incorporated ablative techniques as a standard of care. Patients who are not surgical candidates are not screened further for malignancy. However, with increasing evidence, this approach may eventually be incorporated into clinical practice. As mentioned, surgery carries significant morbidity in spite of its curative effect. Cho et al. conducted a comparative analysis of patients undergoing surgery with those undergoing ablation with ethanol +/− paclitaxel [8]. A total of 620 patients were analyzed, with 310 undergoing EUS-guided pancreatic cyst ablation (EUS-PCA) and 310 undergoing surgical management. Over a 10-year follow-up period, the EUS-PCA group demonstrated a significantly lower cumulative long-term morbidity compared to the surgical group (1.6% vs

33.5%; $P = 0.001$). Similarly, rates of early major adverse events (1.0% vs 8.7%; $P = 0.001$) and late major adverse events (0.3% vs 5.5%; $P = 0.001$) were reduced in the ablation cohort. Patients treated with EUS-PCA also experienced shorter hospital stays (3.5 vs 10.3 days; $P = 0.001$) and a markedly lower incidence of diabetes mellitus (2.2% vs 22.8%; $P = 0.001$), suggesting better preservation of surrounding pancreatic tissue. In contrast, surgical treatment achieved superior complete resolution rates (100% vs 76.5%; $P = 0.001$) and was associated with a lower recurrence rate (0.3% vs 4.6%; $P = 0.001$).

Surveillance ***versus*** *ablation* Song et al. conducted a 10-year comparative study evaluating surveillance versus cyst ablation [12]. The study included 169 patients in the EUS-guided rapid ethanol lavage (EUS-REL) group and 610 patients in the surveillance-only (SO) group, with 159 matched pairs analyzed. The EUS-REL group achieved a radiological complete resolution rate of 74%. Over a 10-year period, the cumulative incidence of progression of branch-duct IPMN was significantly lower in the ablation group compared to surveillance (1.6% vs 21.2%; hazard ratio 12.35; $P = 0.003$). Procedure-related pancreatitis occurred in 13.0% of patients in the EUS-REL group ($n = 22$), with 19 cases classified as mild and 3 as moderate, and no severe adverse events were reported. Additionally, patients undergoing EUS-REL demonstrated a reduced likelihood of requiring surgical resection compared to those under surveillance alone. Despite these differences, both groups showed comparable 10-year overall survival and disease-specific survival rates.

15.3 Patient Selection Criteria for Ablative Therapies

Patient selection is crucial for the success of EUS-guided ablation.

Indications Factors to be considered include—the cyst type, morphology, symptomatology, overall life expectancy from comorbidities, suitability for surgery, and premalignant potential. MCNs harbor the highest risk of malignancy, and proper prognostication of the lesion must be done. Ideally, ablative therapies are best applied to mucinous cysts, unilocular cyst, or oligo-locular cysts (six or less cysts), cysts >1.5 cm (smaller than this are low risk for malignant transformation [13]), and those <3.5 cm have a higher rate of resolution [14] (some suggest cysts up to 6 cm [15, 16]), patients who are not surgical candidates.

Contraindications Multilocular cysts, high-grade dysplasia, or confirmed malignancy are excluded from EUS-guided ablation. Multiseptate cysts present technical difficulties, as a single needle puncture is often inadequate for complete delivery of the ablative agent throughout the cyst. Communication with the main pancreatic duct is a relative contraindication, given the risk that the injected substance may enter the ductal system and precipitate pancreatitis.

15.4 Endoscopic Ultrasound (EUS)-Guided Ablative Techniques

EUS has become a pivotal tool in the management of PCNs, for morphological characterization, biopsy, and for treatment. The main EUS-guided ablative techniques include ethanol ablation, chemotherapeutic injections, and non-injectional methods like radiofrequency ablation (RFA) and photodynamic therapy (PDT). All of these techniques act by causing necrosis of the lesion selectively while preserving the surrounding normal pancreatic tissue [17].

15.4.1 Ethanol Ablation (Table 15.1)

This procedure was first introduced by Gan et al. in 2003 [18]. Their pilot study of 25 patients showed complete resolution of cyst in 35% patients and 8.7% partial resolution (over 1 cm or 75% reduction in the original cyst size), with no complications in any patient up to 1 year follow-up. In this study, they had increased the concentration of ethanol gradually from 5% to 80% with higher benefits. Subsequently, all studies used ethanol concentrations of over 80%. On an average, most studies found a complete cyst resolution rate (CRR) of 25% to 45% [19–22]; the outliers included a study showing a CRR of 9% [23] and another reporting 85% [24]. A systematic review that included eight studies encompassing 207 patients treated with ethanol ablation reported a CRR of 33%. Procedure-related adverse events were observed in 21% of cases, with the most common being abdominal pain (14.5%), followed by fever (3.8%), pancreatitis (2.4%), and intracystic hemorrhage (0.5%). The inconsistency in response is related to the variability of the study designs, the concentration of ethanol used, and the heterogeneity of the cysts in different studies [25].

Mechanism Ethanol induces cell lysis and denaturation of protein and local vascular thrombosis causing cyst resolution [26]. It destroys the epithelium and thus the source of neoplasia. However, its effectiveness varies, with complete resolution rates between 30 and 60%.

Procedure A 22-gauge or 19-gauge needle is used (22-gauge for cysts 2–3 cm, 19-gauge for cysts >3 cm) to aspirate out the cyst content. Then, an almost equal volume of ethanol is injected. For 3–5 min, lavage of the cyst cavity is done. Finally, the cyst cavity is aspirated completely before removing the needle [6, 14] (Fig. 15.1).

Adverse events Reported adverse events include pancreatitis (3–10%), abdominal pain (20–23%), bleeding (0.5–4%), and fever (~4%) [6, 27]. Factors associated with an increased risk of acute pancreatitis include pancreatic cystic lesions located in the uncinate process, the presence of multilocular cysts, possible leakage of ethanol during the procedure, and highly viscous (sticky) cyst fluid [22].

Table 15.1 Studies of EUS-guided ablation using ethanol

Author	No. of subjects	Type of cyst	Average cyst diameter (mm)	Ablative agent	Median follow-up(months)	Complete resolution %	Partial resolution %	Procedure-related adverse events
Gan et al. 2005	25	IPMN (3), MCN (14), SCN (3), PC (1), unknown (2)	19.4	5–80% ethanol	12	35% (8/25)	9%	None
DeWitt et al. 2009	42	IPMN (10), MCN (10), SCN (3), PC (2)	22.4	80% ethanol or saline, followed by ethanol	3–4 months after second lavage	33% (12/36)		10 (abdominal pain), 1 (intracystic hemorrhage), 1 (pancreatitis)
DiMaio et al. 2011	13	IPMN (13)	20.1	80% ethanol	3–6 months	38% (5/13)		1 (abdominal pain)
Caillol et al. 2012	13	MCN (13)	24	99% ethanol	26	85% (11/12)		None
Gomez et al. 2016	23	IPMN (15), MCN (4), non-mucinous (4)	27.5	80% ethanol	40	9% (2/23)	44%	1 (abdominal pain), 1 (pancreatitis)
Park et al. 2016	91	IPMN (9), MCN (12), SCN (33), PC (9), indeterminate (28)	30	99% ethanol	40	45% (41/91)	41%	18 (abdominal pain), 3 (pancreatitis)
Choi et al. 2019	214	IPMN (63), MCN (57), SCN (69), PC (25)	32.2	99% ethanol	immediate	25% (47/190)	44%	10% pancreatitis, 23% abdominal pain, 1% duodenal stricture

IPMN Intraductal papillary mucinous neoplasm, *MCN* Mucinous cystic neoplasm, *SCN* Serous cystic neoplasm, *PC* Pseudocyst

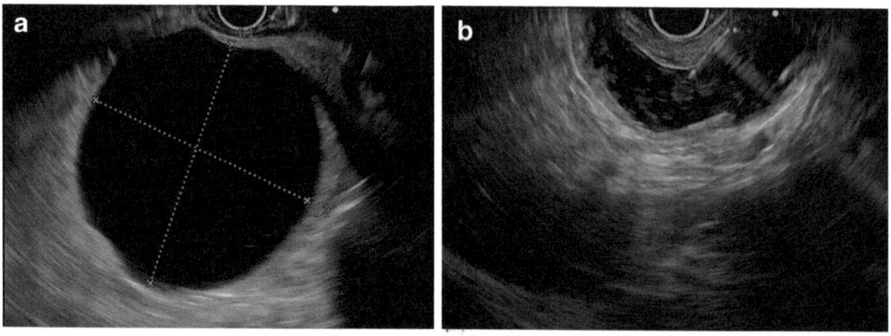

Fig. 15.1 (**a**) : 60 x 57 mm unilocular mucinous cyst. (**b**): Aspiration followed by alcohol lavage

15.4.2 Ethanol and Chemotherapeutic Agents (e.g., Paclitaxel) (Table 15.2)

In order to overcome the limitations associated with ethanol alone, chemotherapeutic agents such as paclitaxel have been incorporated into ablation protocols. Paclitaxel was first used by Oh et al. where they combined paclitaxel injection after ethanol lavage. In the pilot study, 11 out of 14 patients had complete resolution, while 2 had partial resolution at 9 months [28].

Mechanism It was theorized that due to its hydrophobic nature, paclitaxel is less likely to leak from the puncture site and stay within the cyst cavity. The drug inhibits the epithelial layer of cyst for a longer duration by microtubule inhibition [6]. Adding agents like paclitaxel enhances the efficacy of ethanol ablation and leads to higher cyst resolution rates. After the pilot study reporting 79% complete resolution [28], subsequent studies reported CRR range of 50–72% [16, 19, 29, 30]. The long-term follow-up at 6 years reported sustained response, with 98.3% of cysts that achieved complete resolution continuing to remain so [16].

Procedure Following aspiration of the cyst contents, 99% absolute ethanol is instilled into the now-collapsed cyst cavity and maintained with lavage for approximately 3–5 min. During the final round, ethanol is completely re-aspirated, after which a paclitaxel solution is introduced into the cyst, with the injected volume matching the amount of fluid initially aspirated [28]. The administered dose of paclitaxel may range from 1.5 to 24 mg when using a diluted preparation (Taxol; Bristol-Myers Squibb Co., New York, USA) mixed in a 1:1 ratio with 0.9% normal saline, or from 12 to 30 mg when using a nondiluted formulation (Genexol-PM; Samyang Biopharm, Gyeonggi-do, Korea), which is left within the cyst cavity [16, 29]. Before needle withdrawal, 0.5–1 mL of normal saline is used to flush the needle channel to clear any residual paclitaxel solution.

Adverse events These include pancreatitis (2–10%), post-procedure abdominal pain (up to 13%), fever, and abscess formation (<2%). Overall, the combination

Table 15.2 Studies of EUS-guided ablation using ethanol and paclitaxel

Author	No. of subjects	Type of cyst	Average cyst diameter (mm)	Ablative agent	Median follow-up (months)	Complete resolution %	Partial resolution %	No. of procedure-related adverse events
Oh et al. 2008	14	MCN (2), SCN (3), others (9)	25.5	99% ethanol, paclitaxel	9	79% (11/14)	14%	1(pancreatitis), 1 (abdominal pain)
Oh et al. 2009	10	MCN (3), SCN (4), indeterminate cysts (3)	29.5	99% ethanol, paclitaxel	8.5	60% (6/10)	20%	1(pancreatitis)
Oh et al. 2011	47	MCN (9), SCN (15), others (28)	31.8	99% ethanol, paclitaxel	20	62% (29/47)	14%	1 (pancreatitis), 1 (abdominal pain), 1 (fever), 1 (splenic vein obliteration)
DeWitt et al. 2014	22	IPMN (12), MCN (6), SCN (4)	24	99% ethanol, paclitaxel	12	50% (10/20)	25%	1 (peritonitis), 1 (gastric wall cyst), 4 (abdominal pain), 3 (pancreatitis)
Moyer et al. 2016	10	IPMN (2), MCN (7), indeterminate lesions (1)	30	80% ethanol or saline + paclitaxel & gemcitabine	12	Ethanol free 67% (4/6) Ethanol 75% (3/4)		1(pancreatitis)- ethanol arm
Kim et al. 2017	36	MCN (16), branched IPMN (14), SCA (5), pseudocyst (1)	25.8	100% ethanol (n=8) or ethanol + paclitaxel (n=28)	22.3	56% (19/34)	21%	4 (pancreatitis), 4 (abdominal pain), 1 (intracystic hemorrhage)
Moyer et al. 2017	39	IPMN (27), MCN (9), inderterminate (3)	25	80% ethanol or saline + paclitaxel & gemcitabine	12	Ethanol free 67% (14/21) Ethanol 61% (11/18)	Ethanol free 14% (3/21) Ethanol 22% (4/18)	1 (pancreatitis), 4 (abdominal pain)-ethanol arm only
Choi et al. 2017	164	IPMN (11), MCN (71), SCN (16), others (66)	32	99% ethanol, paclitaxel	72	72% (114/158)	20%	6 (pancreatitis), 2 (pseudocyst), 2 (abscess), 1 (intracystic hemorrhage), 1 (pericystic spillage), 1 (pancreatic duct stricture), 1 (splenic vein obstruction), 1 (portal vein thrombosis)

IPMN Intraductal papillary mucinous neoplasm, *MCN* Mucinous cystic neoplasm, *SCN* Serous cystic neoplasm method has reported better safety profiles compared to ethanol alone, with fewer severe adverse events in reported systematic reviews and meta-analysis [25, 29].

15.4.2.1 Large-Surface-Area Microparticle Paclitaxel (Table 15.3)

Large-surface-area microparticle paclitaxel (LSAM-PTX; NanoPac®, CritiTech, Lawrence, KS) is a novel locally acting chemotherapeutic formulation designed to deliver higher concentrations of paclitaxel directly at the target site, thereby enhancing its therapeutic efficacy. Intratumoral injection of LSAM-PTX results in substantially higher local drug levels compared to conventional paclitaxel solutions (concentrations up to 128 times greater). The formulation enables a sustained release of the drug over several weeks, producing prolonged cytotoxic effects before gradually declining to subtoxic levels [31, 32].

In a study by Othman et al., cyst volume reduction ranging from 10% to 78% was observed in 70.6% of patients (n = 10) at 24 weeks [31]. An initial inflammatory response leading to a transient increase in cyst size was noted in some cases, followed by a later necrotic and fibrotic phase associated with reduction in cyst dimensions. These findings supported both the safety and potential effectiveness of EUS-guided fine needle injection (EUS-FNI) of LSAM-PTX in mucinous pancreatic cystic lesions.

In a separate study involving six patients, mean cyst volume reduction ranged between 42% and 89% over a 32-month follow-up period, with one patient experiencing mild pancreatitis as an adverse event [32].

15.4.2.2 Is Alcohol Required for Ablation?

The CHARM trial evaluated whether the use of alcohol is necessary in pancreatic cyst ablation. The hypothesis was that ethanol may be primarily responsible for procedure-related complications, particularly acute pancreatitis [30]. In this prospective, randomized, double-blind pilot study, 10 patients with confirmed

Table 15.3 Studies of EUS-guided ablation using large surface area microparticle paclitaxel

Author	No. of subjects	Type of cyst	Average cyst diameter (mm)	Ablative agent	Median follow-up (months)	Cyst resolution	Procedure-related adverse events
Othman et al. 2022	19	IPMN (19), MCN (2)	27.1	Large surface area microparticle paclitaxel	6	71% decreased in size (35% had >30% reduction)	6% abdominal discomfort, 6% edema, 5% fatigue, 5% headaches
Krishna et al. 2024	6	IPMN (6)	31.8	Large surface area microparticle paclitaxel	32	74% mean surface area reduction	5% pancreatitis

IPMN Intraductal papillary mucinous neoplasm, *MCN* Mucinous cystic neoplasm mucinous pancreatic cysts underwent EUS-guided fine-needle aspiration, followed by lavage using either 80% ethanol or normal saline. Subsequently, both groups received an intracystic combination of paclitaxel and gemcitabine, which was retained within the cyst cavity. They found that cyst reduction was similar in both arms (with and without ethanol), and the only adverse event of pancreatitis was seen in one patient in the ethanol arm. These findings were reinforced by another RCT by the same group [33].

15.4.3 Lauromacrogol Ablation

Linghu et al. evaluated the use of lauromacrogol, a sclerosant agent, for injection into pancreatic cystic lesions [34]. The study included 29 patients, among whom complete resolution was achieved in 11 cases, while 9 patients demonstrated a partial response at 9 months of follow-up. Reported adverse events were limited to mild pancreatitis in two patients and fever in one patient.

In a subsequent study conducted by the same group involving 55 patients treated with this technique, there was a significant reduction in cyst size. The median cyst volume decreased markedly from 11,494.0 mm^3 to 523.6 mm^3 ($P < 0.001$). Post-procedure imaging revealed complete resolution (CR) in 26 patients (47.3%) and partial resolution (PR) in 15 patients (27.3%). Among the 35 patients who were followed for at least 12 months, CR was observed in 18 (51.4%), while 9 (25.7%) showed PR [35].

15.4.4 Radiofrequency Ablation (RFA) (Table 15.4)

Radiofrequency ablation (RFA) is a newer technology that uses electromagnetic energy causing high-frequency alternating currents to produce local heat. This induces coagulation and necrosis and subsequent fibrosis in the targeted area. The pancreatic tissue is thermosensitive, thus making it a more effective therapy [6]. Radiofrequency ablation was first described in porcine models, with the first human application being tried intraoperatively and then percutaneously.

Recent evidence suggests that EUS-RFA may be a safe and potentially effective option for patients with unresectable PDAC. The first human application was described by Song et al. in 2016 in a cohort of six patients with unresectable PDAC, including four with locally advanced disease and two metastatic [36]. In this prospective pilot study, the procedure achieved a technical success rate of 100%, with no serious adverse events; only two patients experienced mild abdominal pain.

Thosani et al. subsequently reported outcomes in 10 patients with PDAC who underwent a total of 22 EUS-RFA sessions (ranging from 1 to 4 sessions per patient) in combination with systemic chemotherapy [37]. Technical success was again 100%, and no major adverse events were observed. Post-procedural abdominal pain occurred in 55% of patients but did not require hospitalization. Among the nine patients who had imaging follow-up, tumor regression was observed in seven

Table 15.4 Studies of EUS-guided ablation using Radiofrequency ablation

Author	No. of subjects with PCN	Type of cyst	Average cyst diameter (mm)	Ablative agent	Median follow-up (months)	Complete resolution %	Partial resolution %	Procedure-related adverse events
Pai et al. 2015	6	4 MCN, 1 IPMN, 1 microcystic adenoma	36.5	RFA	6	33% (2/6)	50%	2 mild abdominal pain
Barthet et al. 2019	17	16 IPMN, 1 mucinous cystadenoma	28	RFA	12	64.7% (11/17) (all mural nodules disappeared)	5.80%	3.50%
Barthet et al. 2021					3 year follow-up of above study	66.6% (all mural nodules disappeared)		
Younis et al. 2022	5	4 IPMN, 1 MCN	36	RFA	7	60% (3/5)	20%	1 mild pancreatitis, 2 abdominal pain

IPMN Intraductal papillary mucinous neoplasm, *MCN* Mucinous cystic neoplasm patients, including a reduction greater than 50% in three cases, while two patients showed disease progression. The median survival was 21 months, with two patients surviving beyond 60 months. The authors proposed several mechanisms underlying these outcomes: direct tumor destruction through coagulative necrosis, enhanced effectiveness of systemic chemotherapy due to increased tumor permeability, and induction of systemic antitumor immune responses following the release of tumor antigens into circulation.

Evidence regarding the use of RFA in PCLs remains limited. In a multicenter study by Pai et al., six PCLs (four mucinous cystic adenomas, one IPMN, and one neuroendocrine tumor) were treated with EUS-RFA [38]. Complete resolution was achieved in two patients, while three others demonstrated a 48.4% reduction in cyst volume. No major post-procedure complications were reported, and only two patients experienced mild abdominal pain.

Another prospective multicenter study evaluated 30 patients (14 pancreatic neuroendocrine tumors, 16 branch-duct IPMNs, and one MCN) who underwent RFA with a follow-up duration of 1 year [39]. At 6 and 12 months, complete resolution of PNETs was observed in 71% and 86% of cases, respectively. Among the 17 PCNs included in the study, resolution rates were 47% at 6 months and 65% at 12 months. The delayed treatment response has been attributed to both local and systemic immune activation following cellular destruction and antigen release, which are subsequently processed by dendritic cells. In a smaller study by Younis et al., involving five PCLs and seven p-NETs, complete radiological resolution was reported in 60% of patients with PCLs [40].

Procedure In the case of p-NETs, the RFA needle can be introduced directly into the lesion under EUS guidance [38]. For PCNs, initially, aspiration of cyst contents is done using a standard FNA needle, or alternatively a 19G needle, leaving only a minimal residual fluid layer. This is followed by advancement of an echogenic EUS-RFA needle, ensuring accurate placement of the tip within the target cyst.

During energy delivery, the formation of echogenic bubbles can be observed within the lesion on EUS imaging. Available EUS-RFA systems are typically monopolar, with variations in design and size. In the study by Barthet et al., an 18G RFA needle (EUS-RA, Starmed, Taewoong, South Korea) was used, delivering energy at 50 W in continuous mode until an impedance of 100 Ohms was reached, indicated by the appearance of hyperechoic bubbles, while ensuring it did not exceed 500 Ohms [39]. The device incorporates an internal cooling mechanism connected to an external pump circulating cold saline. Prior to energy application, EUS Doppler assessment is done to avoid injury to intervening vascular structures. A minimum distance of approximately 2 mm must be maintained between the active tip of the probe and adjacent critical structures such as the common bile duct and the duct of Wirsung. The ablation is complete when echogenic bubbles are seen extending beyond the target lesion along the needle track or when impedance values exceeded 100 Ohms (Fig. 15.2).

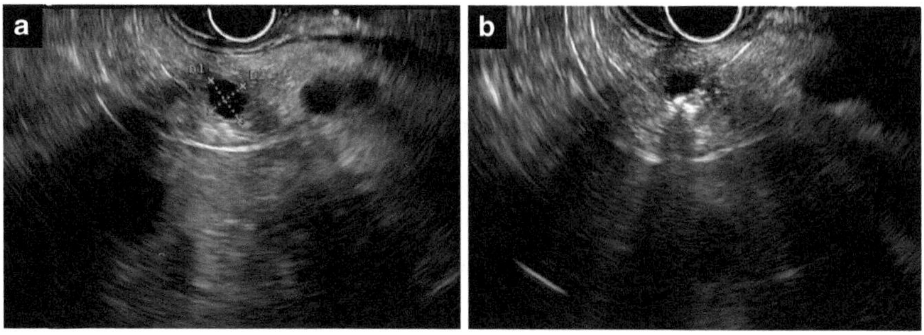

Fig. 15.2 (**a**): 8.7 x 7.2 mm cystic NET. (**b**): Bubbles visualised after RFA application

Safety In the study by Barthet et al., the primary aim was to assess the safety of RFA [39]. Adverse events occurred in 10% of patients, including acute pancreatitis with infection and jejunal perforation. These complications were limited to the initial cases, after which the protocol was modified to include prophylactic measures such as rectal diclofenac, antibiotics, and pre-procedure cyst fluid aspiration. No further adverse events were observed in the remaining 28 patients. One case of pancreatic ductal stenosis occurred and was successfully managed with pancreatic duct stenting. A systematic review of 13 studies involving 134 patients who underwent 165 EUS-RFA procedures for pancreatic lesions (40% NETs, 29% locally advanced PDAC, 31% other lesions) reported complication rates: post-ablation abdominal pain in 10% of cases, pancreatitis in 1%, and perforation or infection in less than 1% [41].

Although higher temperatures may enhance ablation efficacy, temperatures above 90 °C increase the risk of thermal injury, including venous thrombosis, gastrointestinal ulceration, and bleeding. Lower temperatures combined with active cooling are associated with fewer complications [27].

15.5 Which Ablative Technique Is the Best?

As new data and research is advancing, there is increasing innovation and fine tuning of existing techniques. At present, there is more data to suggest ethanol ablation combined with paclitaxel has the best efficacy so far. A meta-analysis including 15 studies with a total of 840 patients undergoing EUS-guided ablation reported an overall complete cyst resolution rate of 44%, with a partial response in 30% of cases [42]. Adverse events occurred in 14% of patients, of which 10% were mild and 4% were severe. Subgroup analysis showed the highest resolution rates with ethanol combined with paclitaxel (70%), followed by lauromacrogol (44%), ethanol alone (32%), and RFA (13%). However, the ethanol-only group had the highest rate of adverse events at 16%.

A position statement by the Asian EUS group and international expert panel provides a detailed summary for further reading about these techniques [15] (Table 15.5) . Figure 5.3 depicts the proposed position of ablative techniques in current practice.

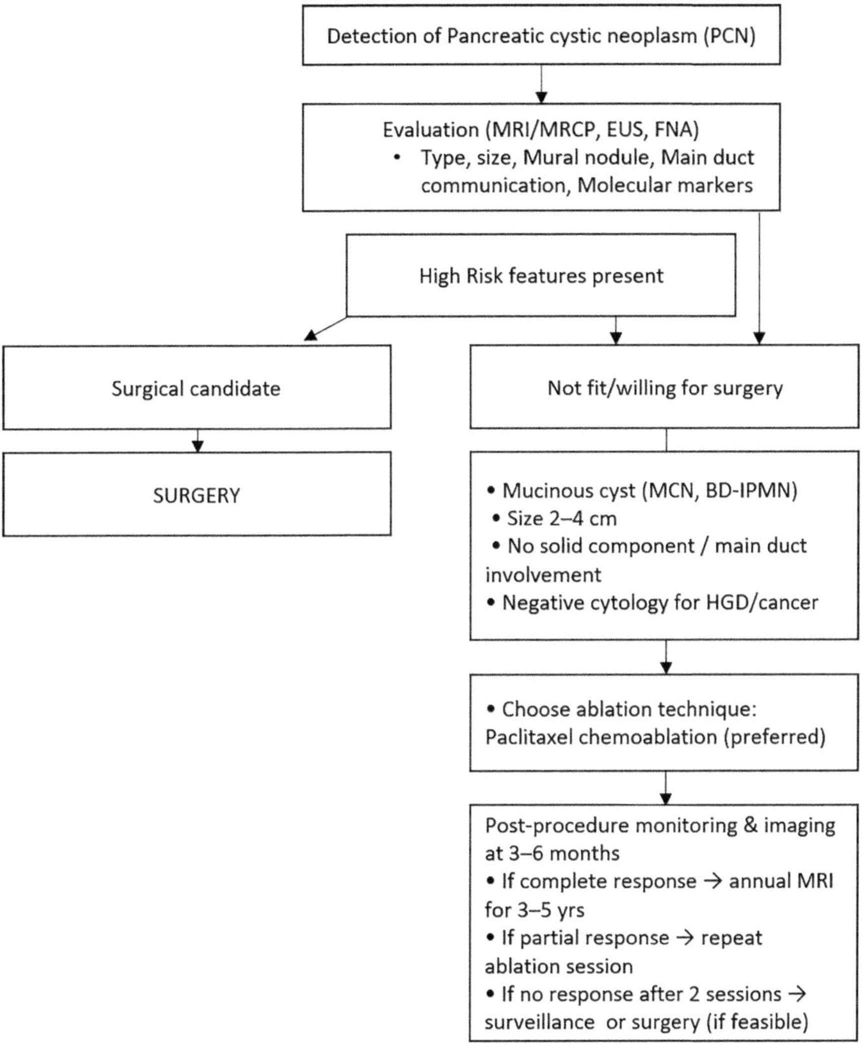

Fig. 15.3 Proposed position of ablative therapies in current practice

Table 15.5 Summary of all the modalities of cyst ablation and surgery

Technique	Mechanism	Complete resolution rate (CRR)	Adverse events (AE)	Best cyst size & type	Key points
Ethanol lavage (EUS-EL)	Chemical necrosis via ethanol-induced epithelial destruction	~25–45% (variable; 9–85% reported)	Pancreatitis 3–10%, abdominal pain 20–23%, fever 4%, bleeding 0.5–4%	Mucinous cysts 2–4 cm; unilocular/≤6 locules	Early technique, inconsistent efficacy, higher AE rate
Ethanol + paclitaxel (EUS-EP)	Ethanol necrosis + paclitaxel microtubule inhibition (retains in cyst)	50–72% (pilot: 79%; long-term 98% sustained CR)	Pancreatitis 2–10%, mild pain/fever <2%	Mucinous cysts 2–4 cm	Best-studied, higher efficacy, fewer severe AEs vs. ethanol alone
Alcohol-free paclitaxel ± gemcitabine (CHARM)	Saline lavage → paclitaxel ± gemcitabine retention	Similar CRR (~60–70%) to ethanol + paclitaxel	Fewer AEs (0% serious adverse events)	Mucinous cysts 2–4 cm	Avoids ethanol-related complications, emerging preferred method
Lauromacrogol ablation	Sclerosant-induced necrosis & fibrosis	~47% CRR; ~27% partial	Mild pancreatitis (~7%), mild fever	Mucinous cysts ≤3.5–4 cm	Simple sclerosant, moderate efficacy
Large surface area microparticle paclitaxel (LSAM/NanoPac)	Sustained-release paclitaxel microparticles	10–78% volume reduction	Mild pancreatitis in (6–7%), fever	Mucinous cysts 2–5 cm	Novel, enhances local dose, promising safety
Radiofrequency ablation (RFA)	Thermal coagulative necrosis	47–65% CRR at 6–12 months (delayed response)	AE ~10% initially; pancreatitis, duct stenosis	Mucinous cysts <4 cm; small NETs	More data in NETs; immune activation benefit
Surgery	Complete excision	100% CR	Morbidity 33%, mortality 2–3%, diabetes 22%	High-risk mucinous cysts, large lesions	Curative but higher morbidity

15.6 Future Directions and Innovations in Ablative Therapies

Emerging technologies and innovative approaches are being explored to improve outcomes:

- *Microwave ablation (MWA)*: MWA offers deeper tissue penetration and uniform heat distribution, and it may be suitable for larger or complex lesions.
- *Cryoablation and laser ablation*: These modalities may provide more precise control over tissue destruction with fewer side effects.
- *Personalized ablation strategies*: Integrating molecular profiling to identify high-risk cysts and tailoring ablation techniques based on cyst subtype and patient-specific factors are anticipated future developments.

15.7 Conclusion

EUS guided ablative therapies for PCNs represent a viable alternative to surgical resection, particularly for patients at high surgical risk. They offer a minimally invasive approach with reasonable efficacy and safety profiles. However, optimizing patient selection, standardizing protocols, and continuing research into newer techniques are essential to further enhance outcomes and expand the role of ablative therapies in clinical practice.

References

1. Guerrero García A, González-Huix F, Levy MJ, García de Paredes AG, Vázquez-Sequeiros E. Ablative therapy in pancreatic cystic lesions. Gastroenterol Hepatol. 2019;42(1):43–50.
2. Brugge WR. Endoscopic ultrasound-guided ablation of pancreatic cysts. Gastroenterol Hepatol (N Y). 2018;14(10):602–4.
3. Vilela A, Quingalahua E, Vargas A, Hawa F, Shannon C, Carpenter ES, et al. Global prevalence of pancreatic cystic lesions in the general population on magnetic resonance imaging: a systematic review and meta-analysis. Clin Gastroenterol Hepatol. 2024;22(9):1798–1809.e6.
4. Ahn DW, Lee SH, Kim J, Yoon WJ, Hwang JH, Jang JY, et al. Long-term outcome of cystic lesions in the pancreas: a retrospective cohort study. Gut Liver. 2012;6(4):493–500.
5. Gaujoux S, Brennan MF, Gonen M, D'Angelica MI, DeMatteo R, Fong Y, et al. Cystic lesions of the pancreas: changes in the presentation and management of 1,424 patients at a single institution over a 15-year time period. J Am Coll Surg. 2011;212(4):590–600; discussion 600–3.
6. Canakis A, Law R, Baron T. An updated review on ablative treatment of pancreatic cystic lesions. Gastrointest Endosc. 2020;91(3):520–6.
7. Choi JH, Lee SH. Endoscopic ultrasound-guided ablation of pancreatic cystic lesions. Int J Gastrointest Intervent. 2022;11(3):119–25.
8. Cho SH, Seo DW, Oh D, Song TJ, Lee SK. Long-term outcomes of endoscopic ultrasound-guided ablation vs surgery for pancreatic cystic tumors. Clin Gastroenterol Hepatol. 2024;22(8):1628–1636.e4.
9. Nemeş R, Curcă T, Paraliov T, Munteanu M, Paşalega M, Dincă N, et al. Cystic tumors of the pancreas. Considerations upon 34 operated cases. Rom J Gastroenterol. 2002;11(4):303–8.

10. Sadot E, Reidy-Lagunes DL, Tang LH, Do RKG, Gonen M, D'Angelica MI, et al. Observation versus resection for small asymptomatic pancreatic neuroendocrine tumors: a matched case-control study. Ann Surg Oncol. 2016;23(4):1361–70.
11. Allen PJ, D'Angelica M, Gonen M, Jaques DP, Coit DG, Jarnagin WR, et al. A selective approach to the resection of cystic lesions of the pancreas: results from 539 consecutive patients. Ann Surg. 2006;244(4):572–82.
12. Song YJ, Huh G, Kim EH, Lee JB, Park DH. Comparison of outcomes of EUS-guided ablation and surveillance only for pancreatic cystic lesions: a propensity score-matching study (with videos). Gastrointest Endosc. 2023;98(4):585–596.e3.
13. Pergolini I, Sahora K, Ferrone CR, Morales-Oyarvide V, Wolpin BM, Mucci LA, et al. Long-term risk of pancreatic malignancy in patients with branch duct Intraductal papillary mucinous neoplasm in a referral center. Gastroenterology. 2017;153(5):1284–1294.e1.
14. Oh HC, Brugge WR. EUS-guided pancreatic cyst ablation: a critical review (with video). Gastrointest Endosc. 2013;77(4):526–33.
15. Teoh AYB, Seo DW, Brugge W, Dewitt J, Kongkam P, Linghu E, et al. Position statement on EUS-guided ablation of pancreatic cystic neoplasms from an international expert panel. Endosc Int Open. 2019;7(9):E1064–77.
16. Choi JH, Seo DW, Song TJ, Park DH, Lee SS, Lee SK, et al. Long-term outcomes after endoscopic ultrasound-guided ablation of pancreatic cysts. Endoscopy. 2017;49(9):866–73.
17. Prete AM, Gonda TA. Endoscopic ultrasound-guided local ablative therapies for the treatment of pancreatic neuroendocrine tumors and cystic lesions: a review of the current literature. J Clin Med. 2023;12(9).
18. Gan SI, Thompson CC, Lauwers GY, Bounds BC, Brugge WR. Ethanol lavage of pancreatic cystic lesions: initial pilot study. Gastrointest Endosc. 2005;61(6):746–52.
19. DeWitt J, McGreevy K, Schmidt CM, Brugge WR. EUS-guided ethanol versus saline solution lavage for pancreatic cysts: a randomized, double-blind study. Gastrointest Endosc. 2009;70(4):710–23.
20. DiMaio CJ, DeWitt JM, Brugge WR. Ablation of pancreatic cystic lesions: the use of multiple endoscopic ultrasound-guided ethanol lavage sessions. Pancreas. 2011;40(5):664–8.
21. Park JK, Song BJ, Ryu JK, Paik WH, Park JM, Kim J, et al. Clinical outcomes of endoscopic ultrasonography-guided pancreatic cyst ablation. Pancreas. 2016;45(6):889–94.
22. Choi JH, Lee SH, Choi YH, You MS, Shin BS, Paik WH, et al. Safety of endoscopic ultrasound-guided ethanol ablation for pancreatic cystic lesions: a single-center experience of 214 patients. Hepatobiliary Pancreat Dis Int. 2019;18(6):562–8.
23. Gómez V, Takahashi N, Levy MJ, McGee KP, Jones A, Huang Y, et al. EUS-guided ethanol lavage does not reliably ablate pancreatic cystic neoplasms (with video). Gastrointest Endosc. 2016;83(5):914–20.
24. Caillol F, Poincloux L, Bories E, Cruzille E, Pesenti C, Darcha C, et al. Ethanol lavage of 14 mucinous cysts of the pancreas: a retrospective study in two tertiary centers. Endosc Ultrasound. 2012;1(1):48–52.
25. Attila T, Adsay V, Faigel DO. The efficacy and safety of endoscopic ultrasound-guided ablation of pancreatic cysts with alcohol and paclitaxel: a systematic review. Eur J Gastroenterol Hepatol. 2019;31(1):1–9.
26. Arshad HMS, Bharmal S, Duman DG, Liangpunsakul S, Turner BG. Advanced endoscopic ultrasound management techniques for preneoplastic pancreatic cystic lesions. J Investig Med. 2017;65(1):7–14.
27. Vargas A, Dutta P, Carpenter ES, Machicado JD. Endoscopic ultrasound-guided ablation of premalignant pancreatic Ccysts and pancreatic cancer. Diagnostics (Basel). 2024;14(5).
28. Oh HC, Seo DW, Lee TY, Kim JY, Lee SS, Lee SK, et al. New treatment for cystic tumors of the pancreas: EUS-guided ethanol lavage with paclitaxel injection. Gastrointest Endosc. 2008;67(4):636–42.
29. Oh HC, Seo DW, Song TJ, Moon SH, Park DH, Soo Lee S, et al. Endoscopic ultrasonography-guided ethanol lavage with paclitaxel injection treats patients with pancreatic cysts. Gastroenterology. 2011;140(1):172–9.

30. Moyer MT, Dye CE, Sharzehi S, Ancrile B, Mathew A, McGarrity TJ, et al. Is alcohol required for effective pancreatic cyst ablation? The prospective randomized CHARM trial pilot study. Endosc Int Open. 2016;4(5):E603–7.
31. Othman M, Patel K, Krishna SG, Mendoza-Ladd A, Verco S, Abidi W, et al. Early phase trial of intracystic injection of large surface area microparticle paclitaxel for treatment of mucinous pancreatic cysts. Endosc Int Open. 2022;10(12):E1517–25.
32. Krishna SG, Ardeshna DR, Shah ZK, Hart PA, Culp S, Jones D, et al. Intracystic injection of large surface area microparticle paclitaxel for chemoablation of intraductal papillary mucinous neoplasms: insights from an expanded access protocol. Pancreatology. 2024;24(2):289–97.
33. Moyer MT, Sharzehi S, Mathew A, Levenick JM, Headlee BD, Blandford JT, et al. The safety and efficacy of an alcohol-free pancreatic cyst ablation protocol. Gastroenterology. 2017;153(5):1295–303.
34. Linghu E, Du C, Chai N, Li H, Wang Z, Sun Y, et al. A prospective study on the safety and effectiveness of using lauromacrogol for ablation of pancreatic cystic neoplasms with the aid of EUS. Gastrointest Endosc. 2017;86(5):872–80.
35. Du C, Chai N, Linghu E, Li H, Feng X, Ning B, et al. Long-term outcomes of EUS-guided lauromacrogol ablation for the treatment of pancreatic cystic neoplasms: 5 years of experience. Endosc Ultrasound. 2022;11(1):44–52.
36. Song TJ, Seo DW, Lakhtakia S, Reddy N, Oh DW, Park DH, et al. Initial experience of EUS-guided radiofrequency ablation of unresectable pancreatic cancer. Gastrointest Endosc. 2016;83(2):440–3.
37. Thosani N, Cen P, Rowe J, Guha S, Bailey-Lundberg JM, Bhakta D, et al. Endoscopic ultrasound-guided radiofrequency ablation (EUS-RFA) for advanced pancreatic and periampullary adenocarcinoma. Sci Rep. 2022;12(1):16516.
38. Pai M, Habib N, Senturk H, Lakhtakia S, Reddy N, Cicinnati VR, et al. Endoscopic ultrasound guided radiofrequency ablation, for pancreatic cystic neoplasms and neuroendocrine tumors. World J Gastrointest Surg. 2015;7(4):52–9.
39. Barthet M, Giovannini M, Lesavre N, Boustiere C, Napoleon B, Koch S, et al. Endoscopic ultrasound-guided radiofrequency ablation for pancreatic neuroendocrine tumors and pancreatic cystic neoplasms: a prospective multicenter study. Endoscopy. 2019;51(9):836–42.
40. Younis F, Ben-Ami Shor D, Lubezky N, Geva R, Osher E, Shibolet O, et al. Endoscopic ultrasound-guided radiofrequency ablation of premalignant pancreatic-cystic neoplasms and neuroendocrine tumors: prospective study. Eur J Gastroenterol Hepatol. 2022;34(11):1111–5.
41. Dhaliwal A, Kolli S, Dhindsa BS, Choa J, Mashiana HS, Ramai D, et al. Efficacy of EUS-RFA in pancreatic tumors: is it ready for prime time? A systematic review and meta-analysis. Endosc Int Open. 2020;8(10):E1243–51.
42. Papaefthymiou A, Johnson GJ, Maida M, Gkolfakis P, Ramai D, Facciorusso A, et al. Performance and safety of EUS ablation techniques for pancreatic cystic lesions: a systematic review and meta-analysis. Cancers (Basel). 2023;15(9). Oid:9661:367851691.

GPSR Compliance

The European Union's (EU) General Product Safety Regulation (GPSR) is a set of rules that requires consumer products to be safe and our obligations to ensure this.

If you have any concerns about our products, you can contact us on ProductSafety@springernature.com

In case Publisher is established outside the EU, the EU authorized representative is:

Springer Nature Customer Service Center GmbH
Europaplatz 3
69115 Heidelberg, Germany

Batch number: 10732090

Printed by Printforce, the Netherlands